Promoting the Health
of Adolescents

ADVISORY BOARD

Promoting the Health of Adolescents

New Directions for the Twenty-first Century

EDITORS

Susan G. Millstein, Ph.D.
University of California, San Francisco

Anne C. Petersen, Ph.D.
University of Minnesota

Elena O. Nightingale, M.D., Ph.D.
Carnegie Corporation of New York

New York   Oxford
OXFORD UNIVERSITY PRESS

Oxford University Press

Oxford   New York   Toronto
Delhi   Bombay   Calcutta   Madras   Karachi
Kuala Lumpur   Singapore   Hong Kong   Tokyo
Nairobi   Dar es Salaam   Cape Town
Melbourne   Auckland   Madrid

and associated companies in
Berlin   Ibadan

Copyright © 1993 by Oxford University Press

First published in 1993 by Oxford University Press, Inc.,
200 Madison Avenue, New York, New York 10016

First issued as an Oxford University Press paperback in 1994

Oxford is a registered trademark of Oxford University Press

Library of Congress Cataloging-in-Publication Data
Promoting the health of adolescents:
new directions for the twenty-first century /
editors, Susan G. Millstein, Anne C. Petersen, Elena O. Nightingale.
p.   cm.   Includes index.
ISBN 0-19-507454-8   ISBN 0-19-509188-4 (pbk.)
1. Teenagers—Health and hygiene.   2. Health behavior in
adolescence.   3. Health promotion.   I. Millstein, Susan G., 1950– .
II. Petersen, Anne C.   III. Nightingale, Elena O.
[DNLM: 1. Adolescence.   2. Adolescent Medicine.
3. Health Promotion.   WS 460 P9655]
RA564.5.P74   1993
613′.0433—dc20
DNLM/DLC   92-22707

2 4 6 8 9 7 5 3 1

Printed in the United States of America
on acid-free paper

FOREWORD

Health Promotion in Historical Perspective

Julius B. Richmond, M.D.

As the editors point out in their introductory chapter to this book, the way in which health has been conceptualized has undergone change at various times in history. In the past, health was viewed in holistic terms, incorporating both ecological and biological issues. This was true even up to the last century. Rudolf Virchow, the founder of modern cellular pathology, laid the scientific basis for much of modern medicine, both conceptually and operationally. Virchow viewed medicine in a social context and saw physicians as the natural attorneys for the poor.

As the natural sciences developed in the latter part of the nineteenth century, however, the focus on specific causes for disease became the dominant motif in medicine. The notion of health tended to move to the background as modern medicine became more and more influenced by the rapid advances in the natural sciences. We then moved into a period in which there was an oversimplification of the concepts used to explain the causes of disease. As modern medicine advanced and became more focused on these concepts, it became harder to highlight some of the positive aspects of health. Even then, however, people such as René Dubos continued to speak with medical audiences about multiple causation in disease and about the relationship of the host and the environment to disease processes. Alan Gregg, vice-president of the Rockefeller Foundation, aptly said:

Almost by definition an organism is an association of organs so intimately related that no part can be changed without changing in some way and in some measure all the others. . . . It is intellectual weakness that prompts us to ascribe a given result to only one sufficient cause. We ignore the value of suspecting that a result may be due to a convergence of several "causes" which separately or in some other sequence will not produce the result we seek to explain. This tendency to overlook convergent or multiple causation seduces us as an unrecognized temptation in our enthusiasm as teachers to make things "clear."[1]

We now seem to have returned to a more comprehensive view of health, considering not only the biology of health, but its social, psychological, and economic aspects as well. George Engel has defined this as a biopsychosocial approach. As we have become more sophisticated about how we conceptualize health, we have become more specific in how we define it as well. The World Health Organization's definition of health is "a state of complete physical, mental and social well-being, not merely the absence of disease and infirmity." Although there remains some ambiguity in our attempts to differentiate disease prevention from health promotion, we are making progress. The ambiguity between these concepts should not become an obstacle to pursuing our goals. Rather, it should be used to encourage further dialogue on the issue, enriching our conceptual models for health. Perhaps we are moving toward a taxonomy of health. A number of years ago, Karl Menninger raised the notion of degrees of wellness and suggested that people could be "weller than well." Clearly, health is not a single entity; in fact, there are probably many different "healths" that deserve consideration in our models. Furthermore, we may also want to consider health as a fluid, dynamic process. Biological, ecological, and psychosocial factors are dynamic interactions that are likely to influence health to different degrees and in different ways as a function of the developmental level of the individual. The present book brings us closer to an understanding of how these dynamic factors operate during adolescence to influence both health behaviors and health status.

Why is health promotion timely now? In the mid-1960s, disease prevention was of little interest to the public or to policymakers. But the beginnings of a movement were emerging with the first report of the Surgeon General's Advisory Committee on Smoking and Health in 1964 and later, in 1979, with the publication of *Healthy People*, the Surgeon General's report on health promotion and disease prevention. As awareness and interest in health promotion grew, we saw a corresponding 35% decline in mortality from heart disease and a 55% decline in mortality from stroke. *Healthy People* also offered measurable and achievable public health goals for each age group in our society. A series of subsequent reports by the Office of Disease Prevention and Health Promotion of the U.S. Public Health Service outlined detailed objectives for the nation by the year 2000.[2]

Today there is a great deal of public interest in disease prevention and health promotion, and high expectations about what can be achieved. The Centers for Disease Control and Prevention and the National Institute for Nursing Research have initiated federal programs on health promotion. Attention to adolescent health promotion and the need to consider the social context in which adolescents live are also evident in the recent report on adolescent health by the congressional Office of Technology Assessment. Professional organizations such as the National Association of School Boards of Education have issued reports for educators on improving the health of adolescents, and the American Medical Association has developed guidelines for adolescent preventive health services. Nonprofit foundations such as Carnegie Corporation of New York, the William T. Grant Foundation, the Kaiser Family Foundation, and others have also contributed to these efforts through their support of innovative programs and their objective to increase public awareness of issues facing adolescents.

This book emerges at a time when the need for knowledge, insight, and creative thinking about adolescent health promotion is deeply felt. To meet the challenge, the editors have brought together an impressive group of scholars and clinicians to discuss the service, research, training, and policy considerations involved in the promotion of adolescent health. This book should serve as a handbook for professionals in the various disciplines caring for adolescents. By consolidating current knowledge on adolescent health promotion from multiple disciplines, the editors are able to present the reader with a broad range of ideas about opportunities for future directions. These carefully considered options will help us achieve the objective of a healthier adolescent population for the next decade and beyond.

Notes

1. See Alan Gregg's *Multiple causation and organismic and integrative approaches to medical education* (Conference on Psychiatric Education, Washington, DC: American Psychiatric Association, 1951).
2. See the Surgeon General's report, sponsored by the United States Department of Health and Human Services, titled *Healthy people: National health promotion and disease prevention objectives* (Washington, DC: U.S. Government Printing Office, 1991).

ACKNOWLEDGMENTS

This volume would not have been possible without the generous support of the Carnegie Corportion of New York and its operating program, the Carnegie Council on Adolescent Development. In particular, we deeply appreciate the contributions of David A. Hamburg, President of Carnegie Corporation, whose vision helped provide the stimulus for this volume and whose continued support made it possible. We also thank Vivien Stewart, Program Chair, The Education and Healthy Development of Children and Youth, and Ruby Takanishi, Executive Director of the Carnegie Council on Adolescent Development for their guidance and foresight throughout the development of the volume. Allyn Mortimer, Program Associate, also provided invaluable assistance for which we are extremely grateful.

We were also exceptionally fortunate to have ongoing guidance and feedback from a distinguished advisory group who gave generously of their expertise during the conceptualization of the book and continued to work with the editors as the volume took shape: Albert Bandura, Michael I. Cohen, Richard Jessor, Denise V. Kandel, Lorraine V. Klerman, Julius B. Richmond, Frederick C. Robbins, and Robert Selman.

The many administrative and editorial tasks associated with the development and production of this book could not have been achieved without the essential contributions of Katharine Beckman, Winifred Bayard, and Annette Dyer at the Carnegie Council on Adolescent Development. Special acknowledgments are also due to Leslie Townsend, whose editorial skills and organizational abilities kept the project moving forward and on schedule. We thank the Division of Adolescent Medicine, Department of Pediatrics, at the University of California, San Francisco, for housing the project.

Our goal of presenting the reader with a multidisciplinary perspective could not have been achieved without the generous contributions of the many professionals from a variety of disciplines who reviewed chapter drafts and provided us with important insights. The contributors to this volume also deserve praise for their willingness to participate in this project in a true spirit of collaboration.

Finally, we express our gratitude to the many other colleagues who stimulated and challenged our thinking about adolescent health promotion over the years.

December 1992
San Francisco, Calif.   S.G.M.
Minneapolis, Minn.   A.C.P.
Washington, D.C.   E.O.N.

CONTENTS

PART II   TOPICAL AREAS FOR PROMOTING HEALTH

Commentary on Part II:
Topical Areas of Interest for Promoting Health

PART III   THE FUTURE OF ADOLESCENT
HEALTH PROMOTION: NEXT STEPS

CONTRIBUTORS

Judith E. N. Albino, Ph.D., President, University of Colorado; Professor, Departments of Psychology and Dentistry, University of Colorado

Amy R. Anson, Research Associate and Doctoral Candidate, Center for Urban Affairs and Policy Research, Northwestern University

Jeanette M. Broering, M.S., R.N., C.P.N.P., Associate Clinical Professor, Department of Pediatrics, University of California, San Francisco

Jeanne Brooks-Gunn, Ph.D., Director, Center for the Development and Education of Young Children and Their Parents, Teachers College, Columbia University

Robert B. Cairns, Ph.D., Cary C. Boshamer Professor, Department of Psychology; Director, Carolina Consortium on Human Development, University of North Carolina

Bruce E. Compas, Ph.D., Associate Professor, Department of Psychology, University of Vermont

Thomas D. Cook, Ph.D., Professor, Departments of Sociology, Psychology, Human Development, and Social Policy, Center for Urban Affairs and Policy Research, Northwestern University

Lisa J. Crockett, Ph.D., Assistant Professor, Department of Human Development and Family Studies, Pennsylvania State University

Felton Earls, M.D., Professor, Departments of Human Behavior and Development and Child Psychiatry, Harvard University

Delbert S. Elliott, Ph.D., Professor, Department of Sociology, Institute of Behavioral Science, University of Colorado

David A. Hamburg, M.D., President, Carnegie Corporation of New York

Ralph Hingson, Sc.D., Professor, School of Public Health, Boston University

Jonathan Howland, Ph.D., M.P.H., Associate Professor, Department of Social and Behavioral Sciences, School of Public Health, Boston University

Charles E. Irwin, Jr., M.D., Professor, Department of Pediatrics; Director, Division of Adolescent Medicine, University of California, San Francisco

Patricia Keeshan, B.S., Doctoral Candidate, Program in Clinical Psychology, Rutgers University

Steven H. Kelder, M.P.H., Research Fellow, School of Public Health, Division of Epidemiology, University of Minnesota

Lorraine V. Klerman, Dr.P.H., Professor and Director, Maternal and Child Health Program, School of Public Health, University of Alabama at Birmingham

Kelli A. Komro, M.A., M.P.H., Research Assistant, School of Public Health, Division of Epidemiology, University of Minnesota

Sandra D. Lawrence, Doctoral Candidate, Program in Clinical Psychology, State University of New York at Buffalo

Howard Leventhal, Ph.D., Professor, Department of Psychology; Chair, Division on Health Policy, Institute for Health, Health Care Policy, and Aging Research, Rutgers University

James A. Mercy, Ph.D., Chief, Epidemiology Branch, Division of Injury Control, National Center for Environmental Health and Injury Control, Centers for Disease Control

Susan G. Millstein, Ph.D., Associate Professor, Department of Pediatrics; Director of Research, Division of Adolescent Medicine, University of California, San Francisco

Allyn M. Mortimer, M.A., Program Associate, Carnegie Corporation of New York

Elena O. Nightingale, M.D., Ph.D., Special Advisor to the President, Carnegie Corporation of New York; Senior Advisor, Carnegie Council on Adolescent Development

Roberta L. Paikoff, Ph.D., Assistant Professor of Psychology in Psychiatry, Institute for Juvenile Research, University of Illinois at Chicago

Cheryl L. Perry, Ph.D., Associate Professor, School of Public Health, University of Minnesota

Anne C. Petersen, Ph.D., Vice-President of Research; Dean, Graduate School, University of Minnesota

Julius B. Richmond, M.D., John D. MacArthur Professor of Health Policy, Emeritus, School of Medicine, Division of Health, Policy, Research and Education, Harvard University

James F. Sallis, Jr., Ph.D., Professor, Department of Psychology, San Diego State University; Assistant Adjunct Professor of Pediatrics, University of California, San Diego

Suzanne B. Walchli, M.B.A., Doctoral Candidate, Department of Marketing, Northwestern University

Promoting the Health
of Adolescents

1

Adolescent Health Promotion: Rationale, Goals, and Objectives

Susan G. Millstein, Anne C. Petersen, and Elena O. Nightingale

> You want to do things . . . to live . . . to get out, have fun, be active. You have to be healthy to work hard . . . to survive in this world. If you're not you might as well be put out on a mountain like they used to do to babies in ancient Greece and let the wolves eat you 'cause you're not going to get anywhere. Thirteen-year-old female (Irwin, 1976)

What is *health promotion?* The term generates different meanings, depending on one's point of view. Whose health are we promoting? Who is defining the construct of health? What is this individual's disciplinary perspective? What is the historical context in which the definition emerges?

Examining historical changes in how health has been conceptualized provides an illustration of the diversity of views about health. The ancient Chinese viewed health as a state of dynamic balance between interrelated biological, psychosocial, and environmental components. Illness occurred when imbalances existed. These imbalances could be caused by factors such as diet and exercise or by disharmonies in family relations. This "ecological" definition of health and illness was later expressed by Hippocrates, whose views formed the basis for much of Western medical science. With the exception of the Early Middle Ages, the model for medical thinking reflected an ecological perspective that considered the human organism within its social and environmental contexts (Noack, 1987).

In the later nineteenth century, a major shift in medical paradigms occurred when attention shifted away from this broad conceptualization and began to focus on the human organism and its physical parts. An emphasis on smaller and smaller components developed. With this change came significant advances in medicine such as the development of germ theory and its influence on the treatment of infectious disease. Illness and disease were viewed as evidence of physiological malfunctioning; the absence of physiological malfunctioning was viewed as evidence of health. The limitations of a strictly biomedical model of illness were recognized, however, when it became clear that disease involved not only infectious agents, but also social and environmental factors such as nutrition and sanitation (Noack, 1987).

In reviewing these historical trends, it should come as no surprise that changing views of illness have also influenced how we think about health. Our ideas about health have shown paradigm shifts similar to those seen with concepts of illness. We have moved from a strictly biological model, with its emphasis on health as the absence of physical dysfunction, to models that incorporate psychological and social-environmental aspects of health. This "biopsychosocial" model considers health in terms of personal experiences of general well-being, the capacity to perform expected roles and tasks, and the fulfilling of one's health potential. As we further integrate ecological perspectives, we move beyond a strictly individual perspective to one that considers the health of our environments and the degree to which our social networks and public policies are health enhancing (Kickbush, 1989). The implications of these conceptual shifts are far-reaching. They include not only how individuals think about health (Chapter 6) and how day-to-day life is organized and experienced (Chapter 5), but also the development of social policy, the allocation of social resources, and the identification of the appropriate players for implementing these policies.

Yet it should also be noted that even in the midst of widespread transformations in our views about health, there remains great diversity in these perspectives. Even as we expand the health construct, it remains couched within specific frameworks. For example, the traditional focus in much of medicine has been the individual. Preventive medicine reflects this focus, with its emphasis on primary prevention of disease among individuals. Public health, which is concerned with populations, focuses on methods of protecting the health of these groups. To the paradigms of disease prevention and health protection we can add a third, overlapping paradigm: that of health promotion, which emphasizes the fulfillment of one's potential for enhanced health. Attempts to draw clear distinctions between these constructs are not likely to be useful; instead, they should be viewed as overlapping, with fluid definitional boundaries.

Defining Goals for Healthy Adolescents

Given our multiple definitions of health, we are still left with the task of defining the healthy adolescent. Here, too, differences of opinion are likely to predominate. The extensive changes that take place during the adolescent years clearly call for qualitatively different expectations about health (Chapter 2). As Chapter 7 notes, alcohol use may be a different risk factor at age 13 than at age 18. Consequently, our goals in relation to alcohol use will vary for adolescents, depending on their stage of development. Goals for younger adolescents, for example, may focus on delaying the onset of normative adult behaviors, while at a later stage goals may need to focus on diminishing the potentially negative consequences of these behaviors. Attempting to delineate one set of goals for all adolescents is not only unrealistic, it is also developmentally inappropriate.

A developmental perspective also suggests that we consider adolescence within the context of the entire life span, and formulate our health promotion goals and priorities with a clear view of the healthy adult in mind. This is not to suggest that we consider only these long-range goals, viewing adolescence as a mere transition to adulthood. Indeed, effective health promotion will require recognition of adolescence as a developmental stage in its own right (Irwin, Commentary on Part I), with consideration of what constitutes healthy *adolescent* development, as well as the multiple paths by which adolescents can make the transition to healthy adulthood (Chapter 2).

Personal beliefs also shape our definitions of the healthy adolescent and generate great divergence of opinion about appropriate health promotion goals. For example, ideological differences about adolescent sexuality influence whether we regard abstinence as the appropriate goal for health promotion or focus on increasing the rate of protected intercourse in order to reduce the negative social, economic, and medical consequences of sexual activity in adolescents. Personal beliefs play a role in less controversial areas as well. Goals in relation to healthy nutrition, for example, may vary among individuals from dissimilar cultural backgrounds (Chapter 10).

Our views are also likely to differ as a function of our experiences in interacting with adolescents. Health care providers who interact with youth in clinical settings are likely to view health in terms of the absence of disease. For teachers, a view of the healthy student often includes attention to the adolescent's learning capacity. The developmental psychologist may think in terms of developmental tasks and their accomplishment, while the employer is concerned about job performance. Parents have a special perspective that probably includes all of these concerns.

These multiple, overlapping perspectives on health suggest that we are unlikely to obtain a consensus about the goals and objectives of health promotion. Yet if interventions are to be successful, they need to be developed with a clear sense of what they hope to accomplish. It will be a challenge to identify these specific goals in such a manner as to reflect careful consideration of these multiple perspectives.

Do Adolescents Need Health Promotion?

By some yardsticks, adolescents appear relatively healthy. If we limit our view of health to physical illness, adolescents fare pretty well. However, as we expand the parameters of the health construct to include psychological, social, and environmental health, significant unmet health needs emerge for this age group. These unmet needs were recognized by the United States Public Health Service (U. S. Department of Health and Human Services, 1991), whose "Year 2000" goals specifically targeted adolescents for special risk reduction efforts in the areas of nutrition, physical activity and fitness, substance use, sexual behavior, violence, unintentional injury, oral health, and mental health.

The rationale for focusing on these particular health issues becomes obvious when one examines the major sources of mortality and morbidity during adolescence, and later in life. Chapters 8 through 14 provide up-to-date, detailed information about many of these topical areas of interest. Overall, the three primary causes of mortality during adolescence are injuries, homicide, and suicide; together, they are responsible for 75% of all adolescent deaths. Major sources of adolescent morbidity include injury and disability associated with the use of motor and recreational vehicles, consequences of sexual activity such as pregnancy and sexually transmitted diseases, and the consequences of substance use. Other significant sources of morbidity include mental disorders, chronic illness, eating disorders, and oral health problems (Gans, Blyth, & Elster, 1990; Irwin, Brindis, Brodt, Bennett, & Rodriguez, 1991; U. S. Congress, 1991; Wetzel, 1987).

The Year 2000 goals also targeted selected subgroups in order to address inequities in health status that exist among subsets of the population defined by factors such as age, gender, economic status, race, and ethnicity. Between early (ages 10–14) and late adolescence (ages 15–19), mortality rates increase by more than 200%. A significant gap in the life expectancy between black and white adolescents exists, with black male adolescents showing the lowest life expectancy. Male adolescents die at a rate more than twice that of their female peers. Age differences in the causes of death also emerge, with a shift toward more violent causes. Among white adolescents, a dramatic increase in suicide occurs during later adolescence, making it the second leading cause of death in this group. For older black adolescents, a different picture emerges, but one that also points toward increases in violence, with homicide ranking as the most likely cause of death. Morbidity rates also vary within the adolescent population. For example, the rate of vehicular injury remains higher for males, while females show higher rates of morbidity on indicators such as utilization of physician services and hospitalization, primarily as a function of reproductive health care needs (Gans et al., 1990; Irwin et al., 1991; U. S. Congress, 1991).

Adolescence: A Special Opportunity for Promoting Health

A life span perspective on health promotion argues against choosing any one life stage as the optimal time for health promotion. The rationale for health promotion at each life stage differs, just as each life stage presents different opportunities for health promotion. What, then, does the adolescent period offer in terms of special opportunities for health promotion?

It is well known that many of the behaviors associated with adult morbidity and mortality begin during the adolescent years. Intervening during adolescence gives us the opportunity not only to prevent the onset of health-damaging behaviors, but also to intervene with health-compromising behaviors that may be less firmly established as part of the lifestyle (Chapter 7). Early intervention also provides an opportunity to introduce, reinforce, and further establish healthy patterns.

Even in the absence of a clear link between specific adolescent actions and adult health outcomes, some behaviors warrant intervention because of their potential for harm during adolescence or because they have irrevocable consequences. Examples include the use of drugs and its negative effects on brain development in adolescents or the potentially lethal combination of substance use and automobile driving.

Finally, there are other reasons for concentrating on this age group. The developmentally based sense of curiosity and interest among adolescents offers an opportunity for health promotion that should not be wasted. Adolescents are extraordinarily receptive to information about themselves and their bodies and anxious to become more autonomous in their decision making. Channeling this energy in productive directions is critical. At the same time, our efforts to recognize the importance of adolescents' participation and our desire to foster individual responsibility for health must avoid the trap of blaming the victim, and should be balanced with an awareness that these behaviors can only emerge within a supportive social context.

Can We Make a Difference?

Identifying adolescents' unmet needs and setting goals for health promotion are important steps that must be taken if we are to maximize the potential for health during this period. The ultimate question, however, is whether we can do anything to meet these needs and reach these goals. Can we make a difference? The answer to this question is a resounding *yes,* we can. The state of the art in health promotion, as illustrated by the authors in this book, clearly indicates the emergence of a set of principles for guiding effective health promotion efforts. What is now required is to set these principles in motion through the efforts of a variety of individuals and institutions.

As the contributors to this book demonstrate, health promotion involves more than a lecture on the consequences of tobacco use, a ban on smoking in schools, a parent's admonition to not smoke, or a query from a physician about one's smoking history. In reality, it requires all of these things and more. Effective health promotion requires enlisting the support of the many individuals and institutions that have contact with or otherwise affect the lives of adolescents. Recent decreases in drunk driving, for example, resulted from multiple interventions that delivered consistent messages designed to change social norms about drunk drivers, creating a social environment in which it was easier to not drive while drunk, and supporting these messages with new legal sanctions (Chapter 14). We have seen numerous examples of successful health promotion using these broad-based strategies, such as the Stanford Heart Disease Prevention Program. Cook, Anson, and Walchli (Chapter 15) describe other successful programs that have been oriented to adolescents.

The recognition that individualized programs are most effective in the context of societal and community change greatly complicates the implementation of health promotion programs. Such a perspective requires not only commitment by individuals to make adolescents a priority, but also cooperation and coordination of complex bureaucratic institutions. Furthermore, as we begin to utilize broader and more diffuse spheres of influence, it becomes increasingly difficult to evaluate the effects of smaller components, such as an individual program.

On the other hand, by not limiting the responsibility for adolescent health to one person or one institution, we create multiple opportunities for promotion to occur. In concert with a widespread commitment to health promotion, small efforts serve to reinforce important themes, thus becoming an integral part of an overall health promotion strategy. A nurse who asks adolescents about tobacco use will have more influence if parents and teachers simultaneously admonish them to abstain. The teacher who educates adolescents about the elements of a healthy diet is reinforced by a school cafeteria that offers healthy choices and a community that provides adolescents with alternatives to fast-food hangouts. Furthermore, an important resource for health promotion that is often overlooked is adolescents themselves. Rather than viewing adolescents as merely the target of health promotion programs, they too should be recruited as important members of the health promotion team.

The Current and Future Status of Adolescent Health Promotion

The publication of the Lalonde report (Lalonde, 1975) ushered in a period of increased attention to prevention. Since then, we have seen an explosion of interest and scientific activity in the area of health promotion in general and adolescent health promotion in particular. During this period, we have seen the emergence of several scholarly journals devoted to adolescence and to health promotion, national goals that incorporate many health promotion principles, national task forces for evaluating the effects of preventive interventions, and various other special efforts by professional organizations, nonprofit institutions, and the federal government. Many of these activities have focused specifically on adolescents, such as the development of guidelines for adolescent preventive services (American Medical Association), the establishment of recommendations and programs to better link adolescent health and education (Carnegie Council on Adolescent Development, National Association of State Boards of Education), and the creation of special programs by the federal government for health promotion and school health (U. S. Public Health Service). Exciting developments in preventive interventions have taken place, and favorable results have emerged.

Against this promising backdrop are certain realities that limit our effectiveness in influencing adolescent health. Many of the most promising scientific developments fail to reach those who interact most often with adolescents, such as health professionals, teachers, and parents. Principles of effective health promotion often remain hidden in scholarly journals. The question "Does anything work?" continues to be asked, with little recognition of the many successful programs that do exist. Furthermore, little interaction appears to take place among investigators who represent different disciplines. Just as adolescent health services are fragmented, so is research on adolescence.

The idea for this book emerged in response to these limitations. Thus, our goals were to bring together the scientific evidence for adolescent health promotion, integrate knowledge from diverse disciplinary perspectives, and translate this knowledge base into a form that would be informative and useful to scientists, practitioners, and others who interact with youth.

The chapters in Part I explore some of the cross-cutting issues of importance in adolescent health and health promotion: biological and psychosocial development; the influence of contextual factors such as economic status, cultural background, and the general social environment; the evolution of individual behaviors into lifestyles; and the importance of considering adolescents' perspectives on health. The chapters in Part II evaluate the state of the art in many areas of interest for adolescent health identified in the Year 2000 objectives: mental health, sexuality, diet and physical activity, oral health, substance abuse, nonviolence, and safety. Commentaries follow each part and provide views of the chapters from the unique perspective of the health care provider in medicine and in nursing. The two chapters in Part III suggest directions we should be taking to develop, implement, and evaluate adolescent health programs, along with options for improving adolescent health today and in the next century.

In this book, we have brought together the collective wisdom of individuals from a variety of disciplines and perspectives. The chapter authors, members of the advisory group, and the many thoughtful reviewers who challenged and stimulated the authors represent a variety of perspectives in terms of their disciplinary focus as well as in their roles as researchers, clinicians, program planners, and administrators. Among the disciplines represented by these individuals are anthropology, dentistry, health education, health policy, human development, medicine, nursing, nutrition, psychology, public health, and sociology. To the extent that this book speaks to others in these disciplines, we will have succeeded in accomplishing an important goal.

Like any book tackling a complex subject, this one has gaps in its coverage. Not all of the issues relevant to adolescent health are discussed. Some topics, such as suicide, are not included as a separate chapter in order to explore more fully topics such as oral health, which typically receive little attention. Our interest in provoking thought about health promotion, and not just illness prevention, is also reflected in our focus on topics such as mental health rather than mental illness.

In considering the needs of multiple adolescent populations, we employ two strategies. Issues of economic status and cultural diversity are treated in separate chapters (3 and 4, respectively). In addition, we asked the authors to address these issues within their own chapters in an attempt to consider more fully the needs of these groups within the mainstream of health promotion. However, not all important groups within the adolescent population receive attention in a separate chapter. The health promotion field would benefit from future efforts to explore in more detail health promotion for special populations such as rural youth; recent immigrants; disabled and chronically ill adolescents; homeless youth; and lesbian, gay, and bisexual youth. Such attention is particularly important in anticipation of changes in the sociodemographic composition of the adolescent population and the implications of those changes for adolescent health, which suggest more, not less, diversity in the adolescent population (Millstein, Irwin, & Brindis, 1990; Chapter 3, this book).

As Richmond notes in the Foreword to this book, the time is ripe for health promotion. We now have well-described conceptual models for guiding our goals and objectives. Although we have not yet lived with these new paradigms long enough to see their widespread diffusion, a foundation for such diffusion exists. This foundation includes a base of scientific principles from which to proceed, examples of programs that work, sophisticated models of implementation and evaluation, and a growing cluster of individuals who are committed to improving the health of adolescents (Hamburg, 1992). Now we need to enlist others as advocates for youth, to apply our knowledge to diverse and needy populations, and to encourage those in decision-making positions to support these efforts.

References

Gans, J. E., Blyth, D. A., & Elster, A. B. (1990). *America's adolescents: How healthy are they?* American Medical Association, Profiles of Adolescent Health Series. Chicago: American Medical Association.

Hamburg, D. A. (1992). *Today's children: Creating a future for a generation in crisis.* New York: Times Books.

Irwin, C. E., Jr. (1976, October). *Towards a new health behavior model for adolescents.* Chicago: Society for Adolescent Medicine.

Irwin C. E., Jr., Brindis, C., Brodt, S., Bennett, T., & Rodriguez R. (1991). *The health of America's youth: Current trends in health status and utilization of health services.* Rockville, MD: Bureau of Maternal and Child Health and Resources Development, Public Health Service.

Kickbush, I. (1989). Self-care in health promotion. *Social Science and Medicine, 29,* 125–130.

Lalonde M. (1975). *A new perspective on the health of Canadians: A working document.* Ottawa: Information Canada, 1–76.

Millstein, S. G., Irwin, C. E., & Brindis, C. (1990). Sociodemographic trends and projections in the adolescent population. In W. R. Hendee & B. Wilford (Eds.), *The health of adolescents* (pp. 1–15). San Francisco: Jossey-Bass.

Noack, H. (1987). Concepts of health and health promotion. In T. Abelin, Z. J. Brzezinski, & V.D.L. Carstairs (Eds.), *Measurement in health promotion and protection* (pp. 5–28). European Series No. 22. Copenhagen: World Health Organization Regional Office for Europe.

U. S. Congress, Office of Technology Assessment (1991, April). *Adolescent health: Volume I: Summary and policy recommendations.* OTA-H-468. Washington, DC: United States Government Printing Office.

U. S. Department of Health and Human Services. (1991). *Healthy people 2000.* Washington, DC: United States Government Printing Office.

Wetzel, J. (1987). *American youth: A statistical snapshot.* Washington, DC: William T. Grant Foundation Commission on Work, Family, and Citizenship.

PART I

The Adolescent, Health, and Society

2

Adolescent Development: Health Risks and Opportunities for Health Promotion

Lisa J. Crockett and Anne C. Petersen

Adolescence is typically viewed as a transitional period between childhood and adulthood, a time during which young people continue to develop the social and intellectual skills that will prepare them for adult roles and responsibilities. During this period, adolescents reach physical and sexual maturity, develop more sophisticated reasoning ability, and make important educational and occupational decisions that will shape their adult careers. These biological, cognitive, and psychosocial changes provide a wealth of developmental opportunities for adolescents to engage in behaviors that lead to health risks, on the one hand, or to develop a healthy lifestyle, on the other. In this chapter, we focus on developmental changes that have implications for the kinds of health risks to which adolescents are exposed, their likelihood of participating in health-risking behaviors, and opportunities for health promotion. *Health* is construed broadly to include physical health, psychological well-being, and social role functioning (Perry & Jessor, 1985). From this perspective, the goal of health promotion is to facilitate the development of young people who are healthy, happy, and prepared to assume their place as adults in society.

The nature of adolescence is strongly determined by the broader sociocultural context. For the most part, the tasks and experiences of adolescence reflect society's organization of the life course in general (Elder, 1985) and, specifically, the cultural structuring of adolescence as a period of preparation for adulthood (Clausen, 1986; Havighurst, 1972). Only the biological fact of puberty is relatively unchanged from culture to culture, and, even so, the social interpretation of and response to pubertal maturation vary (Worthman, 1986). Similarly, within heterogeneous societies such as our own, cultural differences in the experience of adolescence are important to consider. The opportunities, pressures, and resources adolescents confront are influenced by key social, structural, and economic variables related to ethnicity, minority status, gender, and poverty level (Chapters 3 and 7). These differences suggest that health promotion efforts must be tailored to the values, resources, and sociocultural patterns of the target population.

13

It is also important to recognize that adolescent development is shaped by the developmental phases that precede and follow it (Lerner, 1987). The notion of adolescence as a period of preparation for adulthood is key because it emphasizes the developmental challenges toward which the young person is moving and that shape the social pressures and opportunities encountered along the way. The recognition that adolescence follows childhood is equally important: it alerts us to the fact that young adolescents in particular retain much that is childlike and only gradually develop emotional and social maturity. Moreover, the notion of developmental sequence reminds us that prior development affects the vulnerabilities and resources the young person brings to the new challenges of the adolescent period. In sum, adolescent behavior is shaped by prior development in childhood and the future requirements of adulthood, as well as by current expectations and opportunities.

The extended nature of adolescence in Western industrialized nations has led scholars to distinguish three subphases within the adolescent decade (ages 11–20 years): early adolescence (11–14), middle adolescence (15–17), and late adolescence (18–20). These distinctions are quite arbitrary, particularly in terms of the age boundaries identified. Our only point is to delimit three phases of adolescence that may occur at somewhat different chronological ages for different individuals but that have distinct characteristics. Early adolescence is the transition from childhood to adolescence and is characterized primarily by puberty. Middle adolescence is the heart of adolescence, in which there is a dominant peer orientation with all of the stereotypical adolescent preoccupations: adolescent music, attire, appearance, language, and behavior. Late adolescence includes the transition to adulthood and ends when the young person takes on adult work roles, marries, or becomes a parent. This is the period that varies most among individuals in duration and in the chronological ages spanned. Clearly, the opportunities, pressures, skills, and resources available to young people differ during these distinct subphases; consequently, health promotion efforts need to be sensitive to the developmental status of the population of interest.

In contemporary U. S. society, change at adolescence occurs on multiple levels (Petersen, 1987). The individual experiences biological changes related to physical maturation and brain growth, cognitive development, and self-perceptions. Change is also evident in most important social contexts: changes occur in the family system, peer group, and school, and many young people enter the workplace. Often these changes reflect broader changes in social status and role expectations as adolescents move toward adult roles and responsibilities.

These multiple changes have important implications for health risks and health promotion. The changes promote exposure to some new health risks such as alcohol use and sexual activity. In addition, simultaneous change in multiple domains, especially as young people make the transitions from childhood to adolescence and from adolescence to adulthood, may strain the coping capacity of some young people, leading to health-compromising behaviors. On the other hand, some adolescent changes involve increased cognitive and emotional maturity, which can facilitate efforts to promote the adoption of healthy lifestyles. In the following pages, we review the basic individual and contextual changes experienced by adolescents in the United States and discuss the implications of each for health risks and health promotion.

Individual Developmental Change

Biological Development

One of the most fundamental features of the adolescent period is the series of biological changes known collectively as *puberty*. These changes transform the young person physically and physiologically from a child into a reproductively mature adult. This process is a universal feature of human life, linked to fundamental issues of reproduction and continuation of the species. Indeed, puberty is so basic to adolescent development that many scholars identify puberty as the beginning of adolescence (Petersen, 1988).

PUBERTY. Puberty involves a set of biological events that produce change throughout the body (Petersen & Taylor, 1980). The changes fall into two categories: hormonal and somatic. In both sexes, increases in hormone production lead to the development of reproductive capability and a mature physical appearance. Physical changes include pubic hair growth, breast development, and menarche in girls, and genital development, pubic hair growth, voice change, and the emergence of facial hair in boys. A spurt in height and weight occurs in both sexes. (For a detailed discussion of hormonal and somatic changes, see Brooks-Gunn & Reiter, 1990; Petersen & Taylor, 1980; and Reiter, 1987.)

Although all normal adolescents experience the changes of puberty, there are large individual differences in the timing of these changes, as well as in the rapidity with which the changes take place (Eichorn, 1975; Tanner, 1972). In girls, normal puberty may begin as early as age 8 or as late as age 13. Among boys, puberty may begin as early as age 9½ or as late as age 13½. Moreover, some adolescents experience the entire set of changes in as little as 1½ years or as many as 6 years, although the average length of time is about 4 years. These individual differences in timing and tempo mean that youngsters enter the pubertal period with differing levels of preparation and that peers of the same age will show large variation in physical maturity.

Pubertal development influences adolescents' satisfaction with their appearance, with the effects differing for girls and boys. For boys, physical maturation leads to improved body image, probably because increased size and muscular development enhance their social status. For girls, physical maturation leads to greater dissatisfaction with their appearance (Dorn, Crockett, & Petersen, 1988). The normal increase in weight and changes in fat deposition (Frisch, 1983) conflict with cultural norms that emphasize the slender, svelte look (Faust, 1983). Early-maturing girls suffer most because they begin to develop at a time when their age mates still exemplify prepubertal slimness. Unfortunately, the traditional response of women to feeling overweight has been dieting rather than exercise; consequently, teenage girls engage in extensive dieting at a time when nutritional requirements have increased; they may also experience serious eating disorders (Attie, Boooks-Gunn, & Petersen, 1990; Chapter 10).

Although girls appear to be at greater risk for body-image problems and eating disorders, boys are not immune. Boys who participate in sports requiring weight limits may develop eating disorders (Woods, Wilson, & Masland, 1988). There is also evidence that anabolic steroid use among adolescents is motivated by a desire not only to improve athletic performance, but also to improve one's appearance: about one-third of steroid users are not even engaged in sports (Buckley et al., 1988).

Finally, there is some evidence that hormone changes are related to adolescents' emotional states, such as anger and depressed mood (Susman et al., 1987). In addition, some researchers have found a relationship between later pubertal timing and better affective adjustment (Peskin, 1973; Petersen & Crockett, 1985), an effect that persists at least until 12th grade (Petersen, Sarigiani, & Kennedy, 1991). Puberty has been hypothesized to play a role in the etiology of depression (Rutter, 1986), but the hormonal mechanisms that would lead to increased depression at this time have not been identified. A full explanation would have to account for both the general increase in depression at adolescence and the greater increase among girls relative to boys.

BRAIN GROWTH. There is substantial evidence that brain growth continues into adolescence. Although the number of neurons does not increase, there is proliferation of the support cells that brace and nourish the neurons. In addition, myelination (the growth of the myelin sheath around nerve cell axons) continues at least until puberty (Yakovlev & Lecours, 1967), enabling faster neural processing. The number of interconnections between adjacent neurons decreases in the second decade of life (Feinberg, 1987), probably reflecting the disappearance of redundant or inappropriate neural connections. This "fine-tuning" of the neural system coincides with the development of formal operational thought (Graber & Petersen, 1991).

IMPLICATIONS FOR HEALTH PROMOTION. Pubertal development is associated with increased sexual motivation (Udry, Billy, Morris, Groff, & Raj, 1985; Udry, Talbert, & Morris, 1986) and increased sexual attractiveness. Thus, more physically mature adolescents are more likely to be involved in sexual relationships (Udry & Billy, 1987), which increases the risk of pregnancy for girls and the risk of contracting sexually transmitted diseases for both sexes. In addition, a mature appearance may provide entry into older peer groups where behaviors such as sexual intercourse, alcohol use, and drug use are more common (Caspi, Lynam, Moffit, & Silva in press; Magnusson, Stattin, & Allen, 1985). Such a process places early-maturing adolescent girls at particular risk, since they are exposed to health-risking behaviors when they are younger and less likely to have the cognitive and emotional maturity needed for effective coping (Irwin & Millstein, 1986). Consequently, they require special attention.

Despite the increased health risks that appear to accompany adolescent physical development, some aspects of biological development may provide opportunities for health promotion. Most obvious is the possibility that continued brain development leads to enhanced intellectual functioning and improved comprehension of health-related issues. In addition, adolescents' concerns about their physical development and attractiveness (Chapter 6) can provide the impetus for instruction regarding a variety of health-related topics, such as puberty, sexuality, nutrition, exercise, and safe methods of weight control (Carnegie Council on Adolescent Development, 1989).

Cognitive Development

There is ample evidence that during adolescence the capacity for abstract reasoning increases (Keating & Clark 1980); this change has significant implications for health promotion efforts. Between ages 11 and 14, most youngsters become increasingly capable of thinking hypothetically, applying formal logic, and using abstract concepts (Inhelder & Piaget, 1958). Thinking becomes more relative and less absolute, as well as more self-reflective (Turiel, 1989). Adolescents also become increasingly capable of considering an extended time perspective rather than being tied to the here and now (Greene, 1986).

Cognitive capacity as measured by tests is quite different from typical performance, however. Laboratory studies optimize conditions so that maximal performance levels may be attained; everyday situations are usually more time-pressured and often personally stressful (Keating & Clark, 1980). Perhaps for this reason, spontaneous processing, compared to that in the laboratory, is typically less systematic and reflective and depends extensively on prior knowledge (Eylon & Linn, 1988). In particular, thinking on unfamiliar or emotionally arousing topics is likely to be less sophisticated (Linn, 1983). Unfortunately, many of the health-related decisions adolescents confront, such as those surrounding substance use or sexual behavior, involve such "hot" cognitions (Hamburg, 1986). Under such conditions, adolescents (and adults) are less likely to exercise their capacity for abstract, formal reasoning.

DECISION MAKING. Decision-making ability also increases over the adolescent decade (Weithorn & Campbell, 1982). Awareness of possible risks, consideration of future consequences, and the tendency to consult with independent experts show age-related increases over the junior high and high school years (Lewis, 1981). By mid-adolescence, most youngsters are able to reason as well as adults, with similar reasoning flaws (Kuhn, Amsel, & O'Loughlin, 1988).

IMPLICATIONS FOR HEALTH PROMOTION. The cognitive changes adolescents experience should facilitate health promotion efforts, since adolescents become better able to comprehend health risks, reflect on their behavior, and consider the long-term consequences of their actions. Importantly, they should become more responsive to health promotion efforts that require a long-term perspective and attention to symbolic rewards. Of course, the same abilities may make them more susceptible to advertisements that symbolically associate health-compromising products such as cigarettes and alcohol with attractiveness, peer acceptance, and adult status (Steinberg, 1991).

Health promotion programs need to consider developmental differences in reasoning level. In general, younger adolescents require more concrete approaches, whereas older adolescents benefit from more abstract, symbolic approaches. Individual differences in reasoning performance, however, indicate that the most effective strategy may differ even for individuals of the same age. Differences in cognitive experience related to ethnic background, social class, and community resources, for example, may lead individuals of similar age to vary in performance. One possible solution is to use multiple approaches requiring differing levels of abstract reasoning with the same population in order to engage as many individuals as possible.

Health promotion efforts may need to include training in decision making, especially for younger adolescents. Effective decision making can be taught to adolescents as young as age 12 (Mann, Harmoni, Power, Beswick, & Ormond, 1988). Learning to consider alternatives is likely to be a key aspect of this training (Keating, 1990). The optimal approach to training depends on the behavior to be modified, however. Behaviors that are not emotionally charged can probably be handled at a more abstract level, while "hot" issues may need to include experiential components such as role playing. Practice in decision making on these topics should improve performance. In addition, some kinds of beliefs and experience may undermine effective decision making, and such barriers also need to be considered (Adler, Kegeles, Irwin, & Wibbelsman, 1990).

Self and Identity

The development of abstract thought enables a more complex conception of self, greater self-reflection and social comparison, and the development of an extended time perspective. Adolescents can conceptualize themselves in terms of abstract, psychological characteristics, compare themselves to others and to how they might be, and draw conclusions about their future prospects. At the same time, society presses adolescents to begin preparing for the adult roles they will soon enter (Havighurst, 1972). These combined influences have profound implications for a young person's understanding of self.

CONCEPTIONS OF SELF. With the development of formal operational thought, adolescents become able to describe the self more abstractly. Compared to younger children, they are more psychological in their self-descriptions, focusing on personal and interpersonal characteristics, beliefs, and emotional states. They also develop a more differentiated self-concept, recognizing that their behavior and performance vary from setting to setting, but with age they become able to integrate these disparate observations of self into abstract personal characterizations (e.g., sensitive or moody). Harter (1990) notes that this emerging ability to view the self in abstract terms is a liability as well as an advantage. Being less tied to observable behaviors, abstractions are more vulnerable to distortion, resulting in misconceptions of ability. Overestimates of competence may lead to failure, while underestimates may lead to an avoidance of challenges and diminished opportunities for growth.

SELF-ESTEEM. Small gains in self-esteem have been documented during the second decade of life (McCarthy & Hoge, 1982; O'Malley & Bachman, 1983). The improvement, however, may follow an initial decline in self-esteem in early adolescence, particularly among girls (Simmons & Blyth, 1987). Low self-esteem is associated with depression and may contribute to suicidal behavior (Rutter, 1986). Low self-esteem has also been implicated in the development of delinquent behavior and drug use (Kaplan, 1980).

Throughout adolescence, self-esteem appears to be affected by young people's judgments of their competence in certain valued domains (Harter, 1990). Domains identified as important include physical attractiveness, acceptance by peers, and, to a lesser extent, academic competence, athletic ability, and conduct. Physical attractiveness appears to be particularly important for girls (Tobin-Richards, Boxer, & Petersen, 1983). In addition, perceived support from parents and peers is associated with adolescent self-esteem, with peer support taking on increasing importance during this period (Harter, 1990).

Recent work suggests that African-American and white adolescents are similar in self-esteem (Harter, 1990). Different domains of competence, however, may be viewed as important. African-American adolescents may place greater value on nonschool domains where they feel they can excel (e.g., athletics, music, or peer relations) and less on academics.

IDENTITY. The task of identity formation is to develop a stable, coherent picture of oneself that includes an integration of one's past and present experiences and a sense of where one is headed in the future (Erikson, 1968). According to Erikson, this process involves a selective narrowing of choices regarding sexual, occupational, and social roles and a progressive commitment to the choices one makes. Optimally, adolescents have the opportunity to explore a range of possible options in these domains before having to make identity commitments.

Typically, progress toward identity achievement is measured by the status of personal commitments in occupational, social, and ideological domains. Four statuses have been proposed: achievement, moratorium, foreclosure, and diffusion (Marcia, 1966). *Identity-achieved* individuals have made identity commitments after actively exploring possible alternatives; individuals currently engaged in this exploration are in *moratorium*. *Foreclosure* refers to making identity commitments prematurely without exploring alternatives, and *diffusion* refers to a lack of integration in one's sense of self. Developmental research suggests an age-based progression from diffusion to moratorium and identity achievement or, alternatively, from diffusion to foreclosure, although regressions are also possible. In general, the proportion of identity-achieved individuals increases through late adolescence, with achievement occurring earlier in some domains than in others (Waterman, 1985).

Both the content of identity and the progression toward identity achievement may be affected by experiences and opportunities (Ianni, 1989). Research on identity development among minority adolescents highlights these issues. Minority adolescents often score higher on identity foreclosure than do whites, perhaps due to restricted opportunities to explore alternative roles and identities. Diffusion also appears to be more common among minority males than in other groups. In a recent review of this literature, Spencer and Markstrom-Adams (1990) cite several barriers to identity formation in minority youth. These include conflicting values between the minority reference group and the broader society, lack of adult role models who exemplify positive ethnic identity, and inadequate preparation for the stereotyping and prejudice that are frequently experienced.

IMPLICATIONS FOR HEALTH PROMOTION. The changes in self-concept that enable the development of an integrated identity are part of healthy development and should be encouraged. Self-understanding can be fostered through social-cognitive interventions in which adolescents learn to express personal points of view while keeping an open mind to alternative perspectives (Harter, 1990). In addition, active exploration of alternative roles can be supported by vocational internships and apprenticeships. Adolescents should be provided with a broad array of possible role models to increase their chances of finding roles compatible with their interests and abilities. Adult mentors can also promote identity development by providing guidance and support, by serving as role models, and by challenging young people to consider new options and to do their best (Hamilton & Darling, 1989).

To support a healthy sense of self-esteem, adolescents need opportunities to feel competent and successful. This means improving young people's competence in traditionally approved areas such as academics but may also mean supporting areas of competence outside scholastic achievement to engage less academically inclined students (Harter, 1990). The feeling of self-worth is also bolstered by a sense of personal efficacy and potency. Improving life skills (Hamburg, 1989) and providing opportunities for community service (Scales, 1990) should positively affect adolescents' self-esteem. In addition, social support from adults and peers should be enhanced. Support from parents and other important adults can be mobilized through programs that support parent–adolescent communication and engage adults as key players in interventions with youth. Support from peers can be increased through interventions aimed at improving social-cognitive and behavioral skills (Caplan & Weissberg, 1989).

Autonomy

Related to developmental changes in young people's conceptions of self is the process of becoming a self-governing, autonomous individual. Self-reliance, self-control, and the capacity for independent decision making all increase over the adolescent years. Young adolescents perceive themselves as being more independent and self-reliant than do preadolescents and are less likely to report that they rely on their parents for assistance; they also see themselves as more distinct and separate from their parents (Steinberg & Silverberg, 1986). The tendency to make one's own choices rather than conforming to the opinion of others also increases during adolescence, although not in a linear fashion. Conformity to parental opinions decreases steadily, but the tendency to be swayed by peers actually increases before it declines, with peak conformity occurring at around age 13 or 14 (Berndt, 1979). Thus, decreasing conformity to parents is initially counteracted by increasing conformity to peers, with increments in truly autonomous decision making beginning only in midadolescence.

IMPLICATIONS FOR HEALTH PROMOTION. The development of autonomy is a normal and necessary part of becoming a responsible adult. At the same time, many of the choices adolescents face (e.g., regarding unprotected sexual intercourse or drinking and driving) have serious implications. The key, then, is to give adolescents opportunities to develop and exercise their autonomy while minimizing the risk of negative consequences. Risk can be reduced in several ways. One is to make sure that young people are well informed about the possible consequences of various courses of action. Another is to improve decision-making skills by providing practice in considering alternative perspectives. A third is to reduce youngsters' susceptibility to antisocial peer influence by enhancing self-confidence and improving peer resistance skills. A fourth is to reduce opportunities for behaviors having serious negative consequences, perhaps by restricting unsupervised time or monitoring adolescents' behavior. Although this entails some restriction of autonomy, it may at times be necessary.

Finally, it may be possible to capitalize on adolescents' desire for autonomy in health promotion efforts. Health can be presented as something for which the adolescent has personal responsibility. Introducing health in the context of personal choice and control provides an opportunity for young people to exercise their autonomy by committing to health-promoting patterns of behavior such as exercise and proper diet. This should improve adolescents' sense of autonomy and facilitate the adoption of a healthy lifestyle.

Context Changes

It is now well accepted that developmental processes must be viewed in relation to important social contexts (Bronfenbrenner, 1979). During adolescence, key social contexts are the family, peer group, school, and workplace, which are embedded in the local community and the broader society (Hurrelmann, 1989). These contexts and young people's relation to them change over adolescence, creating new opportunities for health-compromising behavior but also new arenas for health promotion. Historical changes in the structure and function of the family, peer group, and school are discussed in Chapter 5. Here we focus on developmental changes in these contexts and their implications for adolescent health.

Family

Changes in the family at adolescence may best be characterized as a transformation in parent–child relationships (Steinberg, 1990), in which the adolescent gradually develops more autonomy from parents and assumes more responsibility in the family. This transformation represents a challenge to family members who must modify their relationships in the direction of greater equality and mutual influence. For parents, this means relinquishing some control.

PARENT–CHILD RELATIONSHIPS. Although relationships between adolescents and their parents were once viewed as inevitably stormy, research has shown that this characterization is largely incorrect (Petersen, 1988). In contrast to the psychoanalytic view (Blos, 1970; Freud, 1958), in most cases individuation and the development of autonomy do not lead to a detachment from parents. Adolescents continue to feel close to their parents (Youniss & Smollar, 1985), to respect them, and to feel they can rely on them (Offer, Ostrov, & Howard, 1981). There is also little evidence of a generation gap. Research has found that parents and adolescents hold similar values with respect to education, religion, and work, with adolescents being more similar to their peers only in areas of "adolescent culture" (e.g., appearance, music preferences) (Kandel & Lesser, 1972; Lerner, Karson, Meisels, & Knapp, 1975).

At the same time, parent–child conflict does increase during adolescence. The increase in conflict occurs in early adolescence and appears to be associated with pubertal development (Hill, Holmbeck, Marlow, Green, & Lynch, 1985; Steinberg, 1981); it reaches a plateau in midadolescence and subsequently declines when the adolescent leaves the parental home (Montemayor, 1983). Although in most families conflict centers on a few mundane topics (e.g., clothing, chores, or schoolwork), in perhaps 15% of families, parent–adolescent relationships are severely troubled and conflict is intense. Intense or pervasive parent–adolescent conflict is not healthy and is related to psychopathology and serious problem behavior (Montemayor, 1983).

Part of the transition at adolescence probably involves a decrease in parental supervision. The current ecology of adolescence is such that young people spend progressively more time away from adults—in their after-school activities, at the shopping mall and video arcades, and at home. On the one hand, this increased autonomy is appropriate given the adolescents' increasing cognitive and emotional maturity; on the other, it provides increased exposure to and opportunities for engaging in health-compromising behaviors such as sexual intercourse or substance abuse and less support for engaging in health-promoting behaviors such as studying. For mature, well-socialized adolescents, there is probably little risk in parents' loosening the reins. For less competent youth, however, decreased supervision may result in more health-risking behaviors; poorly monitored youth are more likely to socialize with deviant peers and to engage in misconduct (Patterson & Stouthamer-Loeber, 1984).

PARENTING STYLE. Parenting style also affects adolescent risk. Steinberg (1990) concludes that both effective conflict resolution (or democracy) and cohesion (or warmth) are important for healthy adolescent development. These provide the basis for "warm relationships in which individuals may express their opinions and assert their individuality" (p. 27). These two characteristics, together with demand-ingness (i.e., expecting mature behavior, setting and consistently enforcing reason-able rules and standards for behavior), are thought to form the components of effective parenting (Maccoby & Martin, 1983). This style, termed *authoritative parenting,* is related to greater psychosocial maturity and better school performance among adolescents (Steinberg, Elman, & Mounts, 1989), as well as less substance abuse (Baumrind, 1991). Recent research with a heterogeneous sample suggests that the relationship between authoritative parenting and school performance holds across ethnic groups (Dornbusch, Ritter, Leiderman, Roberts, & Fraleigh, 1987). In contrast, the style lacking the three components, termed *indifferent* or *uninvolved,* is related to the highest levels of problem behavior and psychological problems (Maccoby & Martin, 1983).

IMPLICATIONS FOR HEALTH PROMOTION. The continued importance of the family during adolescence suggests that parents can be key players in promoting healthy lifestyles. Especially in early adolescence, parents continue to play an important role in setting standards for behavior, instilling values, and providing emotional support. Through these mechanisms, healthy behavior patterns begun in childhood may be maintained and health-risking behaviors either delayed or engaged in more responsibly. Parents can play a crucial role in reinforcing the mes-sages of health-promotion programs and in structuring adolescents' environments and activities so that healthy behavior is supported.

On the other hand, the significance of parents means that adolescents in trou-bled families may be at risk. Adolescents without close ties to parents are more likely to suffer from low self-esteem and to become involved in health-compromis-ing behaviors such as early sexual activity, drug abuse, and delinquency (Monte-mayor, 1983). Changes in family structure, especially those related to divorce and remarriage, also affect the quality of parent–child relationships (Hetherington, 1988), which may in turn increase health risks for some adolescents. Given the importance of parental support and guidance in adolescence, health promotion efforts should seek to strengthen parent–adolescent relationships and facilitate authoritative parenting. The value of emotional warmth, democratic decision mak-ing, appropriate monitoring, and clear standards for behavior should be empha-sized. Where good relationships with parents are not possible, it is important to link youth with other adults who can perform a supportive, mentoring role.

Peers

In adolescence, young people spend more and more time with peers, and the psy-chological importance attached to friendship and peer group relations increases

(Savin-Williams & Berndt, 1990). Change occurs in the structure and size of the peer group, as well as in the qualities of friendship.

CHANGES IN FRIENDSHIP. In early adolescence, young people begin to attach greater importance to intimacy—the capacity to share private thoughts and feelings (Berndt, 1982). From middle childhood to early adolescence, there is an increase in references to intimacy as a basis of friendship (e.g., Buhrmester & Furman, 1987), reported frequency of self-disclosure to friends (Sharabany, Gershoni, & Hofman, 1981), and actual intimate knowledge of one's friends (Diaz & Berndt, 1982). Closeness to friends increases throughout adolescence, surpassing closeness to parents, which remains relatively stable (Youniss & Smollar, 1985). The new emotional closeness and sharing tend to be expressed initially in same-sex relationships, with emotional closeness in cross-sex relationships not approaching that in same-sex friendships until the later years of high school (Sharabany et al., 1981). (For a discussion of cross-sex relationships, see Chapter 9.)

CHANGES IN PEER GROUP STRUCTURE. The structure of the peer network also changes over adolescence. In an early ethnographic study, Dunphy (1963) documented a sequence of peer group changes in which small friendship groups or cliques of same-sex peers prevailed in early adolescence but gave way to heterosexual cliques in midadolescence as dating relationships developed; in the latter phases of adolescence, heterosexual cliques were replaced, in turn, by loose networks of dating couples. More recent work has confirmed the prevalence of cliques in early adolescence (Crockett, Losoff, & Petersen, 1984) and the decrease in clique membership in midadolescence (Shrum & Cheek, 1987). Same-sex friendship groups undoubtedly provide a secure base from which young people can begin to explore issues related to self and identity, as well as the expectations of the adolescent role; they may also provide a safe base for initiating contact with the other sex, as Dunphy (1963) suggested.

A second type of peer group, called the *crowd,* is also common in early and midadolescence. Crowds are typically much larger than cliques and often reflect a particular type of person, such as the "in crowd" or the "jocks." According to Dunphy's (1963) developmental sequence, crowds are groups of cliques that associate at parties and other large-group activities, and their primary purpose is to facilitate the development of cross-sex interaction in a nonintimate setting. More recently, Brown (1989) has argued that crowds are reputation-based rather than interaction-based, with peers assigning adolescents to crowds on the basis of salient characteristics. Based on this view, the function of crowds is to help adolescents organize the large peer system to which they are exposed in secondary school. Crowds also have implications for identity development, since adolescents who are associated with a particular group may come to identify with the norms, values, and characteristics it represents.

CHANGES IN PEER INFLUENCE. The intensification of peer relationships at adolescence increases the potential for peer influence. Peers have been implicated in a variety of health-risking behaviors, including drug and alcohol use, delinquency, and early sexual activity (Brown, 1989). Of course, self-selection into deviant peer groups, as well as peer socialization, may contribute to these relationships (Kandel, 1986). Interestingly, studies of adolescent decision making do not provide evidence of heavy peer influence on risk taking (Furby & Beyth-Marom, 1990).

Peer influence depends on both the intensity of peer pressure and adolescents' susceptibility to this pressure. Studies of perceived peer pressure indicate changes over adolescence, with older adolescents feeling more pressure than younger ones to drink alcohol, have sex, and engage in misconduct (Brown, Clasen, & Eicher, 1986). Reported susceptibility to peer pressure also changes over adolescence, with peak susceptibility occurring in early adolescence (Berndt, 1979). Thus, early adolescence may be a period of heightened vulnerability. Still, it should be noted that for most adolescents, prosocial pressures are greater than antisocial ones and that adolescents report being more swayed by prosocial or neutral pressures than by pressures toward misconduct (Berndt, 1979; Brown, Lohr, & McClenahan, 1986).

MINORITY YOUTH. The importance of peers may be enhanced for minority youth (Spencer & Dornbusch, 1990). These youth become increasingly aware of their parents' lack of power in society and of the disparities between their parents' expectations and those of the dominant culture. This awareness may lead them to turn more to peers for guidance. Unfortunately, this dependence on peers may also prove detrimental. It has been suggested (Fordham & Ogbu, 1986) that for some minority youth, doing well in school may be negatively viewed as a capitulation to "white" society. Peers may, in effect, force some adolescents to choose between their ethnic identity and the values of the dominant culture. This may cut minority youth off from routes to success within the dominant culture.

IMPLICATIONS FOR HEALTH PROMOTION. The positive functions peers seem to serve in healthy adolescent development indicate a need to support these relationships. Loneliness and peer rejection should be targeted for intervention so that the benefits of adolescents' peer relationships are not lost. Social skills training has shown promise for improving adolescents' peer relationships (Caplan & Weissberg, 1989; de Armas & Kelly, 1989). At the same time, the potential contribution of peers to the development of health-risking behaviors needs to be confronted. One approach is to decrease adolescents' susceptibility to peer pressure by increasing their self-confidence and by teaching social skills that enable them to decline invitations to misbehavior effectively (Botvin & Tortu, 1988; Caplan & Weissberg, 1989). Such efforts may be especially useful with young adolescents or other groups (e.g., lower socioeconomic status minority youth) for whom susceptibility to peer pressure appears to be high. Another tactic is to link youngsters to peers with more prosocial values, for example, through cooperative learning situations that bring high-risk adolescents into contact with academically competent, prosocial classmates (Ianni, 1989). Finally, opportunities to engage in antisocial behavior may be curtailed through the introduction of improved monitoring. This might involve adult-supervised after-school activities and weekend programs; such programs provide alternative activities and reduce the pressures on youth to misbehave.

Health promotion efforts are likely to be most successful to the extent that they involve activities that meet adolescents' developmental needs for autonomy, friendship, and group membership. Peer acceptance of the program is probably essential. In addition, peers can become a positive force in health promotion efforts. Older peers, in particular, can encourage healthy behavior by serving as positive role models and promoting pro-health norms in the peer group (Klepp, Halper, & Perry, 1986). Ideally, the value system of the peer network as a whole would be changed to encourage healthy behavior, although this would require a large-scale, communitywide intervention effort (Perry & Jessor, 1985).

School

Throughout the twentieth century in the United States, schooling has become increasingly central in preparing young people for adulthood. Schooling is now essential for a successful future: failure to complete secondary school reduces employment opportunities and the probability of earning an adequate income (W. T. Grant Foundation, 1988). The need for higher skills, and therefore more education, is expected to show a continued increase in the workplace of the twenty first century (Mark, 1987).

CURRENT STATUS. There is ample evidence that schools in the United States are not meeting the needs of adolescents for healthy development. Data on school achievement in the United States compared to other countries demonstrate the pervasive underachievement of our youth. For example, our 13-year-olds score far below their counterparts in other developed countries in science and mathematics achievement (LaPointe, Mead, & Phillips, 1989). Moreover, the U. S. tests designed to chart progress on the most important cognitive skills have found that only 11% of 13-year-olds are adept readers and only 20% write adequate essays (Applebee, Langer, & Mullins, 1986). Minority adolescents seem to fare especially poorly in the current system. Rates of retention in grade school and high school and dropout rates are higher for boys than girls and higher for minority youth than whites. For example, the percentage of 13-year-olds who are at least one grade behind ranges from 22% for white girls to 47% for Hispanic boys, with the rates for blacks falling between those of Hispanics and whites (U. S. Bureau of the Census, 1988). Dropout rates are highest among Hispanic youth.

SCHOOL TRANSITIONS. There is substantial evidence that the transition from elementary school to middle school or junior high school can have negative effects (Eccles & Midgley, 1989). This transition, involving changes in both physical setting and social roles, produces a discontinuity that requires adaptive effort. Academic performance drops with each school transition (Blyth, Simmons, & Carlton-Ford, 1983), with stronger negative effects appearing for adolescents making earlier or multiple, closely spaced transitions (Crockett, Petersen, Graber, Schulenberg, & Ebata, 1989). One study with a heterogeneous urban sample also found negative effects of the transition on girls' self-esteem (Simmons & Blyth, 1987), although studies of suburban middle-class samples found no self-esteem effects (Fenzel & Blyth, 1986).

Studies on the process of school transitions provide important information for understanding these effects. As young adolescents move to junior high school, they have fewer choices and participate less in decision making (Feldlaufer, Midgley, & Eccles, 1988), experience more whole class task organization and less cooperative small group work (Rounds & Osaki, 1982), are evaluated more frequently and formally (Gullickson, 1985), and experience less positive relationships with their teachers (Hawkins & Berndt, 1985). Such studies indicate a less positive school environment after this transition, leading to decreased valuing of school and achievement, especially for those who make the transition with lower achievement (Eccles & Midgley, 1989).

BETTER SCHOOLS. Several studies (Bryk & Thum, 1989; Rutter, Maughan, Mortimore, Ouston, & Smith, 1979) have identified practices and conditions that lead to better student outcomes. These include an orderly social environment, high faculty interest and involvement, high emphasis on academic pursuits, and fewer differences among student courses of study. The Turning Points report (Carnegie Council on Adolescent Development, 1989) focused particularly on middle-grade education, but its findings are highly consistent with those of the studies on effective high schools. The recommendations include (1) creating small learning communities, (2) developing a core academic program, (3) practices that foster achievement rather than those such as tracking that isolate some students, leading to failure and dropping out, (4) appropriate distribution of governance, (5) credentialing of teachers for the middle grades, (6) practices that foster health and fitness, (7) involvement of families, and (8) strengthening connections between schools and communities. Each of these practices is already functioning effectively in some U. S. schools.

The creation of small learning communities is clearly relevant for middle and junior high schools. Youngsters in these schools have just come from more intimate elementary schools but are not yet in specialized classes that might afford increased student–teacher interaction. Small learning communities are defined as groups of no more than 200–300 students linked to a single group of teachers for the duration of middle school. This practice facilitates student–teacher interaction and permits cooperation among teachers with respect to sharing information on students and integrating the curriculum, thus reducing the destructive sense of anonymity (Arhar, Johnson, & Markle, 1989).

IMPLICATIONS FOR HEALTH PROMOTION. Schools are an important context for adolescent health promotion because of the amount of time adolescents spend there, as well as because of the natural opportunities schools provide for health promotion efforts. As noted by the Turning Points report (Carnegie Council on

Adolescent Development, 1989), schools can integrate health issues into a life science curriculum that would capitalize on the intense interest of young adolescents in the changes in their bodies. Curricular integration alone, however, is unlikely to be successful; life skills training (Hamburg, 1989) should be offered by schools as well.

There are limits to what schools can do to ensure the good health of students, particularly with the provision of school health care typically being limited to the school nurse. But schools can begin to meet adolescent health care needs more effectively by ensuring student access to health services and by establishing the school as a health-promoting environment (Carnegie Council on Adolescent Development, 1989). Student access may be enhanced by a school health coordinator and a health advisory team to coordinate referrals to community services, assist with the development of health-related policies for the school, and design health-enhancing activities. School-based health clinics and school-linked health centers are recommended as promising approaches to ensuring student access to health and counseling services (Millstein, 1988).

Schools can be health-promoting environments beyond what they might do in the curriculum. For example, school food services can provide nutritious meals and snacks that meet adolescents' need for healthy physical development. A no-smoking rule also conveys the message that the school is a setting in which everyone understands that smoking is unhealthy. Drug-free schools provide a similar and broader message. Physical fitness is another area in which schools can model healthy behavior; it is important that fitness activities be provided for all students, with the goal of helping students to develop the habit of regular exercise. Finally, schools must be safe environments that teach and use nonviolent methods of conflict management and resolution.

The evidence that the transition from elementary school may be stressful and have negative effects, coupled with the evidence that it is during early adolescence that many youngsters first experiment with health-compromising behaviors, suggests that this transition provides an important opportunity for health promotion efforts (Caplan & Weissberg, 1989; Felner, Gintner, & Primavera, 1982). By middle adolescence, many high-risk youth may no longer be in schools and will have to be reached in community settings.

Work

For the majority of adolescents in the United States today the workplace becomes a fourth important social context. In 1980, roughly two-thirds of high school seniors and one-half of all high school sophomores held part-time jobs (Lewin-Epstein, 1981). Most teenagers are employed in a relatively restricted array of jobs: as workers in restaurants, cashiers, and sales clerks outside of the food industry, clerical assistants in offices, and unskilled laborers. The jobs tend to be monotonous and boring, require little initiative or decision making, and rarely utilize skills learned in school; furthermore, some are highly stressful, requiring work under extreme time pressure (Greenberger & Steinberg, 1986).

Greenberger and Steinberg (1986) speculate about the implications of these work effects for healthy adolescent development. Working seems to promote the development of a work orientation and, among girls, facilitates the development of self-reliance. Nonetheless, adolescent work as it exists today may negatively affect psychological development. The typical adolescent job does not serve as a link to the adult work world, either in providing continuity to the jobs adolescents plan to hold as adults or in linking adolescents to adult co-workers as vocational mentors. Moreover, the routinized nature of the work is neither cognitively stimulating nor related to the role experimentation that is an important part of adolescent identity development. Rather, involvement in work may take time away from other activities that could contribute to identity development. Finally, greater involvement in work leads to fatigue, decreased interest in school, reduced extracurricular involvement, and poorer marks (Steinberg, Greenberger, Garduque, & McAuliffe, 1982). Furthermore, working in excess of 20 hours per week is associated with the development of a cynical attitude toward work, increased acceptance of unethical work practices, and increased drug and alcohol use (Steinberg, Greenberger, Garduque, Ruggiero, & Vaux, 1982). In addition, work is associated with more contact with older peers, decreased adult supervision, and increased discretionary income, which may provide opportunities for health-compromising behaviors such as substance use. Stress on the job also appears to increase the level of substance use (Greenberger, Steinberg, & Vaux, 1981). Although most of the research to date has involved middle-class adolescents working primarily to earn supplementary spending money, a recent study of a heterogeneous sample suggests that many of the negative effects of extensive work involvement hold across socioeconomic and ethnic groups (Steinberg & Dornbusch, 1991).

IMPLICATIONS FOR HEALTH PROMOTION. The typical adolescent job contributes little to personal development and appears to compromise health on a number of dimensions. Detrimental effects are especially likely for adolescents who work more than 20 hours per week. Limiting work involvement to less than 20 hours may help curb the negative effects. A more radical approach would be to upgrade typical adolescent jobs. Low-paying, adult-supervised community service projects would undoubtedly provide a healthier environment than the monotonous and often stressful jobs adolescents usually take, but the appeal of the paycheck may make such alternatives less attractive. Jobs that provide apprenticeship experience relevant to future employment and that link young people to adult vocational mentors might prove especially valuable (Hamilton, 1990), but any job that allows adolescents to develop intellectual and social skills, to have some autonomy, and to feel that their contribution matters will be an improvement.

The Broader Social Context: Community and Society

Adolescents develop within local communities embedded in a broader societal context (Hurrelmann, 1989). The broader society influences adolescent development and health indirectly through the organization of social institutions, the economy, the media, and social policy. The society also provides a dominant set of values or an ideology to which adolescents are exposed, along with expectations concerning adolescent behavior and development. These values and expectations are transmitted through the popular media, as well as through local institutions and the adolescent's social network.

In the United States, adolescence is a time of social redefinition during which young people make the transition from child to adult status. Legally and socially, adolescents have more autonomy than children (although less than adults) and are expected to show more mature, responsible behavior. The greater autonomy granted adolescents is reflected in less adult supervision and in new privileges (e.g., driving, voting) that expose adolescents to more opportunities for health-compromising behaviors. Perhaps inadvertently, we give adolescents more personal control over their health-related choices and then hope they will act wisely, often with little guidance and support. In this sense, we treat them as adults. On the other hand, we restrict adolescents' access to positively valued adult roles (e.g., full-time worker) and attempt to limit their involvement in valued adult behaviors such as sex and drinking. These roles and behaviors thus become attractive symbols of adult status (Jessor, 1984). The social view of adolescents as moving toward adulthood, combined with our desire to limit adolescents' access to valued adult roles and behaviors, may increase the functional value of some health-compromising behavior. The media supports many of these behaviors directly through their portrayals of sex and substance use in television programming, as well as through advertising campaigns directed at youth (Williams, in press).

The local community more directly influences adolescents' motivations and opportunities to engage in health-risking behaviors. Local peer norms reflected, for example, in the rates of teenage childbearing, drug use, and college attendance provide messages about typical and acceptable adolescent behaviors, as well as opportunities for health-compromising behaviors. In addition, adults in the community serve as role models, affecting young people's expectations concerning their likely roles and activities as adults (Erikson, 1968; Ianni, 1989). Communities with a high proportion of well-educated, financially successful adults employed in business and the professions clearly provide a different array of models than impoverished neighborhoods where poor, single-parent households are the norm, illness is chronic, drug abuse is prevalent, and the financially successful adults are involved in illicit activities. Such environmental characteristics affect young people's expectations for the future, their perceptions of how current behavior could jeopardize future chances, and, consequently, their motivation to avoid risky behavior (Dryfoos, 1990). A recent study of neighborhood effects showed that the prevalence of single-mother households and the relative absence of middle-class neighbors affected rates of high school dropping out and teenage childbearing (Brooks-Gunn, Duncan, Kato, & Sealand, 1991).

Obviously, a key aspect of the community environment affecting adolescent risk is its level of economic resources (Chapter 3). Resources also affect opportunities for health promotion, for example, by influencing the quality of local schools and community services. Schools in wealthy areas can provide high-quality education that will increase students' interest in school and their chances of future success. Wealthy communities also provide opportunities for alternative, healthy activities through community clubs and organizations. Thus, community resources influence the quality and quantity of the health risks adolescents face, as well as the local capacity for health promotion.

Conclusions

Adolescence is a period of normal positive growth toward biological, cognitive, and psychosocial maturity. As a period of growth, increased autonomy, and exploration, it also involves risks, with the constellation of risks being dependent on individual strengths and weaknesses and the characteristics of the social environment. The goal of health promotion is to promote positive growth and adjustment throughout this period while helping young people to avoid outcomes that compromise their future health and development. More precisely, our review of adolescent development suggests the following broad goals: (1) to promote physical health and well-being through proper nutrition and exercise, development of a positive body image and healthy sexuality, and adoption of a healthy lifestyle; (2) to promote cognitive maturity, including the capacity for abstract, formal reasoning, social-cognitive skills, and autonomous decision making; (3) to promote self-esteem and a positive sense of personal identity, including positive future goals and a sense of self-efficacy and social responsibility; (4) to promote supportive relationships with family, peers, and other important adults; (5) to provide opportunities for educational and occupational success; and (6) to avoid pitfalls that would interfere with the positive developmental outcomes outlined above. These goals reflect a dual emphasis on promoting health-enhancing behaviors and simultaneously weakening health-compromising behaviors (Perry & Jessor, 1985).

This review suggests that, to be successful, health promotion efforts need to be sensitive to the developmental competencies and needs of the adolescents to be served. Thus, programs geared to the cognitive level of the target population and programs that focus on the challenges and concerns relevant to those adolescents (e.g., physical maturation, peer relations, autonomy, the transition to secondary school) are likely to have greater impact.

Because adolescent development (healthy or otherwise) occurs in a social context defined by family, peers, school, the workplace, and the local community, health promotion efforts need to target not only individual adolescents but also the social contexts in which they live (Dryfoos, 1990). Enhancing self-esteem, for example, may require increasing positive feedback from parents and peers, improving academic skills and performance, and providing additional arenas where young people can succeed. These strategies naturally draw in the family, peer group, school, and workplace. Consequently, one dimension of health promotion with adolescents may include supporting and improving the settings that form the core of their daily lives. This could mean supporting families of adolescents financially and providing services to improve the quality of parent–adolescent relationships and communication. It could mean facilitating friendships with prosocial peers or improving the health-related norms of the local peer network (Chapter 5). Improving the quality of schools and the relevance of the curriculum for adolescents' future goals should be considered, along with establishing the school as a health-enhancing setting (Chapter 5). Finally, the relevance of adolescents' work experience could be improved by providing opportunities for apprenticeships and direct exposure to vocational mentors and possible occupational roles (Hamilton, 1990), as well as by upgrading the typical adolescent workplace. Many of these approaches depend on community and public resources. Local businesses would need to cooperate in enabling adolescents to role-play possible occupations, and school personnel and parents would have to collaborate to enhance the quality of schooling provided. Moreover, the coordination among various settings might need to be improved— for example, that between school and community (Price, Cioci, Penner, & Trautlein, 1990). Thus, successful programs need to have the support and cooperation of community institutions; the most successful ones will target not only individual adolescents also but the key social contexts that structure their daily lives.

References

Adler, N. E., Kegeles, S. M., Irwin, C. E., & Wibbelsman, C. (1990). Adolescent contraceptive behavior: An assessment of decision processes. *Journal of Pediatrics, 116*, 463–471.

Applebee, A., Langer, J., & Mullins, I. (1986). *The writing report card, writing achievement in American schools.* Princeton, NJ: National Assessment of Educational Progress, Educational Testing Service.

Arhar, J. M., Johnson, J. H., & Markle, G. C. (1989). The effects of teaming on students. *Middle School Journal, 20*, 24–27.

Attie, I., Brooks-Gunn, J., & Petersen, A. C. (1990). A developmental perspective on eating disorders and eating problems. In M. Lewis & S. M. Miller (Eds.), *Handbook of developmental psychopathology* (pp. 409–420). New York: Plenum.

Baumrind, D. (1991). The influence of parenting style on adolescent competence and substance use. *Journal of Early Adolescence, 11*, 56–95.

Berndt, T. (1979). Developmental changes in conformity to peers and parents. *Developmental Psychology, 15*, 608–616.

Berndt, T. (1982). The features and effects of friendship in early adolescence. *Child Development, 53*, 1447–1460.

Blos, P. (1970). *The adolescent passage.* New York: International Universities Press.

Blyth, D. A., Simmons, R. G., & Carlton-Ford, S. (1983). The adjustment of early adolescents to school transitions. *Journal of Early Adolescence, 3*, 105–120.

Botvin, G. J., & Tortu, S. (1988). Preventing adolescent substance abuse through life skills training. In R. Price, E. L. Cowen, R. P. Lorian, & J. Ramos-McKay (Eds.), *A casebook for practictioners* (pp. 98–110). Washington, DC: American Psychological Association.

Bronfenbrenner, U. (1979). *The ecology of human development.* Cambridge, MA: Harvard University Press.

Brooks-Gunn, J., Duncan, G. J., Kato, P., & Sealand, N. (1991). *Do neighborhoods influence child and adolescent behavior?* Unpublished manuscript.

Brooks-Gunn, J., & Reiter, E. O. (1990). The role of pubertal processes. In S. S. Feldman & G. R. Elliott (Eds.), *At the threshold: The developing adolescent* (pp. 16–53). Cambridge, MA: Harvard University Press.

Brown, B. (1989). The role of peer groups in adolescents' adjustment to secondary school. In T. J. Berndt & G. W. Ladd (Eds.), *Peer relationships in child development* (pp. 188–216). New York: Wiley.

Brown, B., Clasen, D., & Eicher, S. (1986). Perceptions of peer pressure, peer conformity dispositions, and self-reported behavior among adolescents. *Developmental Psychology, 22,* 521–530.

Brown, B., Lohr, M., & McClenahan, E. (1986). Early adolescents' perceptions of peer pressure. *Journal of Early Adolescence, 6,* 139–154.

Bryk, A. S., & Thum, Y. M. (1989). The effects of high school organization on dropping out: An exploratory investigation. *American Educational Research Journal, 26,* 353–383.

Buckley, W. E., Yesalis, C. E., Friedl, K. E., Anderson, W. A., Streit, A. L., & Wright, J. E. (1988). Estimated prevalence of anabolic steroid use among male high school seniors. *Journal of the American Medical Association, 260,* 3441–3445.

Buhrmester, D., & Furman, W. (1987). The development of companionship and intimacy. *Child Development, 58,* 1101–1113.

Caplan, M. Z., & Weissberg, R. P. (1989). Promoting social competence in early adolescence: Developmental considerations. In B. H. Schneider, G. Attili, J. Nadel, & R. P. Weissberg (Eds.), *Social competence in developmental perspective* (pp. 371–385). Boston: Kluwer.

Carnegie Council on Adolescent Development (1989). *Turning points: Preparing American youth for the 21st century.* Washington, DC: Carnegie Corporation.

Caspi, A., Lynam, D., Moffit, T. E., Silva, C. (in press). Unraveling girls' delinquency: Biological, dispositional, and contextual contributions to adolescent misbehavior. *Developmental Psychology.*

Clausen, J. (1986). *The lifecourse: A sociological perspective.* Englewood Cliffs, NJ: Prentice-Hall.

Crockett, L., Losoff, M., & Petersen A. (1984). Perceptions of the peer group and friendship in early adolescence. *Journal of Early Adolescence, 4,* 155–181.

Crockett, L. J., Petersen, A. C., Graber, J. A., Schulenberg, J. E., & Ebata, A. (1989). School transitions and adjustment during early adolescence. *Journal of Early Adolescence, 9,* 181–210.

de Armas, A., & Kelly, J. A. (1989). Social relationships in adolescence: Skill development and training. In J. Worell & F. Danner (Eds.), *The adolescent as decision-maker: Applications to development and education* (pp. 84–109). San Diego: Academic Press.

Diaz, R., & Berndt, T. (1982). Children's knowledge of a best friend: Fact or fancy? *Developmental Psychology, 18,* 787–794.

Dorn, L. D., Crockett, L. J., & Petersen, A. C. (1988). The relations of pubertal status to intrapersonal changes in young adolescents. *Journal of Early Adolescence, 8,* 405–419.

Dornbusch, S., Ritter, P., Leiderman, P., Roberts, D., & Fraleigh, M. (1987). The relation of parenting style to adolescent school performance. *Child Development, 58,* 1244–1257.

Dryfoos, J. (1990). *Adolescents at risk: Prevalence and prevention.* New York: Oxford University Press.

Dunphy, D. (1963). The social structure of urban adolescent peer groups. *Sociometry, 26,* 230–246.

Eccles, J. S., & Midgley, C. (1989). Stage/environment fit: Developmentally appropriate classrooms for early adolescents. In R. E. Ames & C. Ames (Eds.), *Research on motivation in education (Vol. 3).* New York: Academic Press.

Eichorn, D. H. (1975). Asynchronization in adolescent development. In J. E. Dragastin & G. H. Elder (Eds.), *Adolescence in the life cycle: Psychological change and social context* (pp. 81–96). Washington, DC: Hemisphere.

Elder, G. (1985). *Life course dynamics.* Ithaca, NY: Cornell University Press.

Erikson, E. (1968). *Identity: Youth in crisis.* New York: Norton.

Eylon, B., & Linn, M. C. (1988). Learning and instruction: An examination of four research perspectives in science education. *Review of Educational Research, 58,* 251–301.

Faust, M. S. (1983). Alternative constructions of adolescent growth. In J. Brooks-Gunn & A. C. Petersen (Eds.), *Girls at puberty: Biological and psychosocial perspectives* (pp. 105–125). New York: Plenum.

Feinberg, J. (1987). Adolescence and mental illness [letter]. *Science, 236,* 507–508.

Feldlaufer, H., Midgley, C., & Eccles, J. S. (1988). Student, teacher, and observer perceptions of the classroom environment before and after the transition to junior high school. *Journal of Early Adolescence, 8,* 133–156.

Felner, R. D., Gintner, M., & Primavera, J. (1982). Primary prevention during school transitions: Social support and environmental structure. *American Journal of Community Psychology, 10,* 277–290.

Fenzel, L. M., & Blyth, D. A. (1986). Individual adjustment to school transitions: An exploration of the role of supportive peer relations. *Journal of Early Adolescence, 6,* 315–329.

Fordham, C., & Ogbu, J. (1986). Black students' school success: Coping with the burden of "acting white." *Urban Review, 18,* 176–206.

Freud, A. (1958). *Adolescence: Psychoanalytic study of the child (Vol. 13).* New York: Academic Press.

Frisch, R. (1983). Fatness, puberty, and fertility: The effects of nutrition and physical training on menarche and ovulation. In J. Brooks-Gunn & A. Petersen (Eds.), *Girls at puberty* (pp. 29–49). New York: Plenum.

Furby, L., & Beyth-Marom, R. (1990). *Risk taking in adolescence: A decision-making perspective.* Washington, DC: Carnegie Council on Adolescent Development.

Graber, J. A., & Petersen, A. C. (1991). Cognitive changes at adolescence: Biological perspectives. In K. R. Gibson & A. C. Petersen (Eds.), *Brain maturation and cognitive development* (pp. 253–279). New York: Aldine de Gruyter.

Greenberger, E., & Steinberg, L. (1986). *When teenagers work: The psychological and social costs of adolescent employment.* New York: Basic Books.

Greenberger, E., Steinberg, L., & Vaux, A. (1981). Adolescents who work: Health and behavioral consequences of job stress. *Developmental Psychology, 17,* 691–703.

Greene, A. L. (1986). Future time-perspective in adolescence: The present of things future revisited. *Journal of Youth and Adolescence, 15,* 99–113.

Gullickson, A. R. (1985). Student evaluation techniques and their relationship to grade and curriculum. *Journal of Educational Research, 79,* 96–100.

Hamburg, B. (1986). Subsets of adolescent mothers: Developmental, biomedical, and psychosocial issues. In J. B. Lancaster & B. A. Hamburg (Eds.), *School-age pregnancy and parenthood: Biosocial dimensions* (pp. 115–145). New York: Aldine de Gruyter.

Hamburg, B. (1989). *Life skills training: Preventive interventions for early adolescents.* Washington, DC: Carnegie Council on Adolescent Development.

Hamilton, S. F. (1990). *Apprenticeship for adulthood: Preparing youth for the future.* New York: Free Press.

Hamilton, S. F., & Darling, N. (1989). Mentors in adolescents' lives. In K. Hurrelmann & U. Engel (Eds.), *The social world of adolescents: International perspectives* (pp. 121–139). Berlin: Walter de Gruyter.

Harter, S. (1990). Self and identity development. In S. S. Feldman & G. R. Elliott (Eds.), *At the threshold: The developing adolescent* (pp. 352–387). Cambridge, MA: Harvard University Press.

Havighurst, R. J. (1972). *Developmental tasks and education* (3rd ed.). New York: David McKay.

Hawkins, J., & Berndt, T. J. (1985, April). *Adjustment following the transition to junior high school.* Paper presented at the biennial meeting of the Society for Research in Child Development, Toronto, Canada.

Hetherington, E. M. (1988). Parents, children, and siblings: Six years after divorce. In E. M. Hetherington, R. M. Lerner, & M. Perlmutter (Eds.), *Child development in life-span perspective* (pp. 311–331). Hillsdale, NJ: Erlbaum.

Hill, J., Holmbeck, G., Marlow, L., Green, T., & Lynch, M. (1985). Menarcheal status and parent–child relations in families of seventh-grade girls. *Journal of Youth and Adolescence, 14,* 301–316.

Hurrelmann, K. (1989). Adolescents as productive processors of reality: Methodological perspectives. In K. Hurrelmann & U. Engel (Eds.), *The social world of adolescents: International perspectives* (pp. 107–118). Berlin: Walter de Gruyter.

Ianni, F. (1989). *The search for structure: A report on American youth today.* New York: Free Press.

Inhelder, B., & Piaget, J. (1958). *The growth of logical thinking from childhood to adolescence.* New York: Basic Books.

Irwin, C., & Millstein, S. (1986). Biopsychosocial correlates of risk-taking behaviors during adolescence. *Journal of Adolescent Health Care, 7,* 82–95.

Jessor, R. (1984). Adolescent development and behavioral health. In J. Matarazzo, S. Weiss, J. Herd, N. Miller, & J. M. Weiss (Eds.), *Behavioral health: A handbook of health enhancement and disease prevention* (pp. 69–90). New York: Wiley.

Kandel, D. B. (1986). Processes of peer influences in adolescence. In R. K. Silbereisen & K. Eyferth (Eds.), *Development as action in context* (pp. 203–227). Berlin: Walter de Gruyter.

Kandel, D., & Lesser, G. (1972). *Youth in two worlds.* San Francisco: Jossey-Bass.

Kaplan, H. B. (1980). *Deviant behavior in defense of self.* New York: Academic Press.

Keating, D. P. (1990). Adolescent thinking. In S. S. Feldman & G. R. Elliott (Eds.), *At the threshold: The developing adolescent* (pp. 54–89). Cambridge, MA: Harvard University Press.

Keating, D. P., & Clark, L. V. (1980). Development of physical and social reasoning in adolescence. *Developmental Psychology, 16,* 23–30.

Klepp, K. I., Halper, A., & Perry, C. L. (1986). The efficacy of peer leaders in drug abuse prevention. *Journal of School Health, 56,* 407–411.

Kuhn, D., Amsel, E., & O'Loughlin, M. (1988). *The development of scientific thinking skills.* San Diego, CA: Academic Press.

LaPointe, A. E., Mead, N. A., & Phillips, G. W. (1989). *A world of differences: An international assessment of mathematics and science.* Princeton, NJ: Educational Testing Service.

Lerner, R. M. (1987). A life-span perspective for early adolescence. In R. M. Lerner & T. T. Foch (Eds.), *Biological–psychosocial interactions in early adolescence* (pp. 9–34). Hillsdale, NJ: Erlbaum.

Lerner, R. M., Karson, M., Meisels, M., & Knapp, J. R. (1975). Actual and perceived attitudes of late adolescents: The phenomenon of the generation gap. *Journal of Genetic Psychology, 126,* 197–207.

Lewin-Epstein, N. (1981). *Youth employment during high school.* Washington, DC: National Center for Education Statistics.

Lewis, C. (1981). How adolescents approach decisions: Changes over grades seven to twelve and policy implications. *Child Development, 52,* 538–544.

Linn, M. C. (1983). Content, context, and process in reasoning during adolescence: Selecting a model. *Journal of Early Adolescence, 3,* 63–82.

Maccoby, E., & Martin, J. (1983). Socialization in the context of the family: Parent–child interaction. In E. M. Hetherington (Ed.), *Handbook of child psychology. Vol. 4: Socialization, personality, and social development* (pp. 103–196). New York: Wiley.

Magnusson, D., Stattin, H., & Allen, V. L. (1985). Biological maturation and social development: A longitudinal study of some adjustment processes from mid-adolescence to adulthood. *Journal of Youth and Adolescence, 14,* 267–283.

Mann, L., Harmoni, R., Power, C., Beswick, G., & Ormond, C. (1988). Effectiveness of the GOFOR course in decision-making for high school students. *Journal of Behavioral Decision-Making, 1,* 159–168.

Marcia, J. (1966). Development and validation of ego identity status. *Journal of Personality and Social Psychology, 3,* 551–558.

Mark, J. A. (1987). Technological change and employment: Some results from BLS research. *Monthly Labor Review, 110,* 26–29.

McCarthy, J. D., & Hoge, D. R. (1982). Analysis of age effects in longitudinal studies of adolescent self-esteem. *Developmental Psychology, 18,* 372–379.

Millstein, S. G. (1988). *The potential of school-linked centers to promote adolescent health and development.* Washington, DC: Carnegie Council on Adolescent Development.

Montemayor, R. (1983). Parents and adolescents in conflict: All families some of the time and some families most of the time. *Journal of Early Adolescence, 3,* 83–103.

Offer, D., Ostrov, E., & Howard, K. (1981). *The adolescent: A psychological self-portrait.* New York: Basic Books.

O'Malley, P. M., & Bachman, J. G. (1983). Self-esteem: Change and stability between ages 13 and 23. *Developmental Psychology, 19,* 257–268.

Patterson, G. R., & Stouthamer-Loeber, M. (1984). The correlation of family management practices and delinquency. *Child Development, 55,* 1299–1307.

Perry, C. L., & Jessor, R. (1985). The concept of health promotion and the prevention of adolescent drug abuse. *Health Education Quarterly, 12,* 169–184.

Peskin, H. (1973). Influence of the developmental schedule of puberty on learning and ego development. *Journal of Youth and Adolescence, 2,* 273–290.

Petersen, A. C. (1987). The nature of biological–psychosocial interactions: The sample case of early adolescence. In R. M. Lerner & T. T. Foch (Eds.), *Biological–psychosocial interactions in early adolescence* (pp. 35–61). Hillsdale, NJ: Erlbaum.

Petersen, A. C. (1988). Adolescent development. *Annual Review of Psychology, 39,* 583–607.

Petersen, A. C., & Crockett, L. J. (1985). Pubertal timing and grade effects on adjustment. *Journal of Youth and Adolescence, 14,* 191–206.

Petersen, A. C., Sarigiani, P. A., & Kennedy, R. E. (1991). Adolescent depression: Why more girls? *Journal of Youth and Adolescence, 20,* 247–271.

Petersen, A. C., & Taylor, B. (1980). The biological approach to adolescence: Biological change and psychological adaptation. In J. Adelson (Ed.), *Handbook of adolescent psychology* (pp. 117–155). New York: John Wiley.

Price, R. H., Cioci, M., Penner, W., & Trautlein, B. (1990). *School and community support programs that enhance adolescent health and education.* Washington, DC: Carnegie Council on Adolescent Development.

Reiter, E. O. (1987). Neuroendocrine control processes: Pubertal onset and progression. *Journal of Adolescent Health Care, 8,* 479–491.

Rounds, T. S., & Osaki, S. Y. (1982). *The social organization of classrooms: An analysis of sixth- and seventh-grade activity structures.* (Report EPSSP-82-5). San Francisco: Far West Laboratory.

Rutter, M. (1986). The developmental psychopathology of depression: Issues and perspectives. In M. Rutter, C. Izard, & P. Read (Eds.), *Depression in young people: Developmental and clinical perspectives* (pp. 3–30). New York: Guilford.

Rutter, M., Maughan, B., Mortimore, P., Ouston, J., & Smith, A. (1979). *Fifteen thousand hours: Secondary schools and their effects on children.* Cambridge, MA: Harvard University Press.

Savin-Williams, R. C., & Berndt, T. J. (1990). Friendship and peer relations. In S. S. Feldman & G. R. Elliott (Eds.), *At the threshold: The developing adolescent* (pp. 277–307). Cambridge, MA: Harvard University Press.

Scales, P. (1990). Developing capable young people: An alternative strategy for prevention programs. *Journal of Early Adolescence, 10,* 420–438.

Sharabany, R., Gershoni, R., & Hofman, J. (1981). Girlfriend, boyfriend: Age and sex differences in intimate friendship. *Developmental Psychology, 17,* 800–808.

Shrum, W., & Cheek, N. H. (1987). Social structure during the school years: Onset of the degrouping process. *American Sociological Review, 52,* 218–223.

Simmons, R. G., & Blyth, D. A. (1987). *Moving into adolescence: The impact of pubertal change and school context.* Hawthorne, NY: Aldine.

Spencer, M., & Dornbusch, S. (1990). Challenges in studying minority youth. In S. S. Feldman & G. R. Elliott (Eds.), *At the threshold: The developing adolescent* (pp. 123–146). Cambridge, MA: Harvard University Press.

Spencer, M., & Markstrom-Adams, C. (1990). Identity processes among racial and ethnic minority children in America. *Child Development, 61,* 290–310.

Steinberg, L. (1981). Transformation in family relations at puberty. *Developmental Psychology, 17,* 833–838.

Steinberg, L. (1990). Autonomy, conflict, and harmony in the family relationship. In S. S. Feldman & G. R. Elliott (Eds.), *At the threshold: The developing adolescent* (pp. 255–276). Cambridge, MA: Harvard University Press.

Steinberg, L. (1991). Adolescent transitions and alcohol and other drug use prevention. In E. Goplerud (Ed.), *Preventing adolescent drug use: From theory to practice* (OSAP Prevention

Monograph 8). Rockville, MD: U. S. Department of Health and Human Services, ADAMHA. Alcohol, Drug and Mental Health Administration.

Steinberg, L., & Dornbusch, S. M. (1991). Negative correlates of part-time employment during adolescence: Replication and elaboration. *Developmental Psychology, 27,* 304–313.

Steinberg, L., Elman, J. D., & Mounts, N. S. (1989). Authoritative parenting, psychosocial maturity, and academic success among adolescents. *Child Development, 60,* 1424–1436.

Steinberg, L., Greenberger, E., Garduque, L., & McAuliffe, S. (1982). Adolescents in the labor force: Some costs and benefits to schooling and learning. *Educational Evaluation and Policy Analysis, 4,* 363–372.

Steinberg, L., Greenberger, E., Garduque, L., Ruggiero, M., & Vaux, A. (1982). Effects of working on adolescent development. *Developmental Psychology, 18,* 385–395.

Steinberg, L., & Silverberg, S. (1986). The vicissitudes of autonomy in early adolescence. *Child Development, 57,* 841–851.

Susman, E., Inhoff-Germain, G., Nottelmann, E., Loriaux, D., Cutler, G., Jr., & Chrousos, G. (1987). Hormones, emotional dispositions, and aggressive attributes in young adolescents. *Child Development, 58,* 1114–1134.

Tanner, J. M. (1972). Sequence, tempo, and individual variation in growth and development of boys and girls aged twelve to sixteen. In J. Kagan & R. Coles (Eds.), *Twelve to sixteen: Early adolescence* (pp. 1–24). New York: Norton.

Tobin-Richards, M. H., Boxer, A. M., & Petersen, A. C. (1983). The psychological significance of pubertal change: Sex differences in perceptions of self during early adolescence. In J. Brooks-Gunn & A. C. Petersen (Eds.), *Girls at puberty: Biological and psychosocial perspectives* (pp. 127–154). New York: Plenum Press.

Turiel, E. (1989). Domain-specific social judgments and domain ambiguities. *Merrill-Palmer Quarterly, 35,* 89–114.

Udry, J. R., & Billy, J. O. (1987). Initiation of coitus in early adolescence. *American Sociological Review, 52,* 841–855.

Udry, J. R., Billy, J. O., Morris, N. M., Groff, T. R., & Raj, M. H. (1985). Serum androgenic hormones motivate sexual behavior in adolescent boys. *Fertility and Sterility, 43,* 90–94.

Udry, J. R., Talbert, L. M., & Morris, N. M. (1986). Biosocial foundations for adolescent female sexuality. *Demography, 23,* 217–227.

U. S. Bureau of the Census. (1988). *School enrollment—social and economic characteristics of students: October 1986.* (Current Population Report, Series P-20, No. 429). Washington, DC: U. S. Government Printing Office.

Waterman, A. S. (1985). Identity in the context of adolescent psychology. In A. S. Waterman (Ed.), *Identity in adolescence: Processes and contents* (pp. 5–24). San Francisco: Jossey-Bass.

Weithorn, L. A., & Campbell, S. B. (1982). The competency of children and adolescents to make informed treatment decisions. *Child Development, 53,* 1589–1598.

Williams, J. (in press). Alcohol and tobacco products in the media and the effects on minority adolescents: A review of issues, theory, and empirical studies. In R. M. Lerner (Ed.), *Early adolescence: Perspectives on research, policy, and prevention.* Hillsdale, NJ: Erlbaum.

Woods, E. R., Wilson, C. D., & Masland, R. P. (1988). Weight control methods in high school wrestlers. *Journal of Adolescent Health Care, 9,* 394–397.

Worthman, C. M. (1986). Developmental dyssynchrony as normative experience: Kikuyu adolescents. In J. B. Lancaster & B. A. Hamburg (Eds.), *School-age, pregnancy and parenthood: Biosocial dimensions* (pp. 95–112). New York: Aldine de Gruyter.

W. T. Grant Foundation, Commission on Work, Family, and Citizenship. (1988). *The forgotten half: Pathways to success for America's youth and young families.* Washington, DC: Commission Office.

Yakovlev, P. I., & Lecours, A. R. (1967). The myelogenetic cycles of regional maturation in the brain. In A. Minkowski (Eds.), *Regional development of the brain in early life* (pp. 3–70). Oxford: Blackwell.

Youniss, J., & Smollar, J. (1985). *Adolescents' relations with mothers, fathers, and friends.* Chicago: University of Chicago Press.

3

The Influence of Economic Factors on Health-Related Behaviors in Adolescents

Lorraine V. Klerman

The health of the poor is generally worse than the health of the nonpoor, regardless of age, but poverty is only one of the many factors that affect health status. Genetic endowment, perinatal conditions, the physical and social environments, and medical care are a few others. Poverty appears to influence health both by increasing the likelihood of these factors causing health problems and by influencing health-related behaviors. This chapter will not explore all the ways that poverty can impact adolescent health; instead, it will focus on the *behaviors* of poor adolescents that are likely to compromise their health, such as smoking or using drugs, and on those that are likely to enhance their health, such as using contraceptives or seeking medical care.

Possible Mechanisms of Influence

Why should being poor increase the probability of health-compromising behaviors and reduce the probability of health-enhancing ones?

Income

One reason is obvious. Income that is insufficient to meet basic needs may make particular behaviors difficult—for example, seeking medical care. Other health-promoting activities may require cash, such as participation in some interscholastic athletics or membership in a gym or health club.

In addition, low income often causes families to live in inner-city ghettos. Wilson (1987) has noted that ghetto life provides few role models of health-enhancing behavior (Chapters 4 and 12).

38

Family Environment

Several studies, however, suggest reasons more subtle than inadequate income. Poor adolescents appear less connected to sources that might advocate or model positive behaviors or urge the avoidance of negative ones. These sources include families, schools, and community organizations. Poor adolescents seem greatly influenced by peer groups that may engage in health-compromising activities. Is this because poor adolescents are not receiving adequate emotional support from their families? If so, how does poverty reduce the ability of families to remain close to their adolescents?

Some families live in poverty because they are psychologically or physically handicapped. Such families may be not only unable to earn incomes that would allow them to rise above poverty, but also incapable of providing strong emotional support. Families that do not have such handicaps may react to the stress of their economic circumstances with depression or other responses that distance them from their adolescent children, such as television viewing at best or prostitution or drug dealing at worst. They may try to rise out of poverty by working long hours or having several jobs, again resulting in being unavailable to their adolescents.

Poor families also are less likely to have the formal education or the exposure to various sources of information that would heighten their awareness of the emotional needs of children, especially adolescents. Thus, the effect of poverty on adolescent health and health-related behaviors may be partially mediated by parental education (Mechanic & Hansell, 1987), although much remains to be learned about how education has this effect. (Some research cited in this chapter uses parental education as a measure of poverty and social class.)

Finally, several studies suggest that economic stress may influence adolescent behavior as a function of parental supervision and parental discipline. Many poor adolescents are from households where there is only one parent, usually a mother. Single parents, especially if they are working, may have less time than a parental pair to supervise their children. Adolescents who experience less supervision may become more autonomous, and at earlier ages, than those receiving greater supervision. This may result in the peer group having greater, and sometimes more destructive, influence (Chapters 2 and 5).

Schools and Community Groups

Weakened ties to the family may also affect adolescent health behavior indirectly by lessening the pressure to achieve academically or even to remain in school. Chronic absence or dropping out of school removes the adolescent from one source of information about and support of health promotion. In addition, without strong family pressure, adolescents may not become involved in religious groups or clubs—other potential sources of pressure toward health-enhancing behaviors. Moreover, adolescents who are not in school or engaged in other community activities probably spend less time with adult role models and more time with peers whose influence may lead to health-compromising behaviors.

Psychological Factors

Adolescents may be more likely to practice health-promoting behaviors if they believe that they have the power to influence their future. Alienation or a sense of powerlessness or hopelessness is not conducive to health promotion. Yet a large national study of eighth graders revealed that the perception of personal control over one's life was highest among those in the highest socioeconomic quartile. Those in the lowest quartile were more likely to have a limited sense of personal control and a belief that one reached goals through luck rather than planning or effort (Hafner, Ingels, Schneider, & Stevenson, 1990).

The lengthening of the period prior to the assumption of adult responsibilities has left many adolescents with a sense of rolelessness. This is a problem particularly for those who do not complete high school or seek education beyond it (Nightingale & Wolverton, 1988; Steinberg, 1991). Rolelessness may lessen the adolescent's interest in health-enhancing activities directly, since there is no goal that being healthy will help achieve, and indirectly by making them more dependent on peer approval.

The Concept of Poverty

The federal government classifies individuals and families as poor on the basis of federal poverty guidelines. Families are poor if their incomes are below the federal poverty line and near-poor if their incomes are between 100 and 149% of the line. In 1964, the federal government established the poverty level at three times the cost of the U. S. Department of Agriculture's 1961 Economy Food Plan, because families of three or more persons spent approximately a third of their income on food. Every year since 1964, the poverty level, which varies with family size, has been adjusted for inflation, as measured by the Consumer Price Index, but for nothing else. In 1992, the federal poverty line was $11,570 for a family of three and $13,950 for a family of four. (U.S. Department of Health and Human Services, 1992).

Some experts believe that the federal poverty guidelines are too *high,* that is, that some families below the poverty line are not really poor. This argument is based on the fact that only monetary income is included in the poverty calculations and no allowance is made for Medicaid, food stamps, and other subsidies or for money obtained through the underground economy. Others believe that the guidelines are too *low*—that is, that some families above the poverty line should be defined as poor. A major factor in this argument is the high cost of housing, which now consumes a higher percentage of the income of most poor families than it did in the 1960s. Another problem with the current measure is the absence of adjustment for place of residence, with the exception of Alaska and Hawaii, whose higher costs of living are reflected in the federal guidelines. The cost of living is generally higher in cities than in rural areas, and some areas of the country are more expensive than others even when degree of urbanization is held constant. A 1989 Gallup poll found that Americans defined poverty for a family of four as slightly over $15,000 (DeParle, 1990).

State and federal governments are clearly ambivalent about the appropriateness of the federal poverty guidelines. State programs tend to set a lower standard. For example, in 1992 the maximum monthly benefit for a one-parent family of three under the country's major welfare program, Aid to Families with Dependent Children (AFDC), ranged from 13% of the 1991 federal poverty threshold in Mississippi to 82% in Alaska. Only 14 states provided over 50% of the federal poverty level (U. S. House of Representatives, 1992). These data suggest that most states believe that families can subsist on less than the federal standard. Federal programs, however, often have a higher standard. For example, eligibility for the Special Supplemental Food Program for Women, Infants, and Children (WIC) is 185% of the poverty level and for Medicaid health benefits for children under 6 and pregnant women, 133 percent.

Poverty among Adolescents

Because many low-income families "age out" of poverty, adolescents are less likely to be poor than younger children. Teenage mothers finish school and find employment or marry a man who can provide an income or an additional one. Heads of households with little work experience and, as a result, low-paying jobs, prove their worth and find better-paying ones. Consequently, 23% of children under 6 were below the federal poverty level in 1989 (National Center for Children in Poverty, 1991) compared to 16% of 12- to 17-year-olds (3 million) and 15% of 18- to 21-year-olds (2 million) (U. S. Bureau of the Census, 1990). The Office of Technology Assessment (OTA) estimated that there were 8.27 million adolescents aged 10 to 18 living in poor and near-poor families in 1988 (OTA, 1991b).

Characteristics of Adolescents in Poor Families

Although poverty can be found in all racial/ethnic groups, a higher percentage of adolescents in minority families than in white families are poor. The OTA estimated that in 1988, 27% of all adolescents aged 10 to 18 lived in poor or near-poor families; but the figures were 17% for white, non-Hispanic adolescents compared to 52% for black, non-Hispanic adolescents, 51% for American Indian and Alaskan Native adolescents, 49% for Hispanic adolescents, and 32% for Asian adolescents. Although the minority groups have rates double those of whites, the actual numbers are closer because the white population is so much larger: 3.7 million white adolescents compared to 4.85 million minority adolescents live in poor or near-poor families (OTA, 1991b).

Poverty knows few geographic boundaries. A large percentage of adolescents who live in central cities are poor, but some poor families live in suburbs and many live in rural areas. The South has a higher percentage of adolescents living in poor or near-poor families than the West or the North (OTA, 1991b).

Family composition affects poverty status. Only 15% of adolescents living with both parents are poor or near-poor compared to over a quarter (26%) living with fathers only and over a half (57%) living with mothers only (OTA, 1991b). Although many poor adolescents are in households on welfare, some are in families where one or both parents work, and even work full-time year round (half of poor family householders worked in 1990 and 15% worked year round, full time [U. S. Bureau of the Census, 1991]).

Some adolescents live in homeless families that are often undercounted in the census. The General Accounting Office (1989) estimated that in 1988, approximately 68,000 children under age 16 were members of families that were homeless. (The estimate did not include homeless runaways.) The children were living in urban shelters and hotels, churches, abandoned buildings, cars or public places, and other urban, suburban, and rural settings. An additional 186,000 were "precariously housed," that is, more than one family lived in a single dwelling unit. Twelve percent of the children were 13 to 16 years of age (General Accounting Office, 1989).

Adolescents Outside of Families

Determining the number and characteristics of poor adolescents is further complicated because adolescents who do not live in families usually are not included in the poverty statistics. Many adolescents are in group homes because their parents are unwilling or unable to care for them. Other adolescents are in juvenile detention centers, reception or diagnostic centers, training schools, and other facilities because of delinquency, status offenses, or other reasons. In 1989, the average daily juvenile population in public juvenile detention, correctional, and shelter facilities was over 54,000 (Allen-Hagen, 1991). In 1987, over 30,000 additional youth were in private juvenile custody facilities (Thornberry, Tolnay, Flanagan, & Glynn, 1991). Still other adolescents are in institutions for the retarded or the mentally ill. And many are on the streets, having run away from home or been thrown out by their parents. One million youth are estimated to run away annually (U. S. Department of Health and Human Services, 1990). According to the few studies available, the health and health-related behaviors of these usually uncounted and often forgotten children are poor (Council on Scientific Affairs, 1990; Gans, Blyth, Elster, & Gaveras, 1990; Yates, MacKensie, Pennbridge, & Cohen, 1988), yet few health promotion activities are directed at these out-of-family adolescents.

Limitations of Available Data

The link between economic status and adolescent health is difficult to establish because of significant limitations in the existing data bases. Many sources of information on health, including birth and death statistics and in- and out-patient medical records, do not include economic data such as family income or poverty status. Health interview surveys seldom request economic information from adolescents directly because few know the income of their families and some are even uncertain about their parents' occupations.

In addition to problems with economic data, health data on adolescents may be biased. Many surveys of adolescents are conducted in schools and therefore do not obtain information on those who are absent or who have dropped out—both groups more likely to be poor and in poor health. Much research focuses on other easily studied populations such as those who use public or quasi-public clinics or other health or human service facilities. These studies may produce skewed estimates, since they reflect only those who have sought medical assistance. Also, the poor are more likely to use such facilities than the nonpoor, and these facilities are not uniformly available across the country.

Alternative Ways of Obtaining Economic and Health Information

Researchers often use alternative approaches to obtain information about the economic status of adolescents in relation to their health, such as asking their parents. While parents usually can provide information about the family's economic status, they cannot offer health information from the adolescents' point of view and they may be unaware of their children's health concerns or of their health-related behaviors.

The adolescent health data collected by the ongoing National Health Interview Survey (NHIS) of the National Center for Health Statistics (NCHS) is based on parental reports. The NHIS obtains family income as well as health-related information about each member of the surveyed families. The poverty level is calculated for each family. Unfortunately, the NHIS reports that are published annually, *Current Estimates from the National Health Interview Survey,* report the data by under 18 years, 18–44 years, and age 45 and over. The younger groups are sometimes subdivided into under 5 years, 5–17 years, and 18–24 years, still providing no adolescent age grouping. The NCHS publishes some reports specifically on adolescent health, for example, *Office Visits by Adolescents* (Nelson, 1991) and the section on utilization of health care services by children and adolescents in the 1988 *Current Estimates* (Adams & Hardy, 1989). Moreover, researchers use the NCHS data tapes to perform analyses based on adolescents only. Several published reports based on such analyses are included in this chapter. The NHIS does not include data on institutionalized populations. The NCHS plans to interview adolescents aged 12 to 21 in a Youth Risk Behavior Surveillance supplement to its 1992 NHIS (Kalton, Cannell, Camburn, Oksenberg & Holland, 1991) and as a routine part of NHIS starting in 1995. This will increase significantly the data available on adolescent health-related behavior by economic status.

The National Health and Nutrition Examination Survey (NHANES) examines and interviews adolescents, as well as obtaining information on economic status from parents. This survey, however, is conducted infrequently.

Another approach to determining the economic status of adolescents is the use of proxies. Researchers can infer economic status from area of residence, parental education or occupation, and source of payment for medical care.

Using Race and Ethnicity as Proxies for Economic Status

Race and ethnicity are often used as proxies for economic status because a high percentage of minority adolescents are poor. The relationship between race/ethnicity and poverty, however, is a complex one; determining the independent effects of these factors on health status and health behaviors is extremely difficult because of measurement problems and data inadequacy (Haan & Kaplan, 1985; Miller, 1987; OTA, 1991a).

Some health problems that have a higher incidence among minority populations may be related primarily to race/ethnicity or culture. They include diseases with a genetic component, such as sickle cell anemia, and chronic health conditions that may be associated with culturally variable behaviors, such as eating patterns. Some health problems that minorities experience disproportionately may be a function of economic deprivation, which is higher in these groups. Examples include conditions directly related to insufficient income, such as growth stunting due to inadequate food intake or lead poisoning due to inadequate housing, as well as those due to problems of access to quality health care. The higher rate of vaccine-preventable diseases such as measles among poor children is an example of the latter.

Race/ethnicity and economic status may contribute independently to a health problem, but when both are present, the impact may be particularly large. For example, the high rate of low-birth-weight infants among poor blacks may be due partially to a genetic disposition to produce smaller infants, but the problem is worsened when black pregnant women receive inadequate prenatal care (Baldwin, 1986; Kleinman & Kessel, 1987). Discrimination on the basis of race/ethnicity adds to the health-related problems of all adolescents, but particularly to those of poor ones. As Jessor (1991) has noted, minority status and poverty often have a malignant synergism.

Chapter 4 discusses cultural influences on the health of minority youth; the present chapter examines how economic status affects adolescent health and health behavior. Race will not be used as a proxy for poverty, not only because many minority adolescents are not poor and many majority adolescents are, but also because the chapter's intent is to determine the effect of economic status. While total disaggregation of the effects may be impossible because of their interaction, studies that attempt to determine the relative importance of race/ethnicity and economic status sometimes find that controlling for economic status reduces but does not eliminate differences between the white and minority populations (Lieberman, Ryan, Monson, & Schoenbaum, 1987; Millstein et al., 1992; Wise, Kotelchuck, Wilson, & Mills, 1985).

Length of Time in Poverty

The problem of identifying associations between adolescent health and health-related activities and several economic variables is further complicated by the need to distinguish between the transient poor and a group in long-term poverty, frequently referred to as the *underclass* (Sawhill, 1989). Few health studies are able to make this distinction, and its absence may account for the sometimes modest differences found between poor and nonpoor adolescents. Adolescents whose families are poor for a limited period of time, because of unemployment, divorce, or other reasons, may retain the health status and health-related behaviors that they had when they were not poor, while only those adolescents whose poor economic situation seems intractable may suffer health consequences. The media have spread the image of urban ghettos occupied by delinquent, drug-dealing, sexually promiscuous teenagers. Such adolescents probably comprise a very small percentage of those who will be described as poor in this chapter.

Economic Status and Health Among Adolescents

Respondents in the 1983 and 1984 NHIS reported that 38% of poor adolescents aged 10 to 18 were in excellent health and 7% were in fair or poor health compared to 56% and 2% of adolescents in nonpoor households. Nine percent of poor adolescents had a long-term limitation in their usual activities due to chronic illness or impairment compared to 6% of the nonpoor (Newacheck, 1989a). In 1984, 9% of 10- to 18-year-olds below the poverty line compared to 6% of those above it had a chronic condition that resulted in some loss of ability to conduct the normal activities of adolescence (Newacheck, 1989b).

These data showing higher rates of parental-reported health conditions among poor adolescents are reflected in higher rates of restricted activity days. Between 1985 and 1987, the average number of days spent in bed for 5- to 17-year-olds and 18- to 24-year-olds was 4.8 and 5.0 for whites with family incomes less than $20,000 and 4.0 and 3.4 for those with higher incomes; the rates for blacks were 3.5 and 4.8 compared to 2.7 and 2.2, respectively (Ries, 1990). The reasons for the racial differences are unclear. In 1989, the average number of school-loss days for 15- to 17-year-olds for acute conditions was 5.2 for those with family incomes under $10,000 and 4.1 for those with family incomes of $35,000 or more (Adams & Benson, 1990). In 1988, the rate of hospital discharges among 10- to 18-year-olds also declined as income rose (OTA, 1991b). The NHANES II found that poor 12- to 17-year-olds were shorter, weighed less, and had less caloric intake than nonpoor adolescents, but these differences were statistically significant only for height and weight in white males (Jones, Nesheim, & Habicht, 1985).

The Minnesota Adolescent Health Survey found that for both females and males, self-reported physical abuse was about twice as high in the low parental socioeconomic group as in the middle and upper groups. Sexual abuse also was somewhat higher among females only. Socioeconomic status was based on a combined rating of parents' education level and employment status. Abuse also was associated with low levels of family connectedness and not living with parents (Minnesota Women's Fund, 1990).

Psychological Problems

The 1988 NHIS of Child Health studied three types of parent-reported psychological problems in 12- to 17-year-olds: learning disabilities, emotional or behavioral problems lasting for 3 months or more or requiring psychological help, and delay in growth and development. The percentage of adolescents having any of the three problems ranged from 29% for those with family incomes below $10,000 to 24% for those with family incomes of $40,000 or more. Learning disabilities and emotional or behavioral problems showed a distinct inverse relationship with income. Delay in growth and development did not show such a negative correlation, but was more common among those with incomes under $25,000 than among those above (Zill & Schoenborn, 1990). The authors noted that greater awareness of these psychological problems among more educated parents may have caused an underestimate of the size of the socioeconomic differential.

These findings in regard to psychological conditions were confirmed by a study of rural secondary school students that revealed a direct association between a measure of economic hardship and depression/loneliness. Economic hardship also had an indirect effect on this form of adolescent distress through a strong negative association with parental nurturance and a strong positive association with inconsistent parental discipline (Lempers, Clark-Lempers, & Simons, 1989).

The Minnesota Adolescent Health Survey found that the risk of suicide among females and males decreased slightly as socioeconomic status rose. The risk of suicide was also associated with low levels of family connectedness (Minnesota Women's Fund, 1990).

Teenage Parenthood

A 1979 study of black 13- to 19-year-old unmarried females in Chicago revealed a strong relationship between social class, parental marital status, number of siblings, and rate of pregnancy. Social class was defined on the basis of father's and mother's education, occupational status, labor force and unemployment experience, family income, and housing characteristics. A factor representing these components was produced. The top quartile was classified as upper social class, the two middle quartiles as middle class, and the bottom quartile as lower class. The middle quartiles' pregnancy rate was 53% higher than the upper quartile's and the lower quartile's rate was 95% higher. Neighborhood quality, parental control of behavior, and career aspirations also influenced pregnancy rates. Similar results were found in regard to initial sexual intercourse, with teenagers in the lowest quartile having an initial rate 45% higher than that of the upper and middle quartiles (Hogan & Kitagawa, 1985).

The Minnesota Adolescent Health Survey found that the risk of becoming pregnant was over twice as high among those whose parents were in the lower compared to the upper socioeconomic status group. The risk of making someone pregnant was over 50% higher. Pregnancy risk was also associated with living in a single-parent or no-parent family and with low levels of family connectedness (Minnesota Women's Fund, 1990).

These studies suggest a link between poverty and health status as measured in several ways, a link that may be mediated by family dynamics.

Health-Related Behaviors

Health-compromising behaviors contribute substantially to the rates of pregnancy, illness, injury, disability, and death among *all* adolescents. Only a few studies, however, have examined the question of whether economic status is related to rates of health-related behaviors in adolescence, although studies of adults support such a hypothesis. For example, among adults, 32% of those aged 18 and over with incomes less than $10,000 are current smokers compared to 22% of those with incomes of $50,000 or more (Schoenborn & Boyd, 1989). Other health-related activities associated with income are exercising or playing sports regularly, having a working smoke detector, and wearing seat belts all or most of the time (Schoenborn, 1988).

The epidemiology of adolescent substance abuse, contraceptive use, driving practices, and other potential sources of health problems has been the subject of much research, but only a few studies have analyzed these data by economic variables. Either the research is conducted in relatively homogeneous samples or no measure of family socioeconomic status is included. Both situations suggest a lack of sensitivity among investigators to the importance of this factor or difficulty in obtaining the data. The few studies that provide such data primarily examine substance use and sexual activity.

Health-Compromising Behaviors

Two studies of cigarette smoking indicate a possible relationship to poverty. A 5-year follow-up of a group of adolescents in suburban districts of the Twin Cities metropolitan area who were first studied in seventh grade revealed that drop-outs had the highest rate of smoking, followed by those who had transferred to other schools and those who had been absent at the time of the first survey. Those currently in school had the lowest rate (Pirie, Murray, & Luepker, 1988). Students of low socioeconomic status are more likely to drop out of school (Berman, Lavin, Rudolph, Donoghue, & Hitchcock, 1991), so dropping out may be considered a proxy for poverty. A survey of ninth through twelfth graders in Pittsburgh found that children of professionals were less likely to smoke than children of parents in lower-status occupations. The relationship between occupational class and smoking was not consistent, however (children with parents in semiprofessional occupations were more likely to smoke than those whose parents were semiskilled), and over a quarter of the adolescents did not record their father's occupation (Young & Rogers, 1986).

Although use of illegal drugs is associated in the public mind with poor and usually inner-city adolescents, the research has produced mixed findings. Parental occupation and education were used as proxies in three studies that revealed an association. One Los Angeles area study found a significant association between father's occupation and use of alcohol, illegal drugs, and other mind-altering substances. More abstainers had fathers who were professionals, and more users had fathers in managerial or foreman-type positions. There was no significant correlation between family composition (one- or two-parent home), income, or parental-rated social class (Fawzy, Coombs, Simon, & Bowman-Terrell, 1987).

A study of black and Hispanic male adolescents who lived in economically distressed sections of the District of Columbia revealed no relationship between drug involvement and gender of the head of the household or household fragmentation.

Level of education of the head of the household, however, was associated with adolescent drug involvement. Individuals who used but did not sell drugs and those who both used and sold them were significantly more likely to come from homes where the head of the household had not graduated from high school than were those who neither used nor sold or who sold only (Brounstein, Hatry, Altschuler, & Blair, 1990). Another study of California tenth graders found substance use to be most strongly predicted by friends' marijuana use, but there was also a significant negative association with parents' education (Robinson et al., 1987).

A study of rural secondary students that found no direct association between economic hardship and delinquency/drug use noted that economic hardship increased inconsistent, rejection-oriented parental discipline, which was associated with delinquent and drug abuse behavior (Lempers et al., 1989). This suggests a possible mechanism through which living in an economically stressed, poor household may impact on behavior.

Berman et al. (1991) found higher rates of substance use, including cigarettes, alcohol, and marijuana and other illegal drugs, among dropouts. As already noted, dropping out is associated with socioeconomic status.

Health-Enhancing Behaviors

Appropriate diet, sufficient rest, adequate exercise, use of seat belt and bike/motorcycle helmets, contraceptive use, and medical and dental care are among the behaviors that could have a positive impact on adolescent health. Although the data are meager, those that are available suggest that poor adolescents are less likely than nonpoor ones to engage in these activities. For example, in 1985, 39% of 5- to 17-year-olds wore seat belts all or most of the time. The percentage decreased with age (33% of 10- to 14-year-olds and 31% of 15- to 17-year-olds) but increased with income (Schoenborn, 1988).

The 1988 National Survey of Family Growth showed the relationship between poverty and sexual activity and contraceptive use. Among 15- to 17-year-olds, 42% of those below 200% of the poverty level but only 35% of those above it had ever had sexual intercourse; the corresponding percentages for 18- and 19-year-olds were 81 and 69. Among those who had ever had intercourse, 58% of those in the lower income group compared to 73% of those in the higher income group had used a contraceptive at first intercourse. Twenty-five percent of those at risk for an unintended pregnancy in the lower income group compared to 17% of those in the higher were not using a contraceptive (Forrest & Singh, 1990).

The Chicago study of pregnancy rates among black females found that social class, parents' marital status, and neighborhood quality affected contraceptive use among adolescent females. Forty-one percent of females from the highest social class used contraceptives at first intercourse compared to 17% from the lowest social class. Among males, only social class affected contraceptive use at first intercourse (32% compared to 11%). Career aspirations were of marginal significance for both genders (Hogan, Astone, & Kitagawa, 1985).

Economic status is clearly related to the utilization of health services. In 1988, among those from families with incomes under $10,000, 54% of 12- to 14-year-olds and 46% of 15- to 17-year-olds had visited a physician for routine health care during the past 12 months compared to 63% and 58%, respectively, of those with incomes over $40,000. Having a regular source of routine care usually improves the likelihood of a visit: 83% of 12- to 14-year-olds and 75% of 15- to 17-year-olds in the lowest income group compared to 91% and 87%, respectively, of those in the highest income group had a regular source of care (Bloom, 1990). When 1983–1984 data on medical care were adjusted for perceived health status, the disparity in medical care use between poor and nonpoor adolescents increased as health status worsened. The average number of physician contacts per year for those in excellent health was 1.4 for poor adolescents and 1.8 for nonpoor ones, but for those in fair or poor health it was 5.6 for poor adolescents and 8.8 for nonpoor ones (Newacheck, 1989a).

The limited use of medical care by adolescents is related to their families' insurance status. In 1983 and 1984, the average number of physician visits per year was 1.7 for poor adolescents without Medicaid coverage, 2.8 for poor ones with Medicaid, and 2.4 for nonpoor ones. For those in fair or poor health, Medicaid coverage brought the number of visits for the poor almost to that of the nonpoor (Newacheck, 1989a). In 1988, among those whose family income was below $10,000, 70% of 12- to 14-year-olds and 64% of 15- to 17-year-olds were covered by a health insurance plan or Medicaid compared to 93% and 92%, respectively, of those whose family income was $40,000 or more (Bloom, 1990).

The findings of studies of dental visits are similar (Chapter 11).

Health Promotion for Poor Adolescents

Health promotion for poor adolescents is a greater challenge than for the nonpoor. Conventional sites and approaches should not be ignored, but this group may require radically different approaches and the use of unconventional sites (Price, Cioci, Penner, & Trautlein, 1990).

Schools and Community Groups

Even though their absence and dropout rates are higher, most poor youth, especially younger ones, attend school. A health promotion program designed for middle-class students, however, may not be meaningful to them. In schools with large populations of poor adolescents, health promotion programs such as health classes, peer leadership programs, and youth theater should take into account the students' life situation by using the language with which they are familiar and role models with whom they can identify, and by suggesting forms of behavior that are possible given their economic situation.

Schools can also reach poor youth through health clinics located in or near school sites. Most such clinics currently operate in poverty-stricken areas of large cities and provide basic medical care. These clinics have been successful in increasing adolescent utilization of health services (Lear, Gleicher, St. Germaine, & Porter, 1991). Although their effect on other health-related behaviors is still unproven, clinics have the potential for involving youth in health-enhancing activities in areas such as physical fitness and nonviolent conflict resolution (Carnegie Council on Adolescent Development, 1989). Unfortunately, many clinics have only enough resources to operate in a crisis mode and others must limit their services in important but controversial areas, such as dispensing contraceptives (Dryfoos, 1992).

Several school-based or school-linked projects have claimed success in health promotion with low-income and minority students, although their analyses have not focused on the poverty group. These include Project ALERT in California and Oregon (Ellickson & Bell, 1990), skills training programs in New Jersey and New York (Botvin, Dusenbury, Baker, James-Ortiz, & Kerner, 1989; Botvin et al., 1989), Postponing Sexual Involvement in Atlanta (Howard & McCabe, 1990), and a Baltimore program (Zabin, Hirsch, Smith, Streett, & Hardy, 1986).

Girls Inc. (1991) has demonstrated pregnancy prevention in a program based in a youth-serving group. Other youth organizations also are undertaking a range of health promotion activities. Such programs are particularly important because of the studies linking the absence of parental supervision to health-compromising behaviors. Youth programs should be able to substitute for such supervision and reduce negative peer influences.

Street Workers

Since poor adolescents are more likely to be chronically absent or to drop out of school, another avenue for reaching them is through street workers. Outreach workers who interact with adolescents wherever they congregate are currently being used to combat the use of crack cocaine and to reduce behaviors associated with pregnancy and sexually transmitted diseases, including AIDS. Also, many of the agencies that serve runaways and homeless youth have street outreach programs (National Network of Runaway and Youth Services, 1991).

Access to Health Care

Interactions between poor adolescents and health professionals in conventional and nonconventional settings provide opportunities for discouraging health-compromising behaviors and encouraging health-enhancing ones (Epps & Manley, 1991). The development of special adolescent clinics and reductions in financial barriers would increase the likelihood of such encounters by making health care more accessible. Adolescent clinics within large medical care facilities that serve the poor, such as hospitals and community health centers, are potential sites, although some programs have experienced difficulty attracting many underserved adolescents (Lear, Foster, & Baratz, 1989). School-affiliated clinics in low-income neighborhoods have been more successful (Council on Scientific Affairs, 1989).

Expanded health insurance coverage, particularly Medicaid, also would increase the number of poor adolescents who seek health care. In addition, state implementation of the 1989 federal Early and Periodic Screening, Diagnosis, and Treatment (EPSDT) regulations would encourage utilization.

The health problems of some out-of-home adolescents can be addressed through nontraditional sources of health care such as mobile vans. These have experienced success in attracting high-risk adolescents, including runaways and prostitutes. Some states have developed special programs to provide adequate care for adolescents in foster care (Halfon & Klee, 1991) and in institutions.

Legislation, Regulation, Taxation

Many methods have been used or advocated for making cigarettes and alcohol less available to adolescents. These include restricting their sale by removing cigarette vending machines, raising the drinking age, more strictly enforcing existing laws about the sale of cigarettes and alcohol to minors, and increasing taxes on these substances (Centers for Disease Control, 1991). Some studies indicate that these measures are effective and poor adolescents might be especially sensitive to pricing strategies.

Employment Opportunities and Training

Adolescents who live in impoverished areas may hold a bleak but realistic view of their futures. A perceived lack of opportunity for meaningful employment and participation in the larger society is likely to affect profoundly whether adolescents are willing to invest in that future through health-promoting activities or other means. Thus, increasing job opportunities or increasing adolescents' skills so that they can obtain the jobs that are available probably would improve their health-related activities. Such behaviors are being further encouraged by including health components in job training programs designed for adolescents. Health promotion concepts often stressed in the individual counseling sessions or classes incorporated into such programs include safe sex, appropriate nutrition, exercise, and avoidance of cigarettes, alcohol, and drugs. Examples of such programs include Public/Private Ventures' Summer Training and Education Program (STEP) (1989) and Manpower Demonstration and Research Corporation's New Chance program (Quint, Fink & Rowser, 1991).

Conclusions

Although some studies suggest that poor adolescents engage in fewer health-promoting behaviors than nonpoor ones, the cumulative evidence is barely powerful enough to support the hypothesis that health-related behaviors are a major reason for the poor–nonpoor differential in adolescent health status. Society may again be blaming the victim. Possibly the poorer health status of economically disadvantaged adolescents is not due to anything these adolescents do or do not do, but rather to poverty itself and the inferior housing, nutrition, safety measures, medical care, and other factors associated with low income. Even if behavior is a major cause, the poor adolescent is at a disadvantage. Health promotion requires an individual to make healthful choices. But the ability to make such choices is dependent on information, motivation, skills, and funds. Poverty makes it more difficult to make healthful choices.

Need for Better Data

More research on the behaviors of *poor* adolescents is essential to a better understanding of the dynamics of adolescent health. It is unclear whether a measure of socioeconomic status is omitted from many studies because this variable is thought to be unimportant or because of the difficulty in securing satisfactory family financial data from adolescents. But these data, or relatively valid proxies, can be obtained. Questions can be asked about parental education or occupation, or about eligibility for free or low-cost school meals. Medical records can be checked for the source of payment for medical care. The neighborhoods in which the adolescents live or in which their schools are located can be analyzed by social class variables. One study reported in this chapter used a measure of economic hardship based on changes in the family's style of living such as the mother's becoming employed or the loss of a family car (Lempers et al., 1989). Fortunately, as noted earlier, one major government-sponsored survey, the Youth Risk Survey (Kolbe, 1990), will be the basis for a supplement to the 1992 NHIS and thus will provide data on the economic status of the adolescent's family.

The tendency to depend on school-based studies weakens society's ability to help those who may be most in need: the chronically absent and the dropout. Estimates of smoking and drug and alcohol use are often based on school samples and thus underestimate the size of the problem. Efforts should be made to obtain data on the out-of-school populations through household surveys and street canvassing. The health problems of adolescents in homeless families, juvenile justice facilities, foster care, and on the streets require much more attention.

Need for Theory Testing

The field of adolescent health also needs more studies that test theoretical formulations of why poor adolescents should experience poor health and be less likely to engage in health-promoting activities. Is parental education the most significant factor, as several studies seem to suggest? Or are adverse consequences related to inadequate family resources; to genetic or other parental attributes; to an inadequate parental sense of efficacy, control, or esteem; or to the stresses caused by poverty (Sawhill, 1990)? Do brief episodes of poverty have negative effects on adolescent health and behavior, or can these effects be measured only among those who are in persistent poverty? Can the stresses related to a sudden reduction in family income cause health problems or negative changes in behavior? What factors allow some adolescents to be healthy and to succeed in other ways despite poverty and other risk factors? This latter question is being explored by the MacArthur Foundation Research Network on Successful Adolescent Development among Youth in High-Risk Settings. Clearly, complex issues need to be addressed if interventions are to be successful (Mechanic, 1989).

Need for Health Promotion Activities

The paucity of research on the health-related behaviors of poor adolescents, however, should not be used as an argument against targeted attempts at improving their health-related behaviors. Certainly these should be improved, regardless of whether they are worse than those of the nonpoor. Nor does the lack of conclusive evidence of a differential suggest that attempts to promote healthy behaviors should be the same for poor and nonpoor adolescents.

But, as already noted, health promotion for poor adolescents is likely to be very difficult. First, they often live in environments that are not conducive to health or health promotion. Second, some do not attend school, a frequent site of health promotion activities. Third, they frequently come from families with less ability to supervise their conduct, to promote healthy behaviors, or to control unhealthy ones. Fourth, they may prize membership in peer groups characterized by problem behaviors. Fifth, they may lack the perception of future opportunities that can provide motivation for positive behavior. And finally, for minority adolescents, the interaction of racism and poverty may have such powerful adverse effects that even major efforts to encourage health promotion activities cannot overcome them.

Attempts to better the health status of poor adolescents through health promotion activities should proceed at many levels. Certainly a national policy of economic support for poor families through the welfare system, tax credits, and employment opportunities could reduce poverty and improve adolescent health. Educational reforms that would make school more meaningful for poor adolescents and keep them in school also would have a positive impact. Changes in the health care system that make it more accessible by increasing the availability of facilities attractive to adolescents and reducing economic barriers would aid health promotion activities. These broad-based changes should not preclude directed efforts at the community level; rather, both should proceed concurrently. Efforts to decrease health-compromising behaviors and increase health-enhancing ones should be targeted at poor adolescents in homes, in schools, in the streets, in clubhouses, and through the media. Only through multiple initiatives addressing poor adolescents in many contexts is this country likely to enlist their cooperation and improve their life chances.

Acknowledgments

This chapter was completed while the author was a Scholar-in-Residence with Carnegie Corporation of New York in Washington, DC.

References

Adams, P. F., & Benson, V. (1990). Current estimates from the National Health Interview Survey, 1989. *Vital and health statistics,* Series 10, No. 176. DHHS Publication No. (PHS) 90-1504. Hyattsville, MD: National Center for Health Statistics.

Adams, P. F., & Hardy, A. M. (1989). Current estimates from the National Health Interview Survey, 1988. *Vital and health statistics,* Series 10, No. 173. DHHS Publication No. (PHS) 89-1501. Hyattsville, MD: National Center for Health Statistics.

Allen-Hagen, B. (1991). Public juvenile facilities. Children in custody 1989. *OJJDP update on statistics* (pp. 1–10). Washington, DC: Office of Juvenile Justice and Delinquency Prevention.

Baldwin, W. (1986). Half empty, half full: What we know about low birth weight among blacks. *Journal of the American Medical Association, 255,* 86–88.

Berman, A. M., Lavin, A. T., Rudolph, J. W., Donoghue, A. C., & Hitchcock, J. L. (1991). *The relationship between dropping out and substance abuse: A review of the literature and program implications.* Paper prepared for the Carnegie Corporation of New York.

Bloom, B. (1990). Health insurance and medical care: Health of our nation's children, United States, 1988. *Advance data from vital and health statistics of the National Center for Health Statistics,* No. 188. DHHS Publication No. (PHS) 90-1250. Hyattsville, MD: National Center for Health Statistics.

Botvin, G. J., Batson, H. W., Witts-Vitale, S., Bess, V., Baker, E., & Dusenbury, L. (1989). A psychosocial approach to smoking prevention for urban black youth. *Public Health Reports, 104,* 573–582.

Botvin, G. J., Dusenbury, L., Baker, E., James-Ortiz, S., & Kerner, J. (1989). A skills training approach to smoking prevention among hispanic youth. *Journal of Behavioral Medicine, 12,* 279–296.

Brounstein, P. J., Hatry, H. P., Altschuler, D. M., & Blair, L. H. (1990). *Substance use and delinquency among inner city adolescent males.* Urban Institute Report 90-3). Washington, DC: Urban Institute Press.

Carnegie Council on Adolescent Development (1989). *Turning points. Preparing American youth for the 21st century.* New York: Author.

Centers for Disease Control (1991). State tobacco prevention and control activities: Results of the 1989–1990 Association of State and Territorial Health Officials (ASTHO) Survey. *Morbidity and Mortality Weekly Report, 40,* RR-11.

Council on Scientific Affairs, American Medical Association (1989). Providing medical services through school-based health programs. *Journal of the American Medical Association, 261,* 1939–1942.

Council on Scientific Affairs, American Medical Association (1990). Health status of detained and incarcerated youth. *Journal of the American Medical Association, 263,* 987–991.

DeParle, J. (1990, September 3). In rising debate on poverty, the question: Who is poor? *The New York Times,* pp. 1, 10.

Dryfoos, J. G. (1992). School- and community-based prevention programs. *Adolescent Medicine: State of the Art Reviews, 3,* 241–255.

Ellickson, P. L., & Bell, R. M. (1990). Drug prevention in junior high: A multi-site longitudinal test. *Science, 247,* 1299–1305.

Epps, R. P., & Manley, M. W. (1991). A physician's guide to preventing tobacco use during childhood and adolescence. *Pediatrics, 88,* 140–144.

Fawzy, F. I., Coombs, R. H., Simon, J. M., & Bowman-Terrell, M. (1987). Family composition, socioeconomic status, and adolescent substance use. *Addictive Behaviors, 12,* 79–83.

Forrest, J. D., & Singh, S. (1990). The sexual and reproductive behavior of American women, 1982–1988. *Family Planning Perspectives, 22,* 206–214.

Gans, J. E., Blyth, D. A., Elster, A. B., & Gaveras, L. L. (1990). *Profiles of adolescent health series. Volume I: America's adolescents: How healthy are they?* Chicago: American Medical Association, Department of Adolescent Health.

General Accounting Office (1989). *Children and youth. About 68,000 homeless and 186,000 in shared housing at any given time.* GAO/PEMD-89-14. Washington, DC: Author.

Girls Inc. (1991). *Truth, trust and technology.* New York: Author.

Haan, M., & Kaplan, G. (1985). Socioeconomic position and minority health: A summary of the evidence. In U.S. Department of Health and Human Services, Task Force on Black and Minority Health, *Report of the secretary's task force on black and minority health* (pp. 69–103). Washington, DC: U.S. Government Printing Office.

Hafner, A., Ingels, S., Schneider, B., & Stevenson, D. (1990). *A profile of the American eighth grader: NELS:88. Student descriptive summary.* Washington, DC: U.S. Government Printing Office.

Halfon, N., & Klee, L. (1991). Health and development services for children with multiple needs: The child in foster care. *Yale Law and Policy Review, 9,* 71–95.

Hogan, D. P., Astone, N. M., & Kitagawa, E. M. (1985). Social and environmental factors influencing contraceptive use among black adolescents. *Family Planning Perspectives, 17,* 165–169.

Hogan, D. P., & Kitagawa, E. M. (1985). The impact of social status, family structure, and neighborhood on the fertility of black adolescents. *American Journal of Sociology, 90,* 825–855.

Howard, M., & McCabe, J. B. (1990). Helping teenagers postpone sexual involvement. *Family Planning Perspectives, 22,* 21–26.

Jessor, R. (1991). Personal communication.

Jones, D. Y., Nesheim, M. C., & Habicht, J. P. (1985). Influences in child growth associated with poverty in the 1970s: An examination of HANES I and HANES II, cross-sectional U.S. national surveys. *American Journal of Clinical Nutrition, 42,* 714–724.

Kalton, G., Cannell, C., Camburn, D., Oksenberg, L., & Holland, L. (1991). *Applied research on the conduct of surveys of adolescent health behaviors and characteristics.* Washington, DC: Association of Schools of Public Health.

Kleinman, J. C., & Kessel, S. S. (1987). Racial differences in low birth weight: Trends and risk factors. *New England Journal of Medicine, 317,* 749–754.

Kolbe, L. J. (1990). An epidemiological surveillance system to monitor the prevalence of youth behaviors that most affect health. *Health Education, 21,* 44–48.

Lear, J. G., Foster, H. W., & Baratz, J. A. (1989). The High-Risk Young People's Program: A summing up. *Journal of Adolescent Health Care, 10,* 224–230.

Lear, J. G., Gleicher, H. B., St. Germaine, A., & Porter, P. J. (1991). Reorganizing health care for adolescents: The experience of The School-Based Adolescent Health Care Program. *Journal of Adolescent Health Care, 12,* 450–458.

Lempers, J. D., Clark-Lempers, D., & Simons, R. L. (1989). Economic hardship, parenting, and distress in adolescence. *Child Development, 60,* 25–39.

Lieberman, E., Ryan, K. J., Monson, R. R., & Schoenbaum, S. C. (1987). Risk factors accounting for racial differences in the rate of premature birth. *New England Journal of Medicine, 317,* 743–748.

Mechanic, D. (1989). Socioeconomic status and health: An examination of underlying processes. In J. Bunker, D. Gomby, & B. Kehrer (Eds.), *Pathways to health* (pp. 9–26). Menlo Park, CA: Henry J. Kaiser Family Foundation.

Mechanic, D., & Hansell, S. (1987). Adolescent competence, psychological well-being, and self-assessed physical health. *Journal of Health and Social Behavior, 28,* 364–374.

Miller, S. M. (1987). Race in the health of America. *The Millbank Quarterly, 65,* suppl. 2, 500–531.

Millstein, S. G., Irwin, C. E., Adler, N. E., Cohn, L. D., Kegeles, S. M., & Dolcini, M. M. (1992). Health-risk behaviors and health concerns among young adolescents. *Pediatrics, 89,* 422–428.

Minnesota Women's Fund (1990). *Reflections of risk. Growing up female in Minnesota.* Minneapolis: Author.

National Center for Children in Poverty (1991). *Five million children: 1991 update.* New York: Author.

National Network of Runaway and Youth Services (1991). *To whom do they belong? Runaway, homeless and other youth in high-risk situations in the 1990s.* Washington, DC: Author.

Nelson, C. (1991). Office visits by adolescents. *Advance data from vital and health statistics of the National Center for Health Statistics,* No. 196. DHHS Publication No. (PHS) 91-1250. Hyattsville, MD: National Center for Health Statistics.

Newacheck, P. W. (1989a). Improving access to health services for adolescents from economically disadvantaged families. *Pediatrics, 84,* 1056–1063.

Newacheck, P. W. (1989b). Adolescents with special health needs: Prevalence, severity, and access to health services. *Pediatrics, 84,* 872–881.

Nightingale, E. O., & Wolverton, L. (1988). *Adolescent rolelessness in modern society.* Washington, DC: Carnegie Council on Adolescent Development.

Office of Technology Assessment, U.S. Congress (1991a). *Adolescent health, Volume I: Summary and policy options.* OTA-H-468. Washington, DC: U.S. Government Printing Office.

Office of Technology Assessment, U.S. Congress (1991b). *Adolescent health, Volume III: Cross-cutting issues in the delivery of health and related services.* OTA-H-467. Washington, DC: U.S. Government Printing Office.

Pirie, P. L., Murray, D. M., & Luepker, R. V. (1988). Smoking prevalence in a cohort of adolescents, including absentees, dropouts, and transfers. *American Journal of Public Health, 78,* 176–178.

Price, R. H., Cioci, M., Penner, W., & Trautlein, B. (1990). *School and community support programs that enhance adolescent health and education.* Washington, DC: Carnegie Council on Adolescent Development.

Public/Private Ventures (1989). *Teaching life skills in context.* Philadelphia: Author.

Quint, J. C., Fink, B. L., & Rowser, S. L. (1991). *New Chance: Implementing a comprehensive program for disadvantaged young mothers and their children.* New York: Manpower Demonstration Research Corporation.

Ries, P. (1990). Health of black and white Americans, 1985–87. *Vital and health statistics,* Series 10, No. 171. DHHS Publication No. (PHS) 90-1599. Hyattsville, MD: National Center for Health Statistics.

Robinson, T. N., Killen, J. D., Taylor, C. B., Telch, M. J., Bryson, S. W., Saylor, K. E., Maron, D. J., Maccoby, N., & Farquhar, J. W. (1987). Perspectives on adolescent substance abuse. *Journal of the American Medical Association, 258,* 2071–2076.

Sawhill, I. V. (1989). The underclass: An overview. *The Public Interest. 96,* 3–15.

Sawhill, I. V. (1990). Presentation at a conference, "Meeting Essential Requirements for Healthy Development in the First Few Years of Life," December 17–18, 1990, Carnegie Corporation of New York.

Schoenborn, C. A. (1988). Health promotion and disease prevention: United States, 1985. *Vital and health statistics,* Series 10, No. 163. DHHS Publication No. (PHS) 88-1591. Hyattsville, MD: National Center for Health Statistics.

Schoenborn, C. A., & Boyd, G. (1989). Smoking and other tobacco use: United States, 1987. *Vital and health statistics,* Series 10, No. 169. DHHS Publication No. (PHS) 89-1597. Hyattsville, MD: National Center for Health Statistics.

Steinberg, L. (1991). The logic of adolescence. In P. Edelman & J. Ladner (Eds.), *Adolescence and poverty. The challenge for the 1990s* (pp. 19–36). Washington, DC: Center for National Policy Press.

Thornberry T. R., Tolnay, S. E., Flanagan, T. J., & Glynn, P. (1991). *Children in custody 1987. A comparison of public and private juvenile custody facilities.* Washington, DC: Office of Juvenile Justice and Delinquency Prevention.

U.S. Bureau of the Census. (1991). *Poverty in the United States: 1990.* Current Population Reports, Series P-60, No. 175. Washington, DC: U.S. Government Printing Office.

U.S. Department of Health and Human Services. (1990). *Annual report to the Congress on the Runaway and Homeless Youth Program. Fiscal year 1989.* Washington, DC: Author.

U.S. Department of Health and Human Services (1992). Annual update of the HHS poverty guidelines, *Federal Register 57,* 5455–5457.

U.S. House of Representatives. Committee on Ways and Means (1992). *Overview of entitlement programs.* Washington, DC: U.S. Government Printing Office.

Wilson, W. J. (1987). *The truly disadvantaged.* Chicago: University of Chicago Press.

Wise, P. H., Kotelchuck, M., Wilson, M. L., & Mills, M. (1985). Racial and socioeconomic disparities in childhood mortality in Boston. *New England Journal of Medicine, 313,* 360–366.

Yates, G. I., MacKensie, R., Pennbridge, J., & Cohen, E. (1988). A risk profile comparison of runaway and nonrunaway youth. *American Journal of Public Health, 78,* 820–821.

Young, T. L., & Rogers, K. D. (1986). School performance characteristics preceding onset of smoking in high school students. *American Journal of Diseases of Children, 140,* 257–259.

Zabin, L. S., Hirsch, M. B., Smith, E. A., Streett, R., & Hardy, J. B. (1986). Evaluation of a pregnancy prevention program for urban teenagers. *Family Planning Perspectives, 18,* 119–126.

Zill, N., & Schoenborn, C. A. (1990). Developmental, learning, and emotional problems: Health of our nation's children, United States, 1988. *Advance data from vital and health statistics of the National Center for Health Statistics,* No. 190. DHHS Publication No. (PHS) 91-1250. Hyattsville, MD: National Center for Health Statistics.

4

Health Promotion
for Minority Adolescents:
Cultural Considerations

Felton Earls

A fundamental premise of this chapter is that culture has a high salience for adolescents and that the success of health promotion practices for this age group relies on special attention to cultural considerations. Adolescents are engaged in an active developmental process of evaluating themselves in relation to peers and societal institutions (Feldman & Elliott, 1990; Chapter 2). It is an examination that involves both introspective processes that help form identity and self-esteem, and social processes that position the adolescent in cultural, historical, and political perspectives. This convergence of inner and outer experiences is especially complex and provocative for minority adolescents, those representing geographic origins, racial background, language, history, and customs that are non-European in derivation. It is for these groups, representing some of the culturally diverse segments of American society, that special consideration in regard to health promotion is needed.

Adolescence provides new opportunities to compare and contrast family and local neighborhood cultures with those beyond one's own familiar boundaries. Such encounters have the potential to produce a shift in cultural affiliations and interests or a strengthening of bonds with the original culture. Again, this transition represents a special challenge for minority adolescents, one that many adolescents of the majority culture do not directly encounter.

To answer the question of how to handle cultural diversity in the context of health promotion, some definitions and functions of culture will be reviewed. A few central themes should emerge that can be applied to culturally diverse populations in the United States. A brief overview of the range of groups that make up American diversity will be provided and the characteristics that best distinguish them examined. Finally, a set of principles and objectives of health promotion and their application to culturally diverse groups will be recommended.

Defining Culture

The definition of *culture* in American society requires special attention. Issues related to ethnicity, race, socioeconomic status, and political status all contribute to the meaning of culture in the context of adolescent health. There is no convenient way to disentangle these attributes; indeed, it may be inappropriate to do so in many circumstances. Yet, they each have a signature as part of a pattern of social existence. The point of departure for this chapter is the meaning of this definition for adolescents. Being 16 years old, male, Dominican, Catholic, and poor in the Bronx constitutes a cultural pattern that is likely to be distinctly different from that of a African-American Baptist, of the same age and sex, whose parents migrated from the South to New York and are also poor.

Dimensions of Cultural Diversity

The term *minority* provides a convenient demographic and political term to begin an analysis of cultural diversity in American society. Aside from indexing a group's nondominant size, it often connotes a disadvantage in political power and influence that is directly disproportionate to its size.

Political station in society represents one of many dimensions in American cultural diversity. Racial background, ethnic origin, social class, economic status, gender, religion, language, sexual orientation, and age further describe the mosaic. Such an assortment of attributes can best be understood as a pattern, a pattern that perhaps comes closest to what is meant by culture. Furthermore, the pattern is not static—and it is this pattern that is undergoing tailoring in the context of adolescent development. In subsequent sections of this chapter, consideration will be directed to the need for minority adolescents to find a way to permit dominant and nondominant cultures to coexist in their lives and to the types of adaptations they generate as solutions to this problem. In the final analysis, much of what we consider health promotion for minority adolescents must both acknowledge and incorporate value conflicts in their cultural patterns. Creative solutions to health promotion efforts among minority youth may suggest alternative models for majority youth as well.

Critical Variables That Define Culture in an Open, Dynamic Society

A broad range of characteristics is necessary to provide a frame of reference for describing the different cultural minorities in American society. The list is not intended to be exhaustive, but it is reasonably comprehensive. It includes (1) immigration status, (2) family structure, (3) degree of assimilation or accommodation to the majority culture, (4) language use, (5) child-rearing methods, (6) religious beliefs and practices, (7) health beliefs and practices, including the use of traditional healing, and (8) educational aspirations. Other important characteristics distinguish groups at the community level: quality of housing; the integrity of community institutions, especially schools; and the availability of social support. Attempts have also been made to distinguish groups at the level of individual psychological characteristics such as self-esteem or competitiveness. But this can be a slippery practice, fraught with all the dangers of stereotyping that accompany the misguided impulse to define the character of groups in terms designed to describe individual personality features.

Immigration Status

The decision to migrate is determined by many forces, and few generalizations can be made. The combination of democratic systems, economic opportunity, and political asylum make the United States a desirable objective. The persons choosing to emigrate probably do not represent a random sample of the population. While avoiding a detailed discussion of this complex phenomenon, it is generally accepted that the first wave of immigrants is highly motivated to succeed (Beiser, 1988).

Family Structure

Family structure is typically characterized by the configuration of adults in a household. However, the concept of *household* varies from culture to culture. The majority culture in the United States defines household largely in terms of who resides in the home, but other cultural groups may extend the definition to include people who reside beyond its walls. But for most institutional purposes—legal and social, for example—the majority definition predominates, illustrating how it can be imposed on minority cultures even when it fails to describe or acknowledge their variation accurately.

In the broadest conventional terms, family structure is categorized as either nuclear or extended. The greatest legitimacy has been accorded to the nuclear family, consisting of two biological parents and their children. Extended families are so diverse in their patterns of relatives and near relatives that it is risky to attempt much detailed discussion about their differences (Kellam, Ensminger, & Turner, 1977).

From a large literature on the influences of these two types of families, a few generalizations can be noted. In nuclear families, parent–child relationships are often more intense, with an emphasis on educational achievement and maximizing individual success in the mainstream of society (Modell, 1989). In extended families, there is greater emphasis on group sharing and less focus on competitiveness and individual achievement (Slaughter & Epps, 1987). Because extended families have more generations and larger numbers of children, the traditional culture can be transmitted with greater intensity (Wilson, 1986). The family unit becomes more powerful as an institution and may be more effective in transferring to the local community the values of cooperation and group sharing that it espouses.

By placing emphasis on individual achievement, nuclear minority families may be more likely to foster assimilation into the predominant culture at the expense of losing traditional values. Of course, this discussion greatly simplifies the complexity of structures and functions that are reflected in the variety of American cultures, but it does point to characteristics that are thought to be important in predicting success in middle-class terms. The question is whether or not they have relevance for judging the success of health promotion activities for adolescents.

Contemporary American society is witnessing a weakening of what was once viewed as the ideal nuclear family. This is happening less as a purposive action and more as a reaction to the consequences of divorce and increasing economic pressures on families, with a concomitant rise in women's labor force participation. Children are being partially cared for outside their homes from an early age, school-age children are spending more unsupervised time, more families experience breakup and reconstitution, and more women find themselves the sole breadwinner in their families than ever. (See Chapter 5 for a discussion of the characteristics of family structures in recent decades; see Chapter 3, for a discussion of the economic effects of these changes in family structure.)

Assimilation and Accommodation

Assimilation and accommodation represent two major strategies by which a cultural minority adapts to life within a structure governed by a cultural majority. Individuals can assimilate into the majority culture, relinquishing minority cultural attributes in the process. In the second strategy, accommodation, one learns the rules, values, and habits of the dominant culture while making a conscientious effort to preserve the original culture as well (Ogbu, 1988). These strategies are best conceptualized in multidimensional terms (Olmeda & Padilla, 1978). Individuals may assimilate or accommodate across a variety of domains: language, religion, health beliefs, and educational aspirations.

As a minority group becomes more highly assimilated into the mainstream of American values and customs, changes in health-related attitudes and behaviors may also occur. Acceptance of the predominant values may make such a group more amenable to the conventional strategies used in health promotion. The pattern of diseases characterizing the group may also shift toward that experienced by the majority group (Mendoza et al., 1990). However, behavioral changes may also yield unwanted outcomes. For example, low levels of assimilation are associated with lower rates of completed suicide among Mexican-Americans (Earls, Escobar, & Manson, 1990). In another context, first-generation Mexican-Americans experience lower rates of infant mortality and low birth weight than other groups (Bautista-Hayes, 1990). Later generations appear to lose this advantage, which may be a consequence of adopting the lifestyle and habits (e.g., dietary changes, more sedentary lifestyle, higher rates of smoking) of the dominant culture. Clearly, the degree of assimilation is important to consider in the design of health promotion programs (Andersen, Lewis, Giachello, Aday, & Chiu, 1981; Wells, Golding, Hough, Burnam, & Karno, 1989).

Differentiating between the two modes of adaptation may be quite subtle; yet it carries an important distinction. It is essential to know if minority children and adolescents can be taught to protect their health using strategies readily adopted from work with the majority group. If accommodation is operating, the adoption of such strategies should pose no threat to the child's primary cultural alliances and beliefs. But we must be careful of forcing a process of assimilation at the expense of the minority culture. For example, culturally inclusive materials that depict different ethnic groups in health promotion advertisements may be effective. On the other hand, they may be counterproductive or too simple a model for many lifestyle and behavioral changes to take place.

Ultimately, assimilation can be considered successful only in the absence of discrimination and prejudice. The presence of these biases makes accommodation a more viable alternative. Their impact also provides the fuel to create devices to maintain cultural integrity within an open and dynamic society. Thus global concepts such as *Afrocentricity* (meaning the degree to which traditional African values are conscientiously used by parents or teachers) reflect collective efforts to maintain the abstract and ideal aspects of cultural life, although they need not influence all or nearly all aspects of daily activities.

Language Use

Bilingualism expands the range of expressive capacities but does not restrict or inhibit mastery of the majority language (Diaz, 1983). This point deserves emphasis because for many years bilingualism was thought to be associated with educational disadvantage (Hakuta, 1986). The Indian Bureau made it mandatory that Indian children were to be taught in English only, and that the use of their native languages was to be discouraged at all costs. Variations in languages used include dialect variations as well, such as the many varieties of Spanish spoken in Puerto Rico, Cuba, Mexico, and Nicaragua. Similarly, African-Americans were discouraged from using southern dialects. There is no reason to stifle use of these language forms. Rather, they should be viewed as increasing the range of one's communicative repertoire and reflecting a positive identification with one's heritage. Some types of health promotion activities might well benefit from using such language variations.

Religion

The major function of religion in many minority communities is to enforce conformity to traditional values (Frazier, 1974). It has been shown to be a protective force against deviant and nonconformist behaviors, including tobacco, alcohol and drug use, sexual promiscuity, and violent behavior (Griffith, English, & Mayfield, 1980; Chapter 7). Religious institutions may, in some cases, provide the ideal context in which to introduce and reinforce health promotion concepts and strategies. The multiple roles assumed by the African-American church in America provide a case in point. No institution has been as important in taking on the range of political, social, and behavioral issues that are consistent with the principles of health promotion espoused in the Ottawa Charter (1987). The potential for employing such a community setting for organized health promotion is being examined through endeavors such as Project Spirit (Carnegie Corporation of New York, 1987) but has not been fully exploited.

Health Beliefs

Specific health beliefs of minority cultures may be more vulnerable to the influences of the predominant culture than religious beliefs. This may simply be a consequence of the significant strides that modern medicine has made in preventive and curative practices. Nevertheless, low levels of assimilation may indicate the degree to which the health beliefs of minorities remain intact.

Closely linked to these health beliefs is the use of traditional medicine. Just as in the case of bilingualism, the majority culture believes that the use of traditional medicine is unfortunate and possibly harmful. However, the availability of multiple systems through which to pursue health is more likely to be an advantage than a disadvantage (Neighbors & Jackson, 1984; Snow, 1978). How individuals decide to use one system over or in addition to another may not always be clear, but that in no way invalidates the potential for traditional approaches to be superior to Western approaches for specific conditions. For health promotion to be most effective in cultures still using traditional or non-Western medical systems, efforts will have to be made to understand the differentiated way in which these concepts are evaluated along with those from modern medicine. It is also important for practitioners of Western medicine to share their knowledge with traditional practitioners in an effort to find ways in which multiple systems may actually reinforce good health practices.

Educational Aspirations

Cultures may also differ in the level of formal educational aspirations they espouse. Among the Caribbean nations, for example, Barbados has long been known for its high educational standards. Thus, emigrating Bajians excel academically in African-American communities in the United States (Ogbu, 1987). Similar variations may exist within American Indian, Hispanic, and Asian groups as well (Matute-Bianchi, 1986). Differences in educational aspiration and achievement have important effects on health status (Chapter 3) and should also be considered when designing or evaluating a health promotion program.

Cultural Adaptation in Adolescents

Minority groups are indeed complicated political, economic, and cultural units. The slate of variables described here forms part of a mosaic that attempts to acknowledge formally both the unique and the universal characteristics of such groups in the United States. The full extent to which social and economic forces have eroded the traditional values of these groups must be appreciated. Members of minority groups must simultaneously hold on to their uniqueness and establish a strategy that permits successful negotiation within the dominant group and institutions of society. Adolescents are confronted with both tasks at once. Many of the cultural minorities in the United States value group cohesion and shared responsibilities, values that do not facilitate the striving for individual achievement that characterizes the dominant culture. In confronting such a situation, one may decide not to choose between alternative sets of values, but instead find a way to blend them into a reasonable fabric of more than one reality.

The literature is not very helpful in suggesting how parents might handle the issues of cultural adaptation for adolescents. Of primary concern is how minority parents and teachers of minority youths handle the reality of reduced life opportunities and frail political power that adolescents will face as they make the transition to adulthood. Two strategies, assimilation and accommodation, were discussed earlier. Adults may provide role models of persons who have successfully assimilated into the predominant culture in order to overcome social and economic disadvantages. Alternatively, or concurrently, adults may promote the concepts of accommodation; learning the "white man's game" as a vehicle to success but not as a replacement for existing cultural traditions (Fordham & Ogbu, 1986). Some parents and teachers may not engage their adolescents proactively in either of these strategies, but may use mixed tactics or poorly defined ones. This approach may be problematic to the degree that it sends the adolescent a message that there is no effective way to deal with the "system." In the absence of adult involvement or in the face of contradictory information, adolescents are left to choose for themselves which cultural traditions to adopt.

The Meaning of Diversity

The issue of central concern in this book is the extent to which the boundaries that delineate groups are distinct enough to warrant a modification of generic ideas and programs relevant to health promotion. To the degree that this is required, pluralism becomes a fundamental prerequisite of health promotion.

For example, among Hispanics, while there are commonalities of language and religion, these characteristics go only partway toward delineating the two dozen or more Hispanic cultures present in the United States.

Asian-Americans represent another broad array of over 30 cultural groups, including, for example, Chinese, Filipino, Japanese, East Indian, Korean, and Vietnamese. Like Hispanics, these groups are expanding in size and diversity with ongoing waves of immigration from Southeast Asia.

American Indians, Alaskan Natives, and Native Hawaiians constitute the largest number of cultural groups and perhaps the widest degree of cultural diversity among all minorities in the United States. Some 300 tribes, 278 reservations, and 209 native villages are recognized by the federal government (U.S. Bureau of the Census, 1984a, 1984b).

In considering the varieties of ethnic minority groups that compose American society, a useful concept has been introduced by Ogbu (1985). In his effort to derive a theory of cultural competence, Ogbu maintains that an essential distinction among minorities rests in the circumstances under which they emigrated to the United States. For some minorities, immigration has been voluntary; examples include many of the immigrants from the Far East, Southeast Asia, Latin America, and the Caribbean. For these immigrants, contact is often maintained with the countries of origin. This contact, primarily through kinship systems, serves as a basis for evaluating the extent to which the decision to leave has been beneficial, the degree to which they have prospered in an open and democratic system. It is no accident that these groups often live in geographic areas of the United States that place them in physical, if not psychological, proximity to their native countries.

Involuntary emigrant minorities, on the other hand, are in a more vulnerable state. The circumstances that led to their status have often ruptured bonds with their places of origin and with their traditions. If, as suggested by Ogbu, the motivation to achieve competence is facilitated by the ability to compare levels of educational and economic attainment in the United States with what exists in the country of origin, then involuntary minorities are at an obvious disadvantage in this regard.

African-Americans have long been the largest ethnic minority group in the United States, though given the current demographic transition, they will eventually relinquish that position to Hispanics. While all African-Americans brought to the New World experienced some form of slavery, it is incorrect to assume that this experience created the same imprint on all of black culture. In many Caribbean countries, slavery gave way either precipitously, as in Haiti, or more gradually, as in many of the British colonies, to black governments.

A view of slavery as a catastrophic event that has left an enduring if not indelible mark on African-American life is argued by Patterson (1989). The transition from slavery to racial segregation maintained blacks in a position of powerlessness that continues today. Perhaps even more critical to the health of this group is the enduring fragility of the family. The breakdown of the family and the concomitant relegation of males to a marginal status has seriously weakened the capacity of families to recover a measure of the authority and respect so important in the pursuit of the American ideals of health, wealth, and happiness. The persistent poverty that characterizes this group has made it nearly impossible to differentiate the effects of disadvantaged socioeconomic status from the long-term effects of cultural impoverishment (Wilson, 1987).

Clearly, this within-race distinction among African-Americans is important in understanding the variability of educational and occupational success in the United States (Allen, 1988). Similarly, as new Asian immigrants become settled in the United States, it will be interesting to see if their status as voluntary minorities provides the motivational leverage to facilitate their social and economic progress out of the ranks of minorities.

Ogbu's concept of an involuntary minority group applies with particular gravity to American Indians, Alaskan Natives, and Native Hawaiians. American Indians have experienced a century of policies designed to separate them from their land

and to weaken their cultures. These policies enforce the use of English in education, deny the legitimacy of certain religious practices, and include programs of forced population relocation. It requires no leap of imagination to comprehend how these protracted negative influences have weakened the integrity of family life and led to attitudes and behaviors that are damaging to health. Any program aimed at restoring health must also find ways to overcome the devastation that has been imposed on these cultures. Although Alaskan Natives and Native Hawaiians have not been subject to the forcible removals from their places of origin that many American Indian groups have experienced, many strategies and policies have been devised and successfully implemented to compromise political authority and cultural traditions in these groups as well.

Targeting Health Promotion within Culturally Defined Parameters

A customary approach to targeting health problems for specific subgroups of the population, such as adolescents, is an analysis of vital statistical and survey data. Evidence on the relative extent of violent behavior, intentional and unintentional injury, substance abuse, and teenage pregnancy, diseases, and disorders in various subgroups can be assessed. However, health statistics obtained from large-scale surveys are limited for those interested in health promotion. First, they indicate nothing about the health-sustaining behaviors in these same groups. Second, the condition identified may or may not be the one that the communities themselves would define as the most acute if they were asked. Third, a number of factors operate to limit the accuracy of the rates derived from such methods in minority groups. These range from the varying ways in which critical variables, such as age and ethnicity, may be handled in surveys to biases stemming from the manner in which questionnaires are administered and translated.

The following questions suggest an approach that incorporates cultural issues in adolescent health promotion programs.

1. Are programs that seek to respect local cultural patterns better than those that blur such distinctions? Does efficacy vary from one cultural minority to another, or is it safe to generalize across groups? At issue is the belief that the future success of minority youths is ultimately linked to their capacity to negotiate within the larger society. Successful participation in health promotion, as in education, is probably a function of acquiring both confidence in one's own cultural identity and social competence in the wider society.

   Several programs for American Indian youth take advantage of the integrationist approach. Traditional therapeutic modes such as the four circles (visualizing and analyzing relationships), the talking circle (group therapy), and the sweat lodge (individual prayer and group therapy in a sauna-like setting) have been incorporated in contemporary mental health programs (U. S. Congress, Office of Technology Assessment, 1990). Although not problem free, these efforts have drawn significant participation for services related to child abuse, street youth, and teenage alcoholism. Such culture-specific programs appear to fulfill a need—at least partially—for autonomous control by members of the targeted group.

2. Who are the appropriate cultural role models for health promotion? Borrowing from the potent Hispanic value of *familismo* (familialism, or familism in English) (Marin & Marin, 1991, pp. 22–23), Las Madrinas, a female-to-female mentoring support program, pairs professional Hispanic women with adolescent Hispanic youth in a community setting (Price, Cioci, Penner, & Trautelin, 1990, pp. 45–46). Las Madrinas, or godmothers in Spanish, fulfill the role of fictive kin in an extended family for Ahijadas, or goddaughters. Madrinas join the Ahijadas in a structured 30-week series of activities. This program aims to improve school retention and leadership potential for girls; they learn from each other and from high-achieving adult members of their own community to negotiate their social roles.

3. Should programs be delivered in the language or dialect identified with the culture or in English? Of course, spoken and written language is but one means of conveying information. The use of music, dance, and visual arts should all be considered in enhancing the quality of health promotion messages and material. The general point is a concern for producing messages and defining the adolescent targets of these messages in the most appropriate manner.

4. Given the salience of peers, should health promotion be addressed primarily to groups of adolescents sharing the same culture? If so, or many contexts locations other than schools will need to be identified.

5. What are the most effective ways to empower minority youths? In most cases, a minority community will be economically impoverished. In designing and implementing health promotion programs, it may be useful to consider separating components that cope with poverty from those aimed at cultural issues.

6. The issue discussed in question 5 above is one for which no prescription is available. It does, however, complicate a final and most important issue. How are health promotion objectives integrated into larger programs seeking to increase control over community life?

Each of these problems can be addressed on four levels: (1) public policy, (2) community support, (3) family functioning, and (4) individual behavior and lifestyle. The most successful health promotion programs will seek ways to coordinate activities at all of these levels consistently while giving special attention to the issues of cultural diversity.

Coordinating activities across levels depends on the organization, interest, and commitment of local communities. Families and government both look to the community as a meeting ground. It provides the context to support and sustain families and, at the same time, to implement public policies. Community organization produces leadership, which, in turn, enhances political effectiveness. The result of this is to increase opportunities for participation in the broader society. Such participation should improve the community both physically and socially. It is in this context of empowerment that health behavior and lifestyle are optimally improved (Rapapport, 1987).

The task of improving the quality of life in minority communities is not an easy one. For example, Dalton (1989) gives several reasons why the African-American community has not effectively dealt with the disproportionately high burden of AIDS that it experiences. Ranging from deep-seated mistrust of outsiders to self-deprecating attitudes and feelings of powerlessness, the barriers to inculcating a prevention program tailored to the community have proved formidable.

Health Promotion for Adolescents

What, we might ask, is the role of adolescents in a process that in many minority communities involves fundamental restructuring and a long-range outlook on social change? Foremost, this role places notions of well-being and good health squarely in a political context. This requires that health promotion for adolescents go beyond the mere refinement of educational programs to promote personal skills. Schools, other community agencies, and the adults who work in them must tackle the more difficult problems of teaching minority adolescents to understand how policies are formulated. They should encourage youth to improve both the physical and the social character of their communities.

Already alluded to is the confrontation that minority adolescents must make with both the dominant and the nondominant cultures. In the American system the dominant culture offers opportunities for education and employment that the minority adolescent should be prepared to seize. At the same time, the ethnic culture provides a base of security and personal identity that may either facilitate or hinder the venture beyond local boundaries. Because the dominant culture offers opportunities for social and economic advancement, participation at this level can rival cultural influences derived from the family and the local community. The practice of health promotion will have to give careful consideration to this predicament of the minority adolescent.

In terms of general strategy, two approaches are recommended for health promotion programs designed for minority adolescents: focus groups and adolescent advisory boards. Focus groups represent a way of defining health issues of importance to local groups, while at the same time providing the means to acquire cultural sensitivity. Advisory groups composed of adolescents can facilitate the empowerment of youths to think proactively about their schools and communities. Learning to take such responsibility and having their opinions and decisions taken seriously by adults can be important incentives to take greater responsibility for oneself. It is also through this kind of experience that adolescents can learn how policies shape and control the environments in which they live and learn.

Future Research Directions

As a field for research, adolescent health promotion is new. Its methods are still evolving. Because one of its important contributions may eventually be to minority groups whose health is known to be poorer than that of the dominant group, the issues addressed in this chapter are of fundamental importance in directing this young field.

The first task is to acquire a better understanding of how communities become activated for health promotion. Without leadership and good organization, a community may not be able to initiate a health promotion campaign or respond to an invitation to do so. Research is needed to describe the activation process and to consider what forces inside and outside a community are involved. Some minority communities may be so disorganized that the only way individuals living in them can benefit from health promotion efforts is to go beyond their own communities. This approach is not unlike the reasoning that produced school busing.

Another issue is to know at what intensity, and in what sequence, efforts should be devoted to the four levels of health promotion (policy, community, family, and individual). While coordination at the community level is critical, it is not clear how much investment is required at the other levels to produce a desired change. No doubt this varies with the nature of the health problem to be controlled and the characteristics of the community. But answers to this issue are essential for wise expenditures of funds.

Throughout American history, minority groups have suffered from adverse government policies. Research is needed to examine the extent to which current policies regarding child care, educational reform, family support, health insurance, and the workplace will facilitate or impede family and community-based efforts to sustain cultural practices and institutions that make important contributions to health promotion. Historically, most minority groups have valued group cohesion and shared goals and have resisted wholesale adoption of the majority culture's emphasis on competitiveness and individuality. Public policies can have the effect of weakening the social networks and the interdependence that characterize many minority families and communities.

It is also necessary to study how to involve adolescents in health promotion activities at each of the four levels. Indeed, the contributions that minority adolescents make (for example, through advisory committees) should be an area of research in itself. For example, much of what characterizes the nonparticipation and antipathy of African-American adolescents toward the mainstream American society is reactive in nature (Pierce, 1969; Spencer & Dornbush, 1990). To preserve a sense of dignity, they often feel that they must, as a result of their experience of everyday racism, "fight the power." One way to overcome this attitude is to promote their active participation in improving themselves and their surroundings so that their energies contribute to self-empowerment rather than reacting to an oppressive system.

At the most basic level, it is important to understand the divergent developmental paths that minority adolescents traverse in reaching maturity (Chapter 2). This is an important topic not likely to be exhausted, even with a vigorous research commitment, for many years. Efforts such as the MacArthur Foundation Research Network on Successful Adolescent Development Among Youth in High-Risk Settings (Jessor, 1991) represent an important first step. Discovering the variety of ways in which minority youths learn to cope with the complexities of life in America is as challenging a problem as the social science has to offer.

Final Statement

Throughout this chapter, the importance of the social and cultural contexts in the design and implementation of health promotion programs for minority youths has been stressed. The salience of contextual influences has been a major research theme in developmental and cross-cultural psychology with many practical applications to the field of health promotion (Rogoff, Gauvin, & Ellis, 1984). However, studies have typically stopped short of examining the political circumstances that are as much a determinant of health and human welfare as the traditional psychological and sociological variables studied. An essential contribution of health promotion is to connect the psychological, social, and political levels of reality into a common framework in the pursuit of well-being.

It would seem that the assimilation of minority youths into the larger society is not a viable goal so long as racial and ethnic prejudice and economic discrimination persist. These forms of bias sustain the depreciation of minorities and the communities in which they live, creating both external and internal barriers to success. Since assumptions of personal control and investment in one's future are fundamental to health promotion, these barriers must ultimately be removed if minorities are to attain the level of fitness and survival of the majority.

For the immediate future, health promotion should adopt principles consonant with the concept of cultural accommodation. This approach to program development requires that local cultural influences be integrated into more generic principles, objectives, and methods. There is no formula on how to achieve this, but the most likely model for enduring success will be through a process of community organization and activation. The roles of agencies outside the community are to support these internal processes both morally and economically.

Despite the extraordinary range of diversity and growth in the number of minorities, the predominant ideology of American society continues to emphasize European culture. Nevertheless, progress toward a pluralistic system, described in the 1950s as "reflecting the more or less free, complete, and effective competition of interest groups" (Wilson, 1989, p. 226), has occurred. Given the continued progress of minorities in gaining political representation in the 1990s, there is reason to believe that not all has been lost from the decades of the 1950s and 1960s. For minority youths in particular, direct involvement in health promotion activities is imperative to help counteract attitudes of marginality and resistance to influences from the dominant institutions. Importantly, such involvement provides channels for responsible, health-enhancing behavior.

References

Allen, E. A. (1988). West Indians. In L. Comas-Diaz & E.E.H. Griffith (Eds.), *Clinical guidelines in cross-cultural mental health* (pp. 303–332). New York: Wiley.

Andersen, R., Lewis, A. L., Giachello A. L., Aday, L., & Chiu, G. (1981). Access to medical care among the Hispanic population of the Southwestern United States. *Journal of Health and Social Behavior, 22*, 78–79.

Bautista-Hayes, D. E. (1990). Latino health indicators and the underclass model: From paradox to new policy models. Chicano Studies Research Center, UCLA (draft version).

Beiser, M. (1988). Influences of time, ethnicity, and attachment on depression in Southeast Asian refugees. *American Journal of Psychiatry, 45*, 46–51.

Carnegie Corporation of New York (1987). Black churches: Can they strengthen the Black family? *Carnegie Quarterly, 33*, (½).

Dalton, H. L. (1989). AIDS in blackface. *Daedalus, 118*, 205–227.

Diaz, R. M. (1983). Thought and two languages: The impact of bilingualism on cognitive development. *Review of Research in Education, 10*, 23–54.

Earls, F., Escobar, J. I., & Manson, S. M. (1990). Suicide in minority groups: Epidemiological and cultural perspectives. In S. J. Blumenthal & D. J. Kupfer (Eds.), *Suicide over the life cycle* (pp. 571–598). Washington, DC: American Psychiatric Association Press.

Feldman, S. S., & Elliott, G. R. (1990). *At the threshold: The developing adolescent.* Boston: Harvard University Press.

Frazier, E. F. (1974). *The Negro church in the United States.* New York: Schocken Books.

Fordham, S., & Ogbu, J. U. (1986). Black students' school success: Coping with the burden of "acting white." *The Urban Review, 18*, 176–206.

Griffith, E.E.H., English, T., & Mayfield, V. (1980). Possession, prayer, and testimony: Therapeutic aspects of the Wednesday night meeting in a black church. *Psychiatry, 43*, 120–128.

Hakuta, K. (1986). *Mirror of language: The debate on bilingualism.* New York: Basic Books.

Jessor, R. (1991). MacArthur Foundation Research Network on Successful Adolescent Development Among Youth in High-Risk Settings. *Annual report.* Institute of Behavioral Science, University of Colorado, Boulder.

Kellam, S. G., Ensminger, M. A., & Turner, J. T. (1977). Family structure and the mental health of children. *Archives of General Psychiatry, 34*, 1012–1022.

Marin, G., & Marin, B. V. (1991). *Research with hispanic populations.* Newbury Park, CA: Sage.

Matute-Bianchi, M. E. (1986). Ethnic identities and patterns of school success and failure among Mexican-descent and Japanese-American students in a California high school: An ethnographic analysis. *American Journal of Education, 95*, 233–255.

Mendoza, F. S., Ventura, S. J., Valdez, B., Castillo, R., Saldivar, L. E., Baisden, K., & Martorelli, R. (1990). Selected measures of health status for Mexican-American, mainland Puerto Rican, and Cuban-American children. *Journal of the American Medical Association, 265*, 227–232.

Modell, J. (1989). *Into one's own: From youth to adulthood in the United States 1920–1975.* Berkeley: University of California Press.

Neighbors, H. W., & Jackson, J. S. (1984). The use of informal help: Four patterns of illness behavior in the black community. *American Journal of Community Psychology, 12*, 629–644.

Ogbu, J. U. (1985). A cultural ecology of competence among inner-city blacks. In M. B. Spencer, G. K. Brookins, & W. R. Allen (Eds.), *Beginnings: The social and affective development of black children* (pp. 45–66). Hillsdale, NJ: Erlbaum.

Ogbu, J. U. (1987) Variability in minority school performance: A problem in search of an answer. *Anthropology and Education Quarterly, 18*, 312–334.

Ogbu, J. U. (1988). *Minority youths' school success.* Invited presentation at a Conference on School/College Collaboration, Johns Hopkins University, Baltimore, Maryland, May 8.

Olmeda, E. L., & Padilla, A. M. (1978). Measure of acculturation for Chicano adolescents. *Psychological Reports, 42*, 159–170.

Ottawa Charter for Health Promotion (1987). *Health Promotion, 1,* 3–4.

Patterson, O. (1989). Toward a study of black America. *Dissent,* Fall, 476–486.

Pierce, C. (1969). Violence and counterviolence: The need for a children's domestic exchange. *American Journal of Orthopsychiatry, 39,* 553–568.

Price, R. H., Cioci, M., Penner, W., & Trautelin, B. (1990). *School and community support programs that enhance adolescent health and education.* Working paper prepared for the Carnegie Council on Adolescent Development, Washington, DC.

Rapapport, J. (1987). Can we empower others? The paradox of empowerment. *American Journal of Community Psychology, 15,* 353–373.

Rogoff, B., Gauvin, M., & Ellis, S. (1984). Development viewed in its cultural context. In M. H. Bornstein & M. E. Lamb (Eds.), *Developmental psychology* (pp. 533–571). Hillsdale, NJ: Erlbaum.

Slaughter, D. T., & Epps, E. G. (1987). The home environment and academic achievement of black American children and youth: An overview. *Journal of Negro Education, 56,* 3–20.

Snow, L. F. (1978). Sorcerers, saints, and charlatans: Black folk healers in urban America. *Culture, Medicine and Psychiatry, 2,* 69–106.

Spencer, M. B., & Dornbush, S. M. (1990). Challenges in studying minority youth. In S. S. Feldman & G. R. Elliott (Eds.), *At the threshold: The developing adolescent* (pp. 123–146). Boston: Harvard University Press.

U. S. Bureau of the Census (1984a). *American Indian areas and Alaska Native villages, 1980.* Supplementary Report PC80-51-13. Washington, DC: U. S. Government Printing Office.

U. S. Bureau of the Census (1984b). *A statistical profile of the American Indian population: 1980 census.* Washington, DC: U. S. Government Printing Office.

U. S. Congress, Office of Technology Assessment. (1990). *Indian adolescent mental health* (pp. 50–51). Washington, DC: U. S. Government Printing Office.

Wells, K. B., Golding, J. M., Hough, R. L., Burnam, M. A., & Karno, M. (1989). Acculturation and the probability of use of health services by Mexican Americans. *Health Services Research, 24,* 237–256.

Wilson, J. Q. (1989). *American government.* Lexington, MA: D. C. Health.

Wilson, M. N. (1986). The black extended family. *Developmental Psychology, 22,* 246–258.

Wilson, W. J. (1987). *The truly disadvantaged: The inner city, the underclass and public policy.* Chicago: University of Chicago Press.

5

The Social World of Adolescents: Family, Peers, Schools, and the Community

Cheryl L. Perry, Steven H. Kelder, and Kelli A. Komro

This chapter examines broad changes in the social world of American adolescents that occurred in the 1980s, the implications of these changes for the social health of youth, and promising educational and intervention strategies that appear to promote healthy socialization and may ameliorate some of the health-compromising trends. In the first section, we review Bronfenbrenner's (1979) ecological systems model of development and then highlight its usefulness for understanding health promotion among family, peers, schools, and mass media. The primary concern of this review is the quality of the changes that occurred in the 1980s, particularly as they impacted healthy adolescent socialization. The second section offers potential approaches, solutions, and strategies that also emerged in the past decade and provides, by design, optimism for the 1990s.

The social world—or social environment—provides the opportunities, barriers, role models, and support for the social health of individuals. Social health for an individual is defined as adequate functioning in his or her various social roles (Perry & Jessor, 1985). An adolescent's social roles may include those of son or daughter (or stepson or stepdaughter), sister or brother, student, friend, employee, member of a religious congregation, neighbor, and others. The development of effective, healthy social roles for adulthood is the long-term goal of socialization; and the family, peers, school, community, and the larger society all contribute uniquely to the socialization process (Kandel, 1986; O'Keefe & Reid-Nash, 1987). Socialization, then, is the process of integrating the individual into the social environment, along with the active development of functional social roles. This is complementary to the personal or psychological task of individuation during adolescence and the development of character and personality (Damon, 1983).

One approach to understanding the social world is the ecological perspective (Bronfenbrenner, 1979). According to this approach, the social world may be divided into more proximal and more distal contexts in which the proximal settings are embedded. Bronfenbrenner (1979, 1986) refers to these spheres as *micro-*, *meso-*, *exo-*, and *macrosystems,* respectively.

Microsystems refer to the most proximal contexts in which the young person participates directly, such as the family, the peer group, and the school. All of these socializers have substantial independent influences on the health-related attitudes and behavior of adolescents (Bronfenbrenner, 1986; Brook, Nomura, & Cohen, 1988; Entwisle, 1990; Kandel & Andrews, 1987; Perry & Murray, 1982). Within families, lifestyle patterns such as overeating, cigarette smoking, and exercise habits are modeled by parents, with a resultant influence on their children (Patterson Rupp, Sallis, Atkins, & Nader, 1988; Sallis, Patterson, Buono, Atkins, & Nader, 1988). Similarly, a positive association has been noted between the number of smoking teachers in a school and adolescent smoking rates (Murray, Kiryluk, & Swan, 1984); a lower rate of smoking among students has been associated with a policy that restricted teacher smoking to the staff room, thereby precluding direct modeling (Cooreman & Perdrizet, 1980).

The linkages between these *microsystems* form the next layer of social context, knows as *mesosystems.* A mesosystem is thus a system of microsystems; the consistency or inconsistency of the norms, values, and meanings of particular health-related behaviors among these systems influences the adoption or maintenance of those behaviors (Jessor & Jessor, 1977). The extent to which individuals in one microsystem are involved in other systems determines the strength or "richness" of the mesosystem. Thus, strong interactions between family members and school personnel, which have positive effects on student achievement and school performance (Entwisle, 1990; Epstein, 1987; Stevenson & Baker, 1987), reflect a rich mesosystem. These relationships are precisely what is in jeopardy as school population size increases and as more households consist of two parents in the work force. With the realization that school-based programs would be more effective if reinforced in the home environment, school health campaigns of the 1980s attempted to increase these ties through the use of home-based family participation programs (Perry et al., 1988).

The third layer of social context involves *exosystems:* settings that influence adolescents but in which they do not directly participate. Most influences of the media fall within the exosystem. These influences also include the parents' place of employment, the local school board that sets school policy, or the city council that passes local ordinances affecting adolescents (e.g., curfew or cruising laws).

Community influences are also considered part of the exosystem. These include opportunities for health-enhancing or -compromising behaviors such as through the availability of cigarette vending machines, food selections, the enforcement of alcohol minimum age laws, and the existence of walking/bike trails. Mass media expose adolescents to a multitude of health-related role models, including those that model unprotected sexual behavior (Lowry & Towels, 1989a), alcohol consumption (Strasburger, 1985), and violence (Brown, 1990). Health promotion campaigns have begun to actively counterbalance health-compromising media content with health-enhancing messages.

The most distal system is the *macrosystem,* which consists of culturally based belief systems, economic systems (e.g., capitalism), and the political system. These systems can have profound effects. For example, despite similar rates of sexual activity, European and U. S. adolescents experience different outcomes; cultural attitudes toward sexuality in Europe appear to result in lower teenage pregnancy rates due to increased contraceptive use.

Bronfenbrenner (1979) cautions that systems beyond the microsystems are frequently overlooked, limiting the concept of environment to a single immediate setting containing the subject. Because the various layers of context are systems embedded within each other, what happens at one contextual level can influence what happens at others, and explanations of behavior and developmental patterns cannot be sought at only one level but may need to include several layers of context.

The Social World and Adolescent Behavior: 1990s Update

The American Family

Throughout the 1980s, substantial changes took place within the microsystems of the adolescents' world that had implications for health. The ideal (normative) family, consisting of an employed father, an at-home mother, and two or more school-age children, now accounts for only 7% of American households, compared with 60% in 1955 (Hill, 1987). For example, higher divorce rates and the decision of single women to have children resulted in over half of American children spending part of their childhood in a single-parent family (Stipek & McCroskey, 1989). Correspondingly, many adolescents find themselves in reconstituted families, with stepparental relationships that are just forming at this critical adolescent developmental stage. Hill (1987) notes that the usual or expected transformations in family relations that occur during adolescence do not appear to emerge in reconstituted families.

CHANGES IN FAMILIES. The changes in family structure have also been associated with changes in the work force, where the percentage of mothers who work outside the home has doubled since 1970 (Hoffman, 1989).

The interaction of changes in family structure and employment has resulted in an increase in the amount of time that adolescents spend unsupervised by adults, therefore increasing the time that they spend alone or with peers. The problems with unsupervised time are at least two. First, it provides ample opportunities for adolescents to engage in behaviors that adults might disapprove of or prohibit if they were present. These include behaviors that must be appealing to adolescents, such as alcohol use and sexual intercourse, that are linked to adulthood, maturity, and independence yet are also health-compromising (Perry & Jessor, 1985). The developmental need of adolescents for independence and their desire to attain adult status and maturity provide an incentive for them to engage in what *they* see as adult behaviors. Greater unsupervised time may prematurely grant both independence and emotional emancipation from the family. In contrast, a prolonged supportive environment for adolescents, with gradual steps toward autonomy, appears to be more health enhancing (Irwin & Vaughan, 1988).

ADOLESCENT RELATIONSHIPS WITH ADULTS. A second associated concern with unsupervised time is its lessening of the quantity of time that is available for communication and intimacy with a parent or other supportive adults. Although quantity of time does not guarantee quality, sufficient quantity along with consistent attention is necessary for communication and intimacy. Adolescents who feel close to their parents consistently show more positive psychosocial development, behavioral competence, and psychological well-being (Steinberg, 1989). Adolescents appear to thrive developmentally when the family environment "is characterized by warm relationships in which individuals are permitted to express their opinions and assert their individuality" and where mature behavior is expected (Steinberg, 1989, p. 273). The lack of these relationships may have dire consequences. Reports of loneliness are greater among adolescents than among any other age group (Perlman & Peplau, 1984), especially when parents are separated or divorced (Brennan, 1984). Prolonged loneliness is associated with depression, behavior problems, suicide, and serious illness (Page, 1988; see Chapter 2 for a discussion of gender effects). Additionally, Steinberg (1986) found that the more removed from parental supervision the adolescent was, the more susceptible he or she became to peer influences to engage in health-compromising behavior. This susceptibility was, however, mediated by the extent of parental monitoring and communication of the adolescent's activities during the parent's absence (Steinberg, 1986). Thus, lack of adult supervision may be counterbalanced by consistent and concerned communication. However, when considering adolescents from dysfunctional or abusive families, greater parental contact might be health-compromising (Chapter 8); in those situations, the type and content of communication need to be stressed.

POVERTY. Some segments of society bear a disproportionate burden of the problems associated with unsupervised time, particularly individuals from low-income and poorly educated families. In low-income households, adolescents have less supervised time; they are more likely to have parents working at more than one job, with less flexible work schedules; they are more likely to drop out of high school and to have less income for educational or health-enhancing activities; and they are more likely to experience violence in their home and community. Poor adolescents have fewer opportunities for health-enhancing activities—including supervised time with adults—and greater need for them.

Unsupervised time and decreased opportunities for communication with adults are linked to concerns about the constitution and stability of the American family's microsystem of the 1990s. Over half a million children in the United States are homeless (Children's Defense Fund, 1987), and over 1 million *official* reports of child abuse or neglect are made annually (Emery, 1989). Because the percentage of the total population in poverty increased over the past decade, from 11.6% in 1979 to 14% in 1985, families with children are disproportionally and increasingly represented among the poor (Vanderpool & Richmond, 1990). Children overall are more likely to be poor than *any* other age group, with over half of those in female-headed, single-parent families considered poor. In 1983 nearly a fourth of all children were poor, with children from African-American and Hispanic families at the greatest risk of poverty (Stipek & McCroskey, 1989). As increased poverty is linked to exacerbated physical health risks and poorer adolescent socialization (Hurrelman, 1990), worsening economic trends promise little relief for adolescent–adult relationships under duress in poor households.

Peer Groups

After the family, the microsystem that includes the peer group is of particular importance in an adolescent's social world. An expected social change during adolescence is to value increasingly peer friendships and peer relationships. According to most theorists, peer bonding, with concurrent distancing from the family of origin, constitutes a central task of adolescence (Erickson, 1988; Offer, Ostrov, Howard, & Atkinson, 1988). Adolescents spend more time with their peers than do children. The peer groups are more autonomous and less neighborhood-based, and increasingly include peers of the opposite gender (Brown, 1990). Peers begin to serve as credible sources of information, role models of new social behaviors, sources of social reinforcement, and bridges to alternative lifestyles. These close and supportive friendships appear to have beneficial effects (Savin-Williams & Berndt, 1989). However, adolescents with greater peer than parental identification, especially when peers model and support problem behaviors, are more prone to deviant and health-compromising behaviors (Jessor & Jessor, 1977). Thus the transition to greater peer involvement, like other developmental transitions, indicates a process requiring guidance, skills, and prolonged time to be accomplished optimally. Since adolescents with less adult supervision miss out on the tempering effect of adult values, and at a time when they are developing interpersonal skills to deal with peer pressure, for example, they are more susceptible to peer influences and at a higher risk for poor peer group selection. As the number of single-parent, low-income families and the amount of unsupervised time increased in the 1980s, so has the importance of peers in adolescents' lives (Dornbusch et al., 1985).

Increasing peer influence does lead to questions about its quality and substance. Rather than a single peer culture, multiple peer cultures reflect the diversity of adolescents' values and behaviors (Brown, 1990). Adolescent peer group selection seems to be most strongly influenced by sociodemographic factors and common behavior patterns of, for example, drug use, school achievement, and religious participation. If one's chosen peers have health-enhancing behavior patterns, such as nondrug use, then their influence can be positive for subsequent health-related behavior (Kandel, 1986; Klepp, Halper, & Perry, 1986).

Peers can have positive or negative effects on adolescent behavior. Negative effects have been studied for substance abuse, gang membership, and violence. Positive effects are also possible but have not been studied as much. Examples of positive effects are outcomes for adolescents who share an academic achievement orientation, an environmental commitment, or a commitment to religious youth groups. If peers who have health-enhancing behaviors are selected, the result can be positive. As we view the influence of peers, a reasonable research question is the degree to which peers as well as parents can have positive or negative results.

Schools

The main formal community institution that is responsible for the socialization of adolescents is the educational system. Schooling is expected to structure the social development of children so that they become healthy, competent, well-adjusted adults. This expectation continues even at a time when financial and material support is declining, particularly at the federal level. As the demands increase and resources decrease, the problems within schools appear to intensify.

LACK OF PARENTAL INVOLVEMENT. Ranked as one of the most important problems is the lack of parental involvement in schools. Considerable research has shown that involving parents increases the effectiveness of schools at all levels (Epstein, 1987). One may predict that with the increase in single-parent families, parents will devote less time to involvement in schools. Young people who are living in single-parent families have lower grade point averages and are less likely to complete high school, even after controlling for family income and mother's education (McLanahan & Bumpass, 1988). Disruption of the family unit also increases the difficulty of school transitions and is associated with lower educational attainment (Entwisle, 1990).

PARENTAL AND STUDENT EXPECTATIONS. A cross-cultural comparative study of Asian and American schooling concluded that American parents were the most satisfied with the performance of their local schools even though American children were learning the least academically in these schools. Bishop (1989) speculates that the cause of the lower standards held by American parents is an "uncritical acceptance of institutional arrangements that do not adequately recognize and reinforce student effort and achievement" (p. 7). Bishop also notes that many students have few incentives for working hard in school due to a labor market that fails to reward effort and achievement in high school; peer groups that actively discourage academic effort; and admission to selective colleges that is based not on an absolute or external standard of achievement in high school subjects but rather on aptitude tests. The realization by adolescents that a high school diploma does not provide a secure future in the marketplace, that there is a bleak and uninspiring job market ahead or one in which secondary schooling will have little value, lowers students' morale and may decrease their commitment to achievement in school (Entwisle, 1990).

STRUCTURED LOW ACHIEVEMENT. Another characteristic of schools that may have negative effects is the system of grading, whereby only a few young people reach their potential level of academic success. By design, most adolescents experience some failure in school. Young people whose failures outnumber successes "are compelled to spend a high proportion of their time in an environment in which adult authorities may be transmitting negative evaluations of them" (Simmons, 1987, p. 43). Students' reactions to such an environment may include alienation from school; subgroups of young people may unite and develop countercultures; and they may exhibit antisocial behavior (Simmons, 1987). The process can be more intense for those children from lower social classes attending heterogeneous schools that serve a range of social classes (Simmons, 1987). Students who are not achieving in school are also at highest risk for many health-compromising behaviors that may compound and exacerbate their problems with school performance. Blum (1987) found that youth with below-average grades were two to five times more likely to attempt suicide, smoke cigarettes daily, use alcohol excessively, and be sexually careless than those with above-average grades.

The poor academic preparation and disadvantaged economic backgrounds of young people in minority groups may account for their high dropout rate, rather than life experiences such as greater family disruption or dialect difference (Entwisle, 1990). Scott-Jones (1985) cites, from the High School and Beyond study, the reasons students themselves gave for dropping out of school: dislike of school by white males, poor grades by minority males, marriage and dislike of school by white females, and poor grades and pregnancy for minority females.

DRUG AND ALCOHOL USE. Although the acceleration in adolescent alcohol and drug use declined in the 1980s, the prevalence of use remains unquestionably high. Use of alcohol and drugs affects the functioning of the school because it interferes with learning and is associated with disciplinary problems in the classroom and at school functions. It is also illegal and may involve law enforcement officials with the school. The use of alcohol among high school seniors has remained relatively constant over the past decade, with 92% of the class of 1988 reported having ever used alcohol and 64% reported use within a 30-day period (U. S. Department of Education, 1989). The proportion of seniors who had ever used an illicit drug rose from 55% in 1975 to 66% in 1981. After 1981, the proportion of seniors who had ever used drugs fell, reaching 57% in 1987. There was also a drop in the proportion of seniors who used cocaine, from 17% in 1985 to 12% in 1988 (U. S. Department of Education, 1989).

TEACHERS' VIEWS ON THE SOCIAL ENVIRONMENT OF SCHOOLS. Students' problems and their relationship to school characteristics are important areas of concern. Pallas (1988) surveyed a representative sample of U. S. high school teachers in the spring of 1984 to examine the social environment of the secondary school. The proportion of economically disadvantaged and minority students in school was related to a poorer social environment. For example, a high proportion of minority students was associated with greater administrator involvement, less teacher control over the classroom and school policies, and poorer student behavior. The location of schools was also a factor. Teachers in urban schools reported less control over their classroom and school policies, lower morale, more student disruption, and less consensus on goals than teachers from suburban and rural schools. Another significant characteristic was school size. Relatively small secondary schools enhance personal development and prosocial behavior, although it makes no difference in achievement on standardized tests (Entwisle, 1990). Teachers in high schools with low total enrollment reported better control over classroom and school practices, greater cooperation among staff, better-behaved students, greater consensus on school goals, and higher morale (Pallas, 1988). In contrast, very large schools fared worse on these environmental measures. A student body between 500 and 1,000 now appears to be optimal (Entwisle, 1990). Additional problems mentioned by teachers include lack of parental support, abused/neglected students, student apathy, disruptive classroom behavior, student absenteeism, poor health among students, drugs, alcohol, and violence against students (U. S. Department of Education, 1989).

SCHOOL STRUCTURE. An additional change in the characteristics of schools is their structure. There has been a dramatic decrease in the number of traditional 4-year high schools and a marked increase in the number of junior high schools. In the past two decades, there has been a new movement into the middle school system in which the switch to a new school often precedes adolescence, that is, it occurs in grade 5 or 6 (Simmons, 1987). The timing of school transitions is critical, especially if a developmental mismatch occurs—for example, if the educational environment is not appropriate for the developmental needs of the young adolescent. The social structure of the typical junior high school greatly increases the psychological burden on students at a time when their self-images are both developing and fragile (Entwisle, 1990). Also, the transition into a junior high at ages 12 and 13 couples school change with the rapid bodily changes of puberty. A comparison of seventh graders in a junior high school to those in a K–8 school revealed that the attitudes of junior high school students became more negative: self-esteem and leadership decline for girls; participation in extracurricular activities, grade point averages, and math achievement scores are less high and/or change less favorably for both genders; and levels of victimization (being robbed, threatened, or beaten) are higher for boys (Simmons, 1987).

Whatever the advantages of the K–8 system, there are relatively few K–8 schools in the United States (Simmons, 1987). What is becoming more prevalent is middle schools, with an earlier transition than the junior high school and generally a smaller size. This earlier transition may have an advantage if it precedes pubertal changes. Children could become accustomed to a change in schools before having to cope with the physical and psychological changes of puberty (Simmons, 1987). Also, the structural characteristics of middle schools generally are more similar to those of grade schools than are the characteristics of junior high schools. The transition to middle school appears to be more beneficial if it is gradual (Simmons, 1987).

SCHOOLS' ORGANIZATIONAL CHANGES. In addition to structural changes, complex organizational changes have taken place that have impacted the classroom environments. In her book *Contradictions of Control*, McNeil (1986) analyzes the effects of recent organizational reforms of secondary schools. The reforms that were most often implemented included greater administrative controls over the design and implementation of the curriculum, including student evaluation methods, with an emphasis on restricting teachers' and students' options. Such restrictions may constrain creativity and responsibility in the teaching process and threaten the professional role of educators. Since teachers' actions and attitudes, emphasis on academics, time spent on task, expectations, and classroom structure have all been related to students' academic achievement (Entwisle, 1990), a rigid concentration on curriculum could be counterproductive. Teacher flexibility and student involvement in activities probably are essential for those aspects of cognitive development that are hardest to measure, such as creativity, self-direction, or a student's ability to weigh and use evidence (Entwisle, 1990). Even among schools in poorer communities, the improvement of relations among school staff and between staff and parents, through the introduction of a school-level planning and management team, leads to better academic performance by students (Carnegie Council on Adolescent Development, 1989).

TOTAL SCHOOL ENVIRONMENT. A challenge that remains is how more supportive and positive environments can be promoted in schools (Pallas, 1988). A key element in making a school a positive learning environment appears to be a personal environment that explicitly supports students' physical, emotional, and social well-being in addition to their academic achievement (National Commission on the Role of the School and the Community in Improving Adolescent Health, 1990). Therefore, adolescent health promotion efforts should not only be concerned with the development of programs for specific health behaviors, such as smoking and exercise, but should also consider the total school environment to which young people are exposed to each day.

Mass Media

The pervasiveness of the exosystem of the mass media is the hallmark of the 1990s. The meanings that are communicated through the mass media may be particularly important in adolescence as decisions about adult values and lifestyle are being made and responsibility assumed. The major mass communication system is television, which has undergone significant changes in the past few decades. In the golden age of television (1950s to 1960s), the mostly white, middle-class adolescents on the screen worried about dates, skin blemishes, after-school jobs, and catchers' mitts—images that were relatively innocuous. Now a more inclusive range of television teens agonizes over friends' suicides, a teacher's sexual advance, sexual abuse at home, a friend's pregnancy, or addiction (Strasburger, 1985). Thus, the images present adolescents in crisis and those focused on present rather than future considerations.

Concern over the content of televised messages has grown with the realization that mass media producers and advertisers have very sophisticated techniques of attracting focused attention (Singer, 1985). Bagdikian (1990) notes that "After years of experimenting with various prime-time programs in the late 1940's and early 1950's, commercial broadcasters found the basic way to maintain second-by-second attention: constant violence, gratuitous sex, and deliberate manipulations of split-second change of images and sounds to make an emotional and sensory impact that leaves no time for reflection" (p. 88). Adolescents who are heavy television watchers consistently report viewing the "real" world according to these split-second portrayals on television (Strasburger, 1985). While these ubiquitous violent and sexual images may realistically reflect the social environment for some adolescents, it is questionable how healthy these images are for providing meaning and purpose to adolescent lives or time for assuming responsibility as adults (Gadow & Sprafkin, 1989).

Television youth are portrayed as having no notion of protection, consequences, or social responsibility to one's partner or oneself. In one study of heterosexual relationships in daytime dramas, the ratio of unmarried to married partners was 24 to 1, clearly portraying sexual behavior as more likely to occur outside of marriage rather than within it (Lowry & Towles, 1989a). Lowry and Towles (1989b) also estimate that adolescents watch about 11 sexual behaviors per hour during prime time, and in only 4% of these sexual interactions are the use of contraceptives or the risk of contracting AIDS mentioned. Thus sexuality has been increasingly displayed on television as a casual and carefree activity even in the decade of the emergence of AIDS. In fact, the model of sexuality presented on television focuses on heterosexual relationships between unmarried individuals who have no concern about sexually transmitted diseases or protection; absent is a model that presents a range of sexual options and expression.

Television, films, rock music, videos, and even novels (e.g., Stephen King's *The Dark Half*) increasingly provide images, messages, and role models for violent behavior. Adolescents, on average, view 22 hours of television each week (Strasburger, 1985) and listen to 34 hours of rock music (Brown, 1990). Rock music merges with television on MTV, available on cable television to over half of American households (*Standard & Poor's Industry Surveys*, 1988). In two separate content analyses of MTV videos, over half of the videos were violent, over half of the women were dressed provocatively or were depicted in a condescending manner, and over three-fourths of the videos showed sexual intimacy (Brown, 1990). The result of this exposure to violence through television and music may be a desensitization to violence among adolescent viewers; an increase in the acceptance of aggressive solutions to interpersonal problems, including physical and psychological abuse of females; and subsequent violent and aggressive behavior (Gadow & Sprafkin, 1989; O'Keefe & Reid-Nash, 1987).

The trends of media content are compounded by another significant change: the availability of VCRs and videocassettes in American homes. In 1981, 3% of homes owned televisions with VCRs; by 1988 this figure had risen to 62%—over a 20-fold increase (*Standard and Poor's Industry Surveys*, 1988). With potentially fewer age or content restrictions on what is viewed at home, for the adolescent with substantial unsupervised time the VCR provides greater potential access to violent, X-rated, and pornographic films than was ever possible in the past.

Summary

The social environment of adolescents changed rapidly in the 1980s. Overall, less adolescent time is now spent with parents or adults, leaving greater time unsupervised, and potentially shared time may be compromised by television, VCRs, and cassette tapes—all of which make it increasingly difficult to address concerns of intimacy and communication. Correspondingly, peer groups exert greater influence, perhaps as a way to fulfill functions formerly performed by the family. Schools have been called on to improve academic and social standards, but with the decreasing resources and increasing problems that are a direct reflection of the greater social milieu.

Mass media evolved in the 1980s to the extent that most American homes have VCRs and cable television to augment the attractiveness of television. These mass media images provide solutions to the social questions of adolescents, with seemingly little regard to the socializing role of these images. Adolescents learn about sexuality through almost unlimited exposure to uncritical sexual scenes where protection and responsibility are absent; they learn to control aggression in a context of almost unrestricted viewing of increasingly violent media. The larger culture provides an environment that mirrors these images, with many communities becoming increasingly assaultive. Thus, the American macrosystem—including the micro- and mesosystems of the family, peer group, and schools and their interactions, as well as the exosystems of the mass media and the community—has undergone considerable change in the past decade. This change has unquestionably left numerous challenges for those interested in promoting adolescent health.

Adolescent Health Promotion: Considerations for the Future

Along with the changes in the social environment of the 1980s, increasingly sophisticated approaches to promoting adolescent health have also emerged to provide some optimism and significant guidance for the next decade and beyond. Important progress in conceptualizing health promotion was made in the 1980s as a result of applying social-psychological theory and models to explain population-wide behavior (Bandura, 1986). The use of these models of social behavior, the identification of psychosocial risk factors as the appropriate targets for intervention, and the success of interventions that explicitly sought changes in the social environment and behavior of adolescents were all critical to the progress that has been made.

To guide this discussion, Figure 5.1 provides a conceptual model for adolescent health promotion in the 1990s. The goal of adolescent health promotion encompasses physical, social, psychological, and spiritual well-being, as presented in Perry and Jessor (1985) and elaborated in Irwin and Vaughan (1988) and Noack (1987). The outcomes sought are behaviors that are representative of healthy functioning in these domains: socially competent and prosocial behavior in multiple roles, perceptions of personal well-being and connectedness, positive affect and life involvement, and behavior patterns that promote short- and long-term physical health

Intervention Components

1. Family involvement programs
2. Peer leadership training
3. School-based life skills and social competency curricula
4. Communitywide activities
5. Health-enhancing mass media
6. Healthy public policy promotion

↓

Social Environmental Spheres for Intervention

1. Microsystems—Families, peers, schools
2. Mesosystems—Interactions of families, peers, schools
3. Exosystems—Mass media, community structure
4. Macrosystems—American culture, subcultures

↓

Identification of High-Risk Groups

1. Socioeconomic status
2. Housing and income
3. Parental education and employment
4. Race and gender
5. Family structure

↙ ↓ ↘

Psychosocial Factors as Targets for Intervention

Social Environmental Factors	Individual Factors	Behavioral Factors
Modeling of health-enhancing behaviors by peers, family, and media	Raising the *value* of health, prosocial, and future concerns	Providing *incentives* for adult–adolescent communication and shared activities
Promoting *barriers* to excessive mass media involvement and unsupervised time	Providing experiences to increase *self-efficacy* to manage peer influences	Teaching *social competencies* in developing relationships and discerning the meaning of media images
Providing *opportunities* for adolescent–adult intimacy and communication	Increasing *knowledge* of media images and marketing methods	Changing *intentions* to engage in prosocial activities

Outcomes

Adoption of health-enhancing behaviors
Reduction of health-compromising behaviors

↘ ↓ ↙

Goal   **Adolescent Health Promotion**

Figure 5.1. A conceptual model of adolescent health promotion in the 1990s.

such as nondrug use and low-fat eating habits. Also targeted as outcomes are behaviors that might be diminished since they appear to be health-compromising: limited communication and interaction with healthy adults, perceptions of loneliness and personal crises, antisocial involvement with peers, and behavior patterns that are physically health-compromising such as cigarette smoking or poor eating and exercise habits.

Psychosocial factors that might be targeted for change in health promotion programs include environmental, individual, and behavioral factors that are precursors to or implicators of adolescent behavior. Changes in these psychosocial factors are pragmatic because they address the concerns presented in the previous section on trends and have proven successful in the past (Perry, Klepp, & Sillers, 1989).

Interventions have been and should further be designed for specific microsystems, mesosystems, or exosystems that influence the targeted younger or older adolescents. Several intervention programs for adolescents are proposed below that target changes in the psychosocial risk factors within these systems. These include family involvement programs, peer leadership training, school-based life skills and social competency curricula, communitywide activities, health-enhancing mass media, and healthy public policy promotion. Evidence of the effectiveness of these multiple complementary components comes from adolescent health promotion research of the 1980s (Glanz, Lewis, & Rimer, 1990). The synergetic implementation of these multiple components, at appropriate developmental stages in adolescence and with congruous health messages, is a major challenge of adolescent health promotion for the 1990s.

Family Involvement

There is little argument that, within the micro- and mesosystems of the family and school, positive parental involvement in adolescent health promotion efforts would be beneficial if parents can be recruited, convinced, trained, and maintained (Entwisle, 1990). The question, of course, is, how? Given the already crowded schedules of mostly working parents, another "night out" may not be attractive to them, especially if that means additional unsupervised time for their children (Perry, Crockett, & Pirie, 1987). For parents in some communities, distrust of schools, fear of embarrassing students, and language barriers need to be overcome as well. If the intent of parent education is to encourage healthy involvement, then strategies to increase positive adolescent–adult communication and activity need to be developed and evaluated through the joint efforts of adolescents, parents, teachers, administrators, and researchers.

In the area of physical health promotion, family involvement with young adolescents in regard to eating, exercise, and smoking habits has had both high participation rates and encouraging outcomes (Chapter 10). In these programs, entitled *home team* programs, students are sent weekly packets of stories and activities to complete with family members. For example, to help in changing eating patterns, foods in the refrigerator and cupboards are labeled with stickers as "everyday" or "sometimes" foods by young people and their parents. Alternative snacks are also prepared and evaluated by the family. In the first evaluation of a home team program on eating habits, 86% of the nearly 1,400 families participated and 71% completed the 5-week program (Perry et al., 1988), suggesting that this approach might fit middle-class American lifestyles.

The home team approach also appears possible with families that have lower incomes or speak languages other than English in many areas of the country (Perry et al., 1990). Following programs such as these—carried out at home—with "fun nights" at school also appears to attract a large percentage of families. Fun nights accommodate adults, adolescents, and children and provide experiential opportunities to learn skills through a variety of activity and instructional booths and health-related games (Nader, Sallis, Patterson, Abramson, & Rupp, 1989). For example, young people and their parents learn a short aerobic activity routine from videotapes that the students have prepared. Families taste-test a variety of everyday foods. They play bingo-like games that stress the consequences of cigarette smoking.

The use of home team programs to promote social, psychological, and personal health should be feasible and effective with willing parents and functional families, just as it appears to have been in regard to eating habits and smoking (Stone, Perry, & Luepker, 1989). Because participants see the link with schools, they treat programs as mandated homework and are more likely to participate. The programs require a humorous and attractive motif, appropriate to the content area and appealing to the target group. It seems hopeful, particularly with younger adolescents, that such programs could provide a home-based structure for the acquisition and rehearsal of social skills—such as after-school time management, media literacy, safe sex methods, or alternatives to alcohol use at parties—that have positive health benefits. The programs, however, appear to need school sponsorship and promotion or external incentives to increase participation.

The creation and evaluation of family involvement programs, especially in the area of adolescent socialization, needs broad and careful consideration. Still, a student encouraged to increase communication with an alcoholic or abusive parent might not benefit from such an interaction (Chapter 8). Also, students who live in alternative family structures, whose parents have more than one job, or who are not readily available may not be able to participate completely. In these situations, the teacher or facilitator should be careful to promote teamwork with alternative adults with whom the adolescent is comfortable, such as a neighbor, babysitter, or extended family member. Likewise, conducting such programs within diverse cultural settings requires sensitivity to an incorporation of appropriate social norms and standards of acceptable behavior.

Peer Leadership

In keeping with the notion that multiple consistent messages are most readily acted on, health promotion efforts should capitalize on the potential power of peer influences for health-enhancing outcomes, especially by training emerging adolescent leaders. Peer leaders have been selected and trained to conduct school-based programs, with notable results (Klepp, Halper & Perry, 1986), especially in smoking, alcohol, and drug abuse prevention efforts. Peer leaders generally are elected representatives of classes or whole grade levels, but sometimes they are slightly older youth who conduct cross-age programs. The peer leaders, then, are not academic leaders but popular students who are liked, respected, and seen as role models by their peers.

The task of a peer leader is to serve as a prosocial role model and to provide social information in addition to disseminating information on health-related topics. Compared to school-based programs in which the teacher alone manages the classroom activities, peer leaders enhance the program's capacity by modeling health-enhancing behaviors outside the school setting. Peer leaders are perceived as credible sources of social information, especially on sensitive topics such as sexuality and drug use. As they explicitly support healthier values and lifestyles, they serve to create and reinforce alternative, prosocial norms and behavior patterns.

Peer leaders have been trained by a variety of investigators in the United States and abroad (Perry & Grant, 1988a). The training programs provide scripts to peer leaders for activities within a given program. The trainers present the various peer leader parts in these activities, and then structure both rehearsal and feedback of their performance of these parts. A major goal of the training process is to enhance the leaders' values of social responsibility and the importance of their status as elected representatives in promoting their peers' health.

Activities that peer leaders have been responsible for in health promotion programs include leading small group discussions, reading and giving directions, compiling and reporting their peers' responses to relevant questions, organizing role plays, and leading brainstorming sessions. For example, a peer leader might form a small group of four to five students and then ask each student to write down one reason why people his or her age might begin to smoke, given all the social and health consequences of smoking. She would then listen to the reasons from each member, record them, and report back to the class. In the class of 1989 study, as part of the Minnesota Heart Health Program, 50–60 peer leaders were elected and trained annually during a 5-year period, from sixth to tenth grade, to conduct school-based programs in Fargo, North Dakota, and Moorhead, Minnesota. These programs sought changes in diet, physical activity, tobacco use, alcohol use, drinking and driving, and drug use as part of a communitywide effort to reduce the morbidity and mortality of cardiovascular disease (Blackburn et al., 1984; Perry, Klepp, & Schultz, 1988b). To date, significant reductions in tobacco use have been noted in the class of 1989 (Perry, Klepp, & Sillers, 1989). Significantly, several investigations have suggested that peer leaders might be *necessary* when changes in adolescent social behavior are sought through classroom programs (Botvin et al., 1984; Murray et al., 1984; Perry & Grant, 1988).

Peer leadership training has considerable potential for adolescent health promotion in the 1990s. The research of the past decade has demonstrated its efficacy and the possibilities of implementation even in large-scale projects in diverse settings. Rather than viewing peer leadership as a vehicle of health promotion, it might be useful to consider it as health-enhancing in itself. Adolescents learn group dynamics and management skills as they assume greater responsibility for their own health and for the health of their own generation. Since the training of peer leaders has been quite specific and focused on health-enhancing outcomes, untoward effects such as the use of these leadership skills for antisocial outcomes have not yet been seen.

School-Based Life Skills and Social Competency Curricula

In the 1980s, school-based health promotion programs increasingly were guided by psychosocial behavioral theory for their development and content. For example, instead of learning and relearning the four nutritional food groups, students learned skills in the classroom to select, prepare, and evaluate low-fat foods (Perry, Mullis, & Maile, 1985). Likewise, in smoking and drug abuse prevention programs, instead of focusing on the long-term consequences of use, skills to refuse drugs from peers were presented and rehearsed (Botvin, 1986: Glynn, 1989). In a variety of school health programs, behavior change rather than knowledge acquisition became the desired and acquired outcome. These programs progressively emphasized the requisite intrapersonal and interpersonal skills to enact the targeted behaviors.

Along with this increased emphasis on skills training as a critical component of school health, more generic social competency training for children and adolescents emerged in school and developmental psychology as a strategy to reduce dysfunction and psychopathology and thereby to promote social and psychological health (Chapter 8; Dodge, Pettit, McClaskey, & Brown, 1986; Elias, 1987; Garmezy & Rutter, 1983; Hawkins, Jenson, Catalano, & Lishner, 1988; Spivack & Shure, 1982; Weissberg, Caplan, & Sivo, 1989). Social competency training has also been embedded in the school curricula, with effective programs beginning in preschool and primary grades. In these programs, skills are taught that span multiple behaviors or settings—such as those involved in friendship development, assertiveness training, stress management, impulse control, problem solving, and effective communication. Just as in academic subjects, and certainly as a reflection of the social environment, the social competency skills that are taught in these programs become more interdependent and complex for adolescents than they are for younger children (Schinke & Gilchrist, 1984).

In the 1990s, programs that teach generic social competencies at the microsystem level, as well as skills to change particular behavior patterns, need to be promoted as essential in school curricula for adolescents. Adolescents need skills to manage unsupervised time productively; to select, analyze, and criticize mass media images; to develop and sustain trusting peer relationships; and to communicate more fully with parents and other adults. For adolescents from strongly traditional ethnic families, however, acquiring generic social competencies that disregard cultural differences could create rather than reduce problems at home (Rotheram-Borus & Tsemberis, 1989). In creating school programs, questions of the possible negative consequences for adolescents who acquire mainstream sociocultural behaviors and norms need to be addressed (Chapter 4). For example, some Asian cultures place a high value on group cooperation and shared goals, and have resisted adoption of the majority culture's emphasis on competitiveness and individuality. Therefore, to be effective in diverse ethnic settings, competency training programs need to adapt the mainstream curriculum to better reflect the ethnic group's particular set of norms and values.

Communitywide Activities and Health-Enhancing Mass Media

Because the family and peer groups are the most potent and proximal microsystems in adolescents' lives, considerable attention to parental involvement with home-based programs and peer leadership in school-based social competency curricula will be critical in the 1990s. These approaches will be further strengthened if they are embedded in schools, communities, and cultures that reinforce similar values and norms. Community strategies increase consistency between microsystems and form a more coherent mesosystem. For example, if parents and school programs teach skills to say "no" to alcohol use or precocious sex, yet these same compromising behaviors are modeled by key community role models (such as teachers or football players) or are portrayed on television as acceptable and inconsequential, then the dissonance of these sources weakens the intended message. Alternatively, when programs are designed to be consistent at a community level, change is enhanced considerably. Thus we need to involve various sectors. Even in cases where one element might not make a difference in itself, in combination they may.

A communitywide approach to adolescent health promotion requires agreement on, commitment to, and coordination of the messages to be delivered and the strategies to be developed. The need to organize these efforts carefully requires support from key community leaders representing a variety of sectors. This can be organized in the form of a community advisory board, task forces to work with the various program components, and the training of lay leaders and volunteers (Bracht, 1990). With youth, the existing school district structure and associated parent groups provide an obvious and necessary foundation for community organization. Other youth-serving and social service agencies can be recruited to organize complementary efforts, especially as schools become overburdened with mandates to solve societal problems. These agencies might also be recruited to provide supervision and supplementary programs for adolescents after school—in coordination with school and parental schedules—and as a way to increase adolescent–adult contact and communication (Erickson, 1988; Galambos & Dixon, 1984).

Given the quantity and quality of print and electronic media that are consumed by adolescents, specific strategies that address the socializing role of the mass media need to be given high priority in the 1990s. It is again important that the strategies in this exosystem provide consistent messages and are coordinated with the programs within the other microsystems. The teaching of discriminating mass media skills—or media literacy—has already been suggested as a critical social competency for children and adolescents (Rapaczynski, Singer, & Singer, 1982) and may counterbalance some of the negative messages. A second strategy is to promote and incorporate health-enhancing messages and images in the existing mass media, either directly through planned and produced campaigns or indirectly by providing guidelines for the monitoring and screening of ongoing programs by existing radio and television stations. A third strategy is to limit exposure of adolescents to particular mass media (or to too much mass media) through stronger supervision by parents and adults or by ensuring that excessively violent, sexual, or alcohol-abusing images are not shown during after-school or prime-time hours. These strategies might serve to increase critical thinking about mass media, to prevent excessive exposure to health-compromising images, and potentially to increase pro-social messages.

In the 1980s several communitywide programs to promote cardiovascular health and prevent adolescent drug abuse were initiated in order to test the potency of large-scale change (Blackburn et al., 1984; Farquhar et al., 1984; Pentz et al., 1989). In North Karelia, a formal evaluation of school-based versus school- and communitywide smoking prevention programs was conducted (Vartiainen et al., 1986). Significant differences in smoking onset rates were found between the no-program control students and the school-program-only students, as well as between the school-program-only students and those students in a school program who also reside in communities where nonsmoking and smoking cessation were also being promoted. In the Minnesota Heart Health Youth Program, greater and more sustained behavior change was found when a communitywide approach was used (Perry et al., 1989). Likewise, Flay and Sobel (1983) found that school programs were strengthened by coordinating the content of a program with a short television series as part of prime time news.

Healthy Public Policy Promotion

Concern for adolescent health promotion in the 1990s ultimately involves the recognition of, and involvement with, public policy at the local, state, and national levels. For example, drug abuse prevention programs are currently being expanded due to funds allocated by the U.S. Congress in 1989; the content of these programs is being decided at the state level, programs that are given priority are selected by the local community, and compliant adoption of the programs depends on the support of school administrators and staff. Decisions at each of these levels are guided by policies—laws and rules that govern appropriate behavior, the assignment of priorities, and the allocation of resources (DeLeon & Vandenbos, 1984). Major goals in public policy of the 1990s, then, will be to promote the enactment of laws to raise the priority of adolescent health and health promotion efforts and, correspondingly, to increase the allocation of resources to support these efforts. To do this will require competencies in the legislative process, involvement with and education of elected officials concerning particular adolescent needs, collaboration with news and media representatives to shape the seriousness of problems and possible solutions, and commitment to this lengthy process of change.

Public policy in adolescent health promotion can be directed specifically to the larger systems of opportunities and barriers that support health-related behaviors.

It was recently demonstrated how easily adolescents can purchase tobacco, especially from cigarette vending machines (Forster, Klepp, & Jeffery, 1989). As a result, local ordinances to ban vending machines in several cities in Minnesota have already been enacted and a statewide ban is being considered, thereby considerably reducing access to tobacco for adolescents in Minnesota. Similar access issues might also be addressed in regard to alcohol use and television programming. Public policy that mandates additional school-based educational programs (such as those focusing on media literacy or social competencies) or needed services (such as school-based health clinics or quality latchkey after-school programs) can also be promoted. Public policies that will redirect or enlarge the 2–4% of the national health care dollar that is currently being spent on prevention to specifically increase investment in adolescent health needs can be considered (DeLeon & Vandenbos, 1984). This could also include taxation directed to educational programs or increases in payments for Aid to Families with Dependent Children that might directly aid adolescents who are living in poverty.

Conclusions

A broad and critical look at the socialization of American adolescents in the 1990s is needed. This brief review suggests that increasing proportions of adolescents in the 1980s were raised in poverty, were homeless, and were in homes where there was greater unsupervised time and fewer opportunities for healthy interaction with adults. It also suggests correspondingly greater peer involvement. It points to schools that appear to be struggling with demands to improve academically and, at the same time, to socialize American youth. It suggests that mass media of the 1980s opened the doors to almost unlimited images of alcohol use, violence, and promiscuous sexuality, with cable television, VCR, and popular television programming. Thus the influence of major socializers of youth—families and schools—may be being diminished by the increasing influence of peers and mass media.

A multicomponent approach to adolescent health promotion for the 1990s is considered. This approach proposes greater parental/adult involvement, incorporates peers as leaders in these efforts, teaches social competencies and life skills to cope with and manage the social environment, utilizes mass media and the larger community to reinforce prosocial values and to provide additional support, and encourages involvement in formulating public policies for necessary resources, opportunities, alternatives and restrictions for youth. The promotion of consistent values, messages, and models across the micro-, meso-, exo-, and macrosystems is inherent to these considerations and yet is one of the greatest challenges in enacting successful adolescent health promotion.

Adolescents living in mainstream middle-class America are likely to benefit from the health promotion intervention components that have been evaluated thus far. It is still difficult to imagine how these interventions will be able to achieve the desired and needed impact on adolescents from disenfranchised, poverty-stricken, or dysfunctional families. Surveying the social world of adolescents from the macrosystem perspective directs attention to solutions aimed at the American social structure. While the field of health promotion does not normally address issues of economic and social structure, in general they are relevant to the assignment of priorities and the development of interventions that take into account the strengths and weaknesses of the environmental setting. The promotion of opportunities for improvements in basic human needs such as nutrition, shelter, education, a stable exosystem, social justice, and equity should be considered a salutary development, and one consistent with more global aims of promoting overall adolescent health.

Acknowledgments

The authors would like to thank Maurice Elias, Roger Weissberg, Carolyn Williams, Henry Blackburn, and Hal Faulkner for their helpful suggestions in the preparation of this chapter.

References

Bagdikian, B. H. (1990). Global media corporations control what we watch (and read). *Utne Reader, 40,* 84–89.

Bandura, A. (1986). *Social foundations for thought and action: A social cognitive theory.* Englewood Cliffs, NJ: Prentice-Hall.

Bishop, J. H. (1989). Why the apathy in American high schools. *Educational Research, Jan./Feb.,* 6–10.

Blackburn, H. (1983). Research and demonstration projects in community cardiovascular disease prevention. *Public Health Policy, 4,* 398–421.

Blackburn, H., Luepker, R. V., Kline, F. G., Bracht, N., Carlaw, R., Jacobs, D., Mittelmark, M., Stauffer, L., & Taylor, H. L. (1984). The Minnesota Heart Health Program: A research and demonstration project in cardiovascular disease prevention. In J. D. Matarazzo, S. M. Weiss, J. A. Herd, N. E. Miller, & S. M. Weiss (Eds.), *Behavioral health: A handbook of health enhancement and disease prevention* (pp. 1171–1178). New York: Wiley.

Blum, R. (1987). Contemporary threats to adolescent health in the United States. *Journal of the American Medical Association, 257,* 3390–3395.

Botvin, G. J. (1986). Substance abuse prevention research: Recent developments and future directions. *Journal of School Health, 56,* 369–374.

Botvin, G. J., Baker, E., Renick, N., & Filazzola, A. (1984). A cognitive-behavioral approach to substance abuse prevention. *Addictive Behaviors, 9,* 137–147.

Bracht, N. F. (1990). *Organizing for community health promotion.* Newbury Park, CA: Sage.

Brennan, T. (1984). Adolescent loneliness. In L. A. Peplau & S. E. Goldston (Eds.), *Preventing the harmful consequences of severe and persistent loneliness,* (pp. 83–87 DHHS Pub. No. (ADM) 84-1312. Washington, DC: U.S. Government Printing Office.

Bronfenbrenner, M. (1979). *The ecology of human development: Experiments by nature and design.* Cambridge, MA: Harvard University Press.

Bronfenbrenner, M. (1986). Ecology of the family as a context for human development: Research perspectives. *Developmental Psychology, 22,* 723–742.

Brook, J. S., Nomura, C., & Cohen, P. (1988). A network of influences on adolescent drug involvement: Neighborhood, school peer, and family. *Genetic, Social, and General Psychology Monographs, 115,* 125–145.

Brown, B. B. (1990). Peer groups and peer cultures. In S. S. Feldman & G. R. Elliott (Eds.), *At the threshold: The developing adolescent* (pp. 171–196). Cambridge, MA: Harvard University Press.

Carnegie Council on Adolescent Development (1989). *Turning points: Preparing American youth for the 21st century.* New York: Carnegie Corporation of New York.

Children's Defense Fund (1987). *A children's defense budget, FY 1988.* Washington, DC: Children's Defense Fund.

Cooreman, J., & Perdrizet, S. (1980). Smoking in teenagers: Some psychological aspects. *Adolescence, 15,* 581–588.

Damon, W. (1983). *Social and personality development.* New York: Norton.

DeLeon, P. H., & Vandenbos, G. R. (1984). Public health policy and behavioral health. In J. D. Matarazzo, S. M. Weiss, J. A. Herd, N. E. Miller, & S. M. Weiss (Eds.), *Behavioral health: A handbook of health enhancement and disease prevention* (pp. 150–163). New York: Wiley.

Dodge, K. A., Pettit, G. S., McClaskey, C. L., & Brown, M. M. (1986). Social competence in children. *Monographs of the Society for Research in Child Development, 51,* Serial No. 213.

Dornbusch, S. M., Carlsmith, J. M., Bushwall, P. L., Ritter, P. L., Leiderman, H., Hastorf, A. H., & Gross, R. T. (1985). Single parents, extended households, and the control of adolescents. *Child Development, 56,* 326–341.

Elias, M. J. (1987). Establishing enduring prevention programs: Advancing the legacy of Swampscott. *American Journal of Community Psychology, 15,* 539–553.

Emery, R. E. (1989). Family violence. *American Psychologist, 44,* 321–328.

Entwisle, D. R. (1990). Schools and adolescence. In S. S. Feldman & G. R. Elliott. (Eds.), *At the threshold: The developing adolescent* (pp. 197–224). Cambridge, MA: Harvard University Press.

Epstein, J. L. (1987). Parent involvement: What research says to administrators. *Education and Urban Society, 19,* 119–136.

Erickson, J. B. (1988). Real American children: The challenge for after-school programs. *Child and Youth Care Quarterly, 17,* 86–103.

Farquhar, J. W., Fortmann, S. P., Maccoby, N., Wood, P. D., Haskell, W. L., Taylor, C. B., Flora, J. A., Solomon, D. S., Rogers, T., Adler, E., Breitrose, P., & Weiner, L. (1984). The Stanford Five-City Project: An overview. In J. D. Matarazzo, S. M. Weiss, J. A. Herd, N. E. Miller, & S. M. Weiss (Eds.), *Behavioral health: A handbook of health enhancement and disease prevention* (pp. 1154–1165). New York: Wiley.

Flay, B. R., & Sobel, J. L. (1983). The role of mass media in preventing adolescent substance abuse. In T. J. Glynn, C. G. Leukeford, & J. P. Ludford (Eds.), *Preventing adolescent drug abuse: Intervention strategies* (pp. 5–35). NIDA Research Monograph No. 47. Washington, DC: U.S. Government Printing Office.

Forster, J., Klepp, K. I., & Jeffery, R. (1989). Sources of cigarettes for 10th graders in two Minnesota cities. *Health Education Research, 4,* 45–50.

Gadow, K., & Sprafkin, J. (1989). Field experiments of television violence with children: Evidence for an environmental hazard? *Pediatrics, 83,* 399–405.

Galambos, N. L., & Dixon, R. A. (1984). Toward understanding and caring for latchkey children. *Child Care Quarterly, 13,* 116–125.

Garmezy, N., & Rutter, M. (1983). *Stress, coping, and development in children.* New York: McGraw-Hill.

Glanz, K., Lewis, F. M., & Rimer, B. (1990). *Health behavior and health education: Theory, research, and practice.* San Francisco: Jossey-Bass.

Glynn, T. J. (1989). Essential elements of school-based smoking prevention programs: Research results. *Journal of School Health, 59,* 181–188.

Hawkins, J. D., Jenson, J. M., Catalano, R. F., & Lishner, D. M. (1988). Delinquency and drug abuse: Implications for social services. *Social Service Review, 61,* 258–284.

Hill, J. P. (1987). Research on adolescents and their families: Past and present. In C. E. Irwin, Jr. (Ed.), *Adolescent social behavior and health.* (pp. 13–32). San Francisco: Jossey-Bass.

Hoffman, L. W. (1989). Effects of maternal employment in the two-parent family. *American Psychologist, 44,* 283–292.

Hurrelman, K. (1990). Health promotion for adolescents: Preventive and corrective strategies against problem behavior. *Journal of Adolescence, 13,* 231–250.

Irwin, C. E., & Vaughan, E. (1988). Psychosocial context of adolescent development. *Journal of Adolescent Health Care, 9,* 115–195.

Jessor, R., & Jessor, S. L. (1977). *Problem behavior and psychosocial development. A longitudinal study of youth.* New York: Academic Press.

Kandel, D. B. (1986). Processes of peer influences in adolescent drug use: A developmental perspective. *Advances in Alcohol Substance Abuse, 4,* 139–163.

Kandel, D. B., & Andrews, K. (1987). Processes of adolescent socialization by parents and peers. *The International Journal of the Addictions, 22,* 319–342.

Klepp, K. I., Halper, A., & Perry, C. L. (1986). The efficacy of peer leaders in drug abuse prevention. *Journal of School Health, 56,* 407–411.

Lowry, D. T., & Towles, D. E. (1989a). Soap opera portrayals of sex, contraception, and sexually transmitted diseases. *Journal of Communication, 39,* 76–83.

Lowry, D. T., & Towles, D. E. (1989b). Prime time TV portrayals of sex, contraception and venereal diseases. *Journalism Quarterly, 66,* 347–352.

McLanahan, S. S., & Bumpass, L. (1988). Comment: A note on the effect of family structure on school enrollment. In G. D. Sandefur & M. Tienda (Eds.), *Divided Opportunities* (pp. 195–201). New York: Plenum.

McNeil, L. M. (1986). *Contradictions of control: School structure and school knowledge,* New York: Routledge & Kegan Paul.

Murray, D. M., Johnson, C. A., Leupker, R. V., & Mittlemark, M. B. (1984). The prevention of cigarette smoking in children: A comparison of four strategies. *Journal of Applied Social Psychology, 14,* 274–288.

Murray, M., Kiryluk, S., & Swan, A. V. (1984). School characteristics and adolescent smoking. Results from the MRC Derbyshore Smoking Study of 1974–8 and from a follow-up in 1981. *Journal of Epidemiology and Community Health, 38,* 167–172.

Nader, P. R., Sallis, J. F., Patterson, T. L., Abramson, I. S., & Rupp, J. W. (1989). A family approach to cardiovascular risk reduction: Results from the San Diego Family Heart Project. *Health Education Quarterly, 16,* 229–244.

National Commission on the Role of the School and the Community in Improving Adolescent Health (1990). *Code blue: Uniting for healthier youth.*

Noack, H. (1987). Concepts of health and health promotion. In *Measurement in Health Promotion and Protection.* WHO publication, European Series. Alexandria, VA: National Association of State Boards of Education.

Offer, D., Ostrov, E., Howard, K. I., & Atkinson, R. (1988). *The teenage world: Adolescents' self-image in ten countries.* New York: Plenum Medical Book Co.

O'Keefe, G. J., & Reid-Nash, K. (1987). Socializing function. In C. R. Berger & S. H. Chaffee (Eds.), *Handbook of communication,* (pp. 419–445). Newbury Park, CA: Sage.

Page, R. M. (1988). Adolescent loneliness: A priority for school health education. *Health Education,* June/July, 20–22.

Pallas, A. M. (1988). School climate in American high schools. *Teachers College Record, 89,* 541–554.

Patterson, T. L., Rupp, J., Sallis, J., Atkins, C., & Nader, P. (1988). Aggregation of dietary calories, fats, and sodium in Mexican American and Anglo families. *American Journal of Preventive Medicine, 4,* 75–82.

Pentz, M. A., Dwyer, J. H., MacKinnon, D. P., Flay, B. R., Hansen, W. B., Wang, E. Y., & Johnson, D. A. (1989). A multicommunity trial for primary prevention of adolescent drug abuse. *Journal of the American Medical Association, 261,* 3259–3266.

Perlman, D., & Peplau, L. A. (1984). Loneliness research: A survey of empirical findings. In L. A. Peplau & S. E. Goldston (Eds.), *Preventing the harmful consequences of severe and persistent lone-*

liness (pp. 13–46). DHSS Pub. No. (ADM) 84-1312. Washington, DC: U.S. Government Printing Office.

Perry, C. L., Crockett, S. J., & Pirie, P. (1987). Influencing parental health behavior: Implications of community assessments. *Health Education, 18,* 68–77.

Perry, C. L., & Grant, M. (1988). Comparing peer-led to teacher-led youth alcohol education in four countries. *Alcohol Health and Research World, 12,* 322–336.

Perry, C. L., & Jessor, R. (1985). The concept of health promotion and the prevention of adolescent drug abuse. *Health Education Quarterly, 12,* 169–184.

Perry, C. L., Klepp, K. I., & Schultz, J. (1988). Primary prevention of cardiovascular disease: Community-wide strategies for youth. *Journal of Consulting and Clinical Psychology, 56,* 358–364.

Perry, C. L., Klepp, K. I., & Sillers, C. (1989). Community-wide strategies for cardiovascular health: The Minnesota Heart Health Program Youth Program. *Health Education Research, 4,* 87–101.

Perry, C. L., Luepker, R. V., Murray, D. M., Kurth, C., Mullis, R., Crockett, S., & Jacobs, D. J. (1988). Parent involvement with children's health promotion: The Minnesota Home Team. *American Journal of Public Health, 78,* 1156–1160.

Perry, C. L., Mullis, R. M., & Maile, M. C. (1985). Modifying the eating behavior of young children. *Journal of School Health, 55,* 399–402.

Perry, C. L., & Murray, D. M. (1982). Enhancing the transition years: The challenge of adolescent health promotion. *Journal of School Health,* May, 307–311.

Perry, C. L., Stone, E. J., Parcel, G. S., Ellison, R. C., Nader, P., Webber, L. S., & Luepker, R. V. (1990) School-based cardiovascular health promotion: The Child and Adolescent Trial for Cardiovascular Health (CATCH). *Journal of School Health, 60,* 443–447.

Rapaczynski, W., Singer, D. G., & Singer, J. (1982). Teaching television: A curriculum for young children. *Journal of Communication, 32,* 46–55.

Rotheram-Borus, M. J., & Tsemberis, S. J. (1989). Social competency training programs in ethnically diverse communities. In G. W. Albee and J. M. Joffe (Eds.), *Primary prevention of psychopathology, Volume XII* (pp. 297–318). Newberry Park, CA: Sage.

Sallis, J. F., Patteron, T. L., Buono, M. J., Atkins, C. J., & Nader, P. (1988). Aggregation of physical activity habits in Mexican American and Anglo families. *Journal of Behavioral Medicine, 11,* 31–41.

Savin-Williams, R. C., & Berndt, T. J. (1989). Friendship and peer relations. In S. S. Feldman & G. R. Elliott (Eds.), *At the threshold: The developing adolescent* (pp. 277–307). Cambridge MA: Harvard University Press.

Schinke, S. P., & Gilchrist, L. D. (1984). *Life skills counseling with adolescents.* Baltimore: University Park Press.

Scott-Jones, D. (1985). *Assessing American education: Shrinking resources, growing demands.* Paper commissioned by the National Center for Education Statistics.

Simmons, R. G. (1987). Social transition and adolescent development. In C. E. Irwin Jr. (Ed.), *Adolescent social behavior and health* (pp. 33–62). San Francisco: Jossey-Bass.

Singer, D. G. (1985). Alcohol, television and teenagers. *Pediatrics, Sex, Drugs, Rock 'n Roll Supplement,* 668–674.

Spivack, G., & Shure, M. B. (1982). The cognition of social adjustment: Interpersonal cognitive problem-solving thinking. In B. B. Lahey & A. E. Kazdin (Eds.), *Advances in clinical child psychology: Volume 5* (pp. 323–372). New York: Plenum.

Standard & Poor's Industry Surveys. (1988). *Cable television: Excellent operating outlook continues for cable.* New York: Standard and Poor Corporation.

Steinberg, L. (1986). Latch-key children and susceptibility to peer pressure: An ecological analyses. *Developmental Psychology, 22,* 433–439.

Steinberg, L. (1989). Autonomy, conflict and harmony in the family relationship. In S. S. Feldman & G. R. Elliott (Eds.), *At the threshold: The developing adolescent* (pp. 255–276). Cambridge MA: Harvard University Press.

Stevenson, D. L., & Baker, D. P. (1987). The family–school relation and the child's school performance. *Child Development, 58,* 1348–1357.

Stipek, D., & McCroskey, J. (1989). Investing in children: Government and workplace policies for parents. *American Psychologist, 44,* 416–423.

Stone, E. J., Perry, C. L., & Luepker, R. V. (1989). Behavioral research for cardiovascular health promotion with youth. *Health Education Quarterly, 16,* 155–169.

Strasburger, V. C. (1985). Television and adolescents. *Pediatric Annals, 14,* 814–820.

U.S. Department of Education, Center for Education Statistics (1989). Elementary and secondary education. In *Digest of education statistics* (pp. 39–158). Washington, DC: National Center for Education Statistics.

Vanderpool, N. A., & Richmond, J. B. (1990). Child health in the United States: Prospects for the 1990's. *Annual Review of Public Health, 11,* 185–205.

Vartiainen, E., McAlister, A., Puska, P., Viri, L., Tossavainen, K., Niskanen, E., & Pallonen, U. (1986). *Short-term effects of school and community-based programs to prevent smoking and alcohol abuse among adolescents.* Unpublished manuscript. Department of Epidemiology, National Public Health Institute, Kuopio, Finland.

Weissberg, R. P., Caplan, M. Z., & Sivo, P. J. (1989). A new conceptual framework for establishing school-based social competence promotion programs. In L. A. Bond & B. E. Compas (Eds.), *Primary prevention and promotion in the schools* (pp. 225–296). Newbury Park, CA: Sage.

6

A View of Health
from the Adolescent's Perspective

Susan G. Millstein

Many authors, including those in this book, have suggested that more attention be paid to the phenomenological aspects of adolescent health and development. Such an approach would examine health from the adolescent's perspective, exploring the meaning of health to the adolescent, motivations for health-related behaviors, how health communications are interpreted and acted on, and how health behaviors are experienced. This type of research inquiry is customary in disciplines such as anthropology and education but is infrequently employed as a scientific tool in psychology or medicine. There are, however, compelling arguments for extending our research on adolescent health issues to include phenomenological inquiries.

One such argument concerns the role of belief systems in health behavior. Perhaps the best illustration of how individuals' perceptions and belief systems influence behavior can be seen in the behavioral variations associated with cross-cultural differences in social mores and customs (Weidman, 1988). Even within more homogeneous cultural milieus, perceptions and belief systems influence individuals' health behaviors. Through cognitive processes, individuals interpret health-related information that they use in making decisions regarding future actions. Beliefs about personal vulnerability and the capacity to perform specific behaviors are also associated with a variety of health and illness behaviors such as utilization of health services, keeping appointments, complying with treatment, and engaging in preventive activities (for reviews see Becker & Maiman, 1983; Cleary, 1987; Kirscht, 1983; Wallston & Wallston, 1984). These beliefs and decision-making processes become increasingly important to recognize during adolescence, when young people are given further personal responsibility for health and health-related decisions.

To the extent that we view adolescent health behaviors as motivated and purposive, it is also important to be aware of the motivations that underlie specific behaviors. As Chapter 12 notes, interventions are unlikely to be successful if they are developed without a sense of the reasons why people engage in the behavior. This is especially true when we intend to offer alternatives to unhealthy behaviors. An understanding of the underlying motivations should form the basis for choosing such alternatives.

97

Finally, exploring adolescents' perspectives has the potential for facilitating communication between adults and adolescents. Communication between patients and health care providers is known to increase adherence and patient satisfaction (DiNicola & DiMatteo, 1984). Adolescents themselves consider communication an important component of the health care visit (Giblin & Poland, 1985; Resnick, Blum, & Hedin, 1980), and there is little reason to think that the effects of effective communication would be different for adolescents than for adults.

This chapter will present a view of health from the adolescent's perspective, reviewing research on the conceptual frameworks that adolescents use to think about health and their specific health concerns. Beliefs, attitudes, and expectations that are likely to play an important role in adolescents' health behaviors are also examined, including health knowledge and beliefs about personal vulnerability, health risks, health promotion, and social contexts for promoting health. The potential utility of this information for health promotion programs is discussed at the conclusion of the chapter.

Conceptual Frameworks for Health and the Health Concerns of Adolescents

Definitions of Health and Illness

Adolescents define health using criteria similar to those of adults: health means being able to live up to one's potential; being able to function physically, mentally, and socially; and experiencing positive affective states (Eiser, Patterson, & Eiser, 1983; Millstein, Adler, & Irwin, 1981; Natapoff, 1978; Radius, Dillman, Becker, Rosenstock, & Horvath, 1980). Although "not being sick" is a common theme in adolescents' (as well as adults') health concepts, most of the content in adolescents' health conceptions focuses on other aspects of health, especially functional status and prevention (what one can do to *enhance* and *maintain* health; Millstein & Irwin, 1987). Adolescents' definitions fit the health paradigm described by Perry and Jessor (1985), which consists of four dimensions: physical health, mental and emotional health, social health (including interpersonal and role functioning), and personal health (reflecting the realization of one's potential).

Concepts of health and illness seem to develop according to a fairly predictable course that is consistent with the predictions of Piaget's theory of cognitive development (Burbach & Peterson, 1986: Campbell, 1975). Young children view health and illness in relatively simplistic terms; they describe vague feeling states and rely extensively on the judgment of others to determine when they are ill. They generally have difficulty defining the concept of health except vis-à-vis illness. In early adolescence, relatively concrete thinking about illness still predominates, usually related to specific diseases and disorders. Concepts of health show a similar lack of abstraction, often focusing on the absence of illness.

As adolescents mature, their concepts of both illness and health become more inclusive and more abstract. The older adolescent is more likely to recognize psychological, affective, and social components relevant to health and illness, such as issues related to coping abilities, emotional health, and interpersonal relations. Older adolescents are also more likely to recognize personal behavior as a factor in health, acknowledging the role that individuals play in maintaining, damaging, or restoring their health. The onset of formal operational thinking in some youth is also associated with the ability to view health and illness in hypothetical terms (Chapter 2).

Perceptions of Health Status

The accuracy with which adolescents perceive their health status has been viewed in contradictory terms. On the one hand, adolescents are seen as minimizing their symptoms through denial and failing to respond to symptoms appropriately. On the other hand, they are also viewed as exaggerating and dwelling on symptoms due to greater self-consciousness, introspection, and attention to body states (Mechanic, 1983; Millstein & Litt, 1990). Of course, both types of behavior may characterize a given individual at different times. In terms of perceptions of health status, however, the data more strongly suggest the latter.

While adolescents generally report themselves as being healthy (Parcel, Nader, & Meyer, 1977; Sobal, Klein, Graham, & Black, 1988), they view their health as being poorer than do physicians who examine them or their parents (National Center for Health Statistics, 1977). It is not clear whether the differences that emerge are a function of heightened self-consciousness in adolescents, or whether they reflect differences in how adolescents and adults define good health. Variations in the definition of good health for adolescents and adults could reflect scaling or calibration differences (Furby & Beyth-Marom, 1990), differences in understanding of scaling terms (Cohn, Macfarlane, & Yanez, 1991), or differences in knowledge about what constitutes good health.

Health Concerns

Adolescents identify a variety of health concerns reflecting common medical problems as well as psychosocial issues. Common concerns include those related to appearance (height, weight, acne), emotional states (depression, anxiety), interpersonal relationships (parents, friends, and other adults), school (schoolwork and career), and physical complaints (headaches, stomach aches, vision problems, dental problems). Adolescents also recognize the health issues most frequently identified by professionals: substance use, sexual behavior, birth control, sexually transmitted diseases, and pregnancy (Alexander, 1989; Giblin & Poland, 1985; Marks, Malizio, Hoch, Brody, & Fisher, 1983; Parcel et al., 1977; Sternlieb & Munan, 1972).

Although adolescents clearly acknowledge a wide range of concerns, only a few issues consistently rank highly. These include issues pertaining to school, dental health, acne, interpersonal relationships, and mental health (American School Health Association [ASHA], 1989; Sternlieb & Munan, 1972). Concerns related to substance use, sexual behavior, nutrition, and exercise rank lower in most samples

(Eme, Maisiak & Goodale, 1979; Feldman, Hodgson, Corber, & Quinn, 1986; Sobal et al., 1988). However, one must always be aware of the potential for bias when adolescents are asked about sensitive issues such as sexuality or substance use. These issues may rank low not because they are of little concern, but because they are more difficult to disclose.

MENTAL HEALTH AND SOURCES OF STRESS   Mental health concerns consistently rank highly among adolescents (ASHA, 1989; Benedict, Lundeen, & Morr, 1981; Parcel et al., 1977; Sternlieb & Munan, 1972). Like adults, adolescents define mental health primarily in terms of subjective well-being and feelings of contentment and happiness (Chapter 8). Departures from these positive feelings are common; between 10% and 30% of adolescents report distress about sadness, depression, or anxiety (Marks et al., 1983; Parcel et al., 1977; University of Minnesota, 1989). Adolescents may find it difficult to raise these concerns and discuss them with others. In a suburban sample of 649 adolescents, almost 10% acknowledged having concerns about emotional upsets and depression but did not discuss these issues with their physician (Marks et al., 1983).

Sources of stress identified by adolescents include peer and family relationships, academics, athletics, job-related concerns, and personal adequacy issues (Armacost, 1989; Burke & Weir, 1978; Greene, 1988; Porteus, 1979). Other, less frequently studied but recognized sources of stress include racial prejudice and tension (Armacost, 1989). Like other aspects of the adolescent experience, sources of stress have usually been defined from the perspective of the adult. Lists of stressful life events are typically presented to the adolescent, with instructions to note whether or not a particular event took place. A few studies have attempted to assess the degree to which these presumably stressful events were, in fact, stressful to the adolescent (Siddique & D'Arcy, 1984); even fewer have asked the adolescent to define *a priori* the events that he or she perceives as stressful.

Individual and Contextual Differences in Concerns

Although there are differences in health concerns as a function of developmental level, gender, race, ethnicity, and socioeconomic factors, in many ways the similarities are more striking than the differences. Nevertheless, a number of important and consistent differences have emerged. These are discussed below.

DEVELOPMENTAL FACTORS.   Cross-sectional studies have shown differences in the health concerns of younger and older adolescents, differences that are consistent with the developmental tasks they face. A study of over 5,000 children and adolescents found increasing interest among them in topics such as growth and development, preventive health behaviors, mental health, and social-emotional development as children moved into the early adolescent years (Byler, Lewis, & Totman, 1969).

Among younger adolescents (e.g., those between the ages of 11 and 13), concerns about growth and development, especially pubertal processes, are common

(Byler et al., 1969). Concern about how one compares with others emerges (Levenson, Morrow, Johnson, & Pfefferbaum, 1983), as do concerns about how one is viewed by the opposite sex. Shyness is a common concern (Porteus, 1979; Millstein et al., 1992). Concerns about smoking and drug use also appear to be more common among younger adolescents (Byler et al., 1969; Levenson et al., 1983; Violato & Holden, 1988), perhaps as a reflection of anticipatory anxiety among a group with little experience with substance use.

The middle adolescent years (e.g., ages 14 to 15) are usually marked by the transition from middle school or junior high school to high school. With this transition, adolescent concerns show an increasing emphasis on the peer group, including the world of the opposite sex. Concerns about peer group acceptance and relationships with friends are heightened. For females, concerns about appearance become paramount (Eme et al., 1979; University of Minnesota, 1989; Violato & Holden, 1988). Issues regarding self-esteem also loom large (Levenson et al., 1983).

As adolescents mature further, their concerns begin to focus increasingly on school and grades, as well as on future career plans (Eme et al., 1979; Violato & Holden, 1988). Not surprisingly, college-bound adolescents express the highest degree of concern about career and grades. Independence, an issue among early adolescents, reemerges as a major concern for late adolescents (Eme et al., 1979). Concerns about emotional health (e.g., depression, nervousness) and birth control also increase (Parcel et al., 1977), especially among females (Feldman et al., 1986).

Sources of stress show similar developmental patterns. In early adolescence, stress related to families appears to have more negative effects on adolescents' psychological functioning than other sources of stress. In middle adolescence, stressors related to peers appear to be more significant. In late adolescence, academic stress becomes paramount (Wagner & Compas, 1990).

Studies have not examined differences in the health concerns of adolescents early and late in development, relying instead on chronological age as a measure of developmental status. This is a serious limitation, since chronological age and pubertal status differentially predict interests in certain topics (Ryan, Millstein, & Irwin, 1988). For example, adolescents who show early physical maturation evidence earlier onset of concerns about the opposite sex than do late-developing adolescents.

Although surveys can identify whether a particular concern exists, differences in the meaning or interpretation of the concern cannot be extracted. Thus, while most adolescents express interest and concerns relative to various aspects of reproductive health, the quality of their concerns differs dramatically over the adolescent decade. In younger adolescents, reproductive health issues often center on the meaning of puberty, menstruation, and physical differences between the sexes. Interest in sexual behavior emerges fairly early, but it shifts from interest in why sexual attraction takes place and the mechanics of sexual activity to more complex questions about ethical issues, societal mores, negotiating sexual relationships, and the relationship of intimacy to sex (Metropolitan Life Foundation, 1988). Similarly, interest in mental health and illness exists throughout the adolescent years but shifts over time from a general interest in mental illness to more personal concerns about one's own mental health. This shift to a more personal interest may be responsible for the increased concern noted about mental health issues in the older group.

GENDER DIFFERENCES. Many studies have reported gender differences, both in the number and types of health concerns reported by adolescents. Across studies representing a diversity of samples, females consistently report thinking more about their health, having more health concerns, and experiencing more health problems than do males (Alexander, 1989; Brunswick & Josephson, 1972; Feldman et al., 1986; Parcel et al., 1977; Porteus, 1979; Radius et al., 1980; Sobal et al., 1988; University of Minnesota, 1989; Violato & Holden, 1988). Although some of the gender differences can be accounted for by sex-linked concerns such as menstruation and pregnancy, girls are also more likely than boys to have concerns about appearance (Alexander, 1989; Eme et al., 1979; Feldman et al., 1986; Levenson et al., 1983; Parcel et al., 1977; Violato & Holden, 1988), emotional states (Feldman et al., 1986; Millstein et al., 1992; Parcel et al., 1977; Sobal, 1988), and interpersonal relationships (Parcel et al., 1977). Interpersonal stressors of particular salience to female adolescents include acceptance by the opposite sex (Burke & Weir, 1978) and by peers (Greene, 1988). Greater stress from interpersonal sources among females is thought to result from female adolescents' strong dependence on families and peers for emotional support and expression of personal problems (Siddique & D'Arcy, 1984).

Males, on the other hand, are more likely to have concerns in the areas of sports and future vocational plans (Parcel et al., 1977; Porteus, 1979) and also report more stress in relation to these concerns (Armacost, 1989). Although some studies show increased concern about school performance in males (Porteus, 1979), others report increased school concerns in females (Eme et al., 1979; Violato & Holder, 1988). Some of the variance may reflect a gender–age interaction, with earlier concerns about school performance typical of females and later concerns typical of males (University of Minnesota, 1989).

The differences in the types of concerns emphasized by males and females may also account for some of the difference in the perceptions of health status noted earlier. Alexander (1989) found that perceptions of health status in eighth-grade females were dependent on concerns about emotional and social issues, while for males health status was defined more strongly in terms of physical concerns. This could explain why females perceive themselves as having poorer health and more health problems. Since physical problems during adolescence are minimal, males, who primarily use these as defining health, would be expected to perceive themselves as being in better health.

Gender differences in health concerns appear to be increasing over time and may partially reflect the increasing concern among females regarding weight issues. Feldman et al. (1986) note that the gender differences in weight concerns they found are larger than those reported earlier by Sternlieb and Munan (1972) and suggest that we are seeing an increase in this sex difference as cultural forces change. This explanation would also be consistent with increases in eating disorders among female adolescents that have taken place over the past years (Chapter 10).

In examining gender differences, it is also important to keep in mind the different rates at which males and females mature. Some of the differences attributed to gender may in fact be developmentally driven (Alexander, 1989). Careful analyses of gender–age interactions are needed to tease out these effects.

RACIAL AND ETHNIC VARIATION. Few studies have examined differences in health concerns as a function of race or ethnicity, and even fewer have disentangled the effects of social class in their analyses. The limited research available shows that in comparison with white adolescents, black adolescents rate their health as poorer (Alexander, 1989; Brunswick, 1969), think more about their health (American Cancer Society, 1979; Sobal et al., 1988), have more health concerns (Sobal et al., 1988), are more concerned about future illness (American Cancer Society, 1979), and believe they are more susceptible to specific diseases, such as cancer (Price, Desmond, Wallace, Smith, & Stewart, 1988). Hispanic youth also report feeling less healthy than their white peers (Brunswick, 1969) and, in one study, less healthy than black adolescents (Parcel et al., 1977).

Differences also emerge in the nature of the specific concerns. Black adolescents are more concerned about substance use than white adolescents (Alexander, 1989). They also rank school concerns higher than white adolescents (Alexander, 1989; Sobal et al., 1988). Concerns about mental health may show a different pattern, with white adolescents reporting mental health concerns more often than Hispanic or black adolescents (Parcel et al., 1977).

Actual differences in health status among white, black, and Hispanic youth could explain some of these perceptions. Since health status is closely tied to economic status and since minorities are generally economically disadvantaged (Chapter 3), it is not clear whether these racial-ethnic differences would persist or new ones would emerge in studies controlling for economic status.

SOCIAL CLASS AND ECONOMIC STATUS. Little is known about how economic conditions influence adolescents' perceptions about the world (see Bloom-Feshbach, Bloom-Feshbach, & Heller, 1982 for a review). In a Canadian sample, Feldman et al. (1986) found no variation in adolescent health concerns by social class. It is possible that the absence of social class effects in this sample may reflect the availability of universal health care in Canada. However, at least two American studies reported no differences in perceived vulnerability to health problems as a function of socioeconomic status (Gochman & Saucier, 1982; Michielutte & Diseker, 1982).

As in other areas of adolescents' lives, sources of stress vary as a function of the context in which the adolescent lives. Adolescents living in different situations would be expected to report different types of stressors. For example, stress related to material deprivation has been reported in a British sample (Porteus, 1979) but has been less frequently studied in this country. Given the striking increases in poverty among youth in the United States, such investigations would probably show high rates of stress in this regard.

Limitations of Current Research on Adolescents' Health

Studies on adolescent health typically present the adolescent with a preconstructed list of health issues and ask the adolescent to identify those concerns that apply to him or her. This may not be the best way to ascertain the concerns that are actually salient to adolescents, particularly vis-à-vis other life concerns. Bias may emerge in either direction, highlighting concerns of little actual relevance or obscuring others of high relevance. For example, concerns about sports injuries, which were acknowledged by 20% of adolescents in one sample (Feldman et al., 1986), had not emerged previously as a source of concern, perhaps because this issue had not been included on the list of concerns used in most studies. Similarly, a recent study that specifically examined issues such as violence and interpersonal aggression found that a large majority of adolescents feared theft of their personal belongings, and a modest percentage (19%) feared actual violence (Armacost, 1989). The lack of consistency among studies in what is included on the lists of concerns makes it extremely difficult to compare studies.

The use of questionnaires also fails to capture the richness of experience that other data collection approaches such as interviews can generate. An example of this is provided by Porteus's (1979) study of 15-year-old British adolescents. Consistent with other studies, "interpersonal concerns" ranked highly as issues of importance. But the in-depth interviews provided additional information about the meaning of this descriptive label. Interpersonal issues were evident in relation to peers, family, and self–other relationships. Peer concerns included the ability to make and keep friends, issues regarding bullying and peer aggression, shyness, and relationships with the opposite sex. Relationships with family members were also of concern, particularly issues regarding communication with parents, arguments with parents, arguments between parents, and issues of control and trust. Aspects of self–other relationships that emerged included self-consciousness in relation to others, being criticized unfairly, not being listened to, and difficulties in speaking up for oneself. This brief description of adolescents interpersonal concerns goes far beyond what most studies have reported.

Health Knowledge and Beliefs

Health Knowledge

Adolescents often have misperceptions about health issues (Centers for Disease Control, 1988; Morrison, 1985), although with enough exposure, such as in the case of information on AIDS, their knowledge increases (Brown & Fritz, 1988; DiClemente, Zorn, & Temoshok, 1986; Strunin & Hingson, 1987). As one would expect, younger adolescents possess less factual knowledge about a variety of health topics than do older adolescents (Morrison, 1985).

Studies on racial and ethnic differences in knowledge have generally not controlled for social and economic class differences. With this caveat in mind, studies show that in comparison to their white peers, black adolescents have less knowledge about sexuality, contraception, AIDS, and cancer (American Cancer Society, 1979; DiClemente, Boyer, & Morales, 1988; Eisen, Zellman, & McAlister, 1985; Morrison, 1985; Price et al., 1988). It is probable that much of the racial-ethnic variance in knowledge can be attributed to differences in economic status, given the relationship of economic status and education (Chapter 3). Cultural factors may also play a role via erroneous beliefs held by a particular culture, or because beliefs characterizing minority cultures may be viewed as wrong by the majority culture (Chapter 4).

Knowledge is generally viewed as a necessary but insufficient condition for health-related behaviors to occur. Although it is often assumed that more knowledge is better, this may not always be the case. Some facts may simply be irrelevant, given the motivations of the individual. For example, knowledge about the health effects of tobacco use is important only if health is a motivating factor for a given individual. Even where a motivation for health does exist, some types of knowledge may be more important than others in actual decision making. For example, knowledge that smoking constricts blood vessels may be less relevant than knowledge that smoking causes heart attacks or makes it more difficult to exercise. A major task in making decisions is to sort through vast amounts of information and to determine what is pertinent to a particular decision and what is not. For adolescents who have limited experience with these complex decisions, this may appear to be an overwhelming task. This may explain why 34% of adolescents say they are very concerned about making the wrong decisions about their future and about not being able to change them (American Home Economics Association [AHEA], 1988). Perhaps we could facilitate interventions for this age group by recognizing which elements of knowledge are most critical to informed decision making and by not overexposing youth to irrelevant facts.

Cognitive biases that influence the interpretation of educational information have been identified for adults, but little research has focused on the adolescent population (Furby & Beyth-Marom, 1990). There has been almost no discussion, for example, about how adolescents interpret the health information to which they are exposed. The assumption seems to be that the message we intend to convey is in fact the message that the adolescent receives. Not only is this likely to be erroneous, it also may be dangerous. For example, AIDS prevention messages that counsel adolescents to "know your partner" could be counterproductive if the adolescent interprets this as meaning "someone you have known for a few weeks." Differences in interpretation within the adolescent population as a function of factors such as developmental level, cultural background, and education are also likely to exist.

Perceptions of Vulnerability to Health Problems

A widely held belief about adolescents is that they perceive themselves as being invulnerable to harm as a direct result of their level of cognitive development. Despite frequent references to this adolescent invulnerability and its developmental basis in both professional and popular literature, no empirical work supports the assertion (Melton, 1988). Adolescents, like adults, evidence significant bias when asked to estimate their personal vulnerability to harm. Informal comparisons of the degree of optimistic bias in studies of adolescents and adults suggest that differences between these groups are not significant (Millstein, in press). Furthermore, some research suggests that perceptions of personal susceptibility to health problems may be a stable personality trait (Gochman, 1985). While clinical observations of youth have suggested differences in the awareness of personal susceptibility, these observations have not been followed by careful examination of the observed differences and their source.

Perceptions of vulnerability have been shown to vary as a function of race/ethnicity, and show that black and Hispanic adolescents feel more susceptible to a variety of health outcomes (such as cancer, pregnancy, and AIDS) than do their white peers (Eisen et al., 1985; Michielutte & Diseker, 1982; Price et al., 1988). DiClemente et al. (1988) found that racial/ethnic differences in vulnerability were primarily a function of knowledge. Research on the role of socioeconomic factors has failed to show an association between these factors and perceived vulnerability (Gochman & Saucier, 1982; Michielutte & Diseker, 1982).

Perceptions of Health Risks

Adolescents generally recognize as potential health threats personal behaviors such as substance use, sexual activity, and risks related to the use of recreational and motor vehicles. Brunswick (1969) found the primary health threats adolescents identified to be behavioral, including lack of exercise, lack of sleep, not eating properly, and smoking cigarettes. Environmental threats to health were also identified, such as air pollution and nuclear war (Brunswick, 1969; Millstein & Irwin, 1985). Adolescents also identified health threats that fall outside constrictive definitions of health, including family and peer relations and school problems (Benedict et al., 1981; Marks et al., 1983; Parcel et al., 1977; Sternlieb & Munan, 1972). Differences emerge when adolescents are asked about general threats to youth versus personal factors that place them at risk. Like adults, adolescents probably underestimate the potentially negative consequences of their personal behavior. Adolescents also anticipate, sometimes incorrectly, that the risks associated with certain behaviors will diminish with increased age (Millstein & Irwin, 1985).

Factors that moderate the perception of risks are not well understood. However, the National Adolescent School Health Survey reported that the frequency of use of substances such as alcohol and marijuana was a factor in how risky adolescents perceived these behaviors to be (ASHA, 1989). An understanding of how the adolescent defines occasional versus regular use is thus important.

Perceptions of Health Promoting Behaviors

Interestingly, only a few studies have examined adolescents' perceptions about factors that are health promoting. Three separate interview studies of younger adolescents have been conducted, with similar findings. Behaviors most often identified as health-enhancing included proper nutrition, exercise, getting enough sleep, and seeing the doctor or dentist. Other health-enhancing factors mentioned were maintaining personal hygiene, dressing properly for the weather, avoiding temperature extremes, taking vitamins, avoiding injury, staying away from sick people, having a positive attitude, and avoiding negative feelings (Altman & Revenson, 1985; Korbin & Kahorik, 1985; Millstein & Irwin, 1986). Older adolescents ranked the most important behavior to be brushing teeth, followed by staying clean, getting enough sleep, keeping emergency numbers by the telephone, watching one's weight, wearing warm clothing, exercising, and seeing the dentist (Millstein & Irwin, 1986).

Differences Between Adolescent and Adult Perceptions

Adolescents' views about health and health problems and those of adults do not always correspond (Levenson, Morrow, Gregory, & Pfefferbaum, 1984; National Center for Health Statistics [NCHS], 1977). Adults not only underestimate the degree of concern adolescents report about their health (Sobal et al., 1988), they also have misperceptions about adolescents' level of knowledge about specific topics. One study, for example, found that physicians underrated the amount of factual knowledge adolescents had on AIDS, as well as underestimating the obstacles perceived by the adolescent in taking preventive action (Manning & Balson, 1989). Instances in which adults overestimate adolescents' knowledge are also likely to exist.

Adults also fail to recognize some of the specific health concerns of adolescents. An example occurs in regard to dental and oral health. Across studies, adolescents consistently rank dental concerns as being of great importance (Parcel et al., 1977; Sobal et al., 1988; Sternlieb & Munan, 1972). Yet this topic rarely receives attention in discussions of adolescent health. Sobal et al. (1988) also found that adults failed to recognize the strong concern among high school students in relation to school problems, dental problems, and their relationships with adults. In a study of older children and young (sixth-grade) adolescents, Greene (1988) found that the death of a pet was the most frequently mentioned stressor (69%). Other stressors included grades, illness/injury, moving to a new home, interpersonal conflict, and lost possessions.

As noted earlier, some of the differences between adolescents and adults may reflect a scaling or calibration issue, although this remains to be investigated. However, it is unlikely that scaling issues explain all of the variance, particularly since adults themselves differ in their perceptions of adolescents' concerns. Levenson, Morrow, and Pfefferbaum (1984) found that in comparison with physicians, for example, teachers and nurses tended to view peer acceptance as more important to adolescents.

An analysis of data from the Health Examination Survey on health-related behavior and attitudes in pairs of adolescents and parents indicated that the degree of correspondence between the perceptions of parents and adolescents was higher in females, older adolescents, white adolescents, and those from families with higher income (NCHS, 1977).

Contexts for Promoting Adolescent Health

As noted by many authors in this book, a variety of settings provide opportunities for promoting adolescent health. Proximal, interpersonal contexts for health promotion include families and peers. Institutional contexts include schools and health care settings. More distal influences include the mass media (Chapters 2 and 5). Few studies have examined adolescents' perceptions about these social contexts. Yet these perceptions could be useful in assessing the strengths and weaknesses of using particular contextual settings for the delivery of health promotion programs. As we shall see, depending on the topic, adolescents have preferences for certain sources of information. Consistent with social psychological research on source credibility, adolescents view the information from these sources with different degrees of confidence.

SCHOOLS. School is a critical avenue for health promotion efforts, both because of the emphasis on learning and because it is a place where adolescents congregate (Chapter 5). Adolescents are generally interested in health education classes (Metropolitan Life Foundation, 1988) and are receptive to school settings as a source of health information (University of Minnesota, 1989). Areas in which adolescents believe schools should provide more education include stress management; dealing with major events that affect families such as death, divorce, and unemployment; and self-esteem (AHEA, 1988; Metropolitan Life Foundation, 1988).

Teachers in particular represent major sources of interaction for adolescents. However, a number of studies suggest that teachers are not looked upon as major sources of support (Metropolitan Life Foundation, 1988; Porteus, 1979; University of Minnesota, 1989). In the Minnesota sample, fewer than 45% of adolescents believed that their teachers cared about them, with steady declines between grades 7 and 12. It seems unlikely that adolescents will be open to discussing their concerns, especially sensitive ones, with individuals they perceive as nonsupportive.

Other important issues for which the adolescent perspective would be valuable include how much they depend on and trust the information they receive from school and their willingness to be influenced by teachers. It would also be useful to explore adolescents' perceptions about contradictions between what they are taught in school about health promotion (e.g., proper nutrition) and the message promoted by the actual school environment (e.g., the presence of unhealthy foods in school cafeterias).

HEALTH CARE SETTINGS. Health care providers are generally viewed by adolescents as credible information sources about health; they are the preferred adult sources for health information (Levenson, Morrow, & Morgan, 1986). Adolescents' preferences for receiving health information from providers does not necessarily mean that they want such counseling to take place in a face-to-face encounter. Manning and Balson (1989) note that while adolescents report a preference for learning about AIDS from health care providers, they also prefer to learn about sensitive topic areas in anonymous group settings. This suggests a potentially important role for health care providers in school health education activities that take place in group settings such as classrooms.

Adolescents' preferences for certain types of provider characteristics are similar to the preferences of adults. In three studies using different methodologies, the qualities that adolescents identified as desirable included compassion and understanding, an ability to communicate with the adolescent, and a willingness to be straightforward and honest (Giblin & Poland, 1985; Hodgson, Feldman, Corber, & Quinn, 1986; Resnick et al. 1980). Other qualities frequently mentioned were competence, kindness, and warmth. Adolescents reported disliking providers who treat them in a patronizing manner and those who appear unfriendly or impersonal. Again, most adults would dislike these characteristics in their providers as well.

The issue of confidentiality of visits, particularly that parents not be informed, appears to be an especially important issue to adolescents (Giblin & Poland, 1985; Resnick et al., 1980), more so when sensitive issues such as sexuality are involved. Marks et al. (1983) found that adolescents were unwilling to seek health care in relation to sensitive topics if their parents knew about the visit. Although many states have provisions for confidential care of these sensitive problems, adolescents demonstrate significant misperceptions about whether and where they can receive confidential health care (ASHA, 1989).

Beyond the issue of individual providers, adolescents also appear to have preferences for certain types of health care systems. Characteristics of health care settings that adolescents view as desirable include clean and comfortable waiting areas, the availability of the same provider across visits, having enough time with the provider, and convenience. Other considerations include reasonable cost and the availability of specific services. Adolescents also prefer youth-oriented health care facilities to those oriented to adults or young children. Adolescents report disliking the childish appearance that is typical of many pediatric settings (Hodgson et al., 1986) and the presence of mothers and small children (Resnick et al., 1980). Adolescents appear to view providers in adolescent-oriented settings as being more attuned to them, while in traditional settings, providers are viewed as cold, aloof, and inconsiderate of adolescent patients (Resnick et al., 1980). Although studies specifically comparing adolescents' willingness to utilize different sites for health-related services have not been done, there appears to be fairly strong willingness to use school-based clinics among youth, especially when sensitive health problems such as depression are involved (Institute for Health Policy Studies, 1987; Riggs & Cheng, 1988). Studies from school-based health centers report that adolescents like the positive staff attitudes, helpfulness, and communication abilities; the services offered; confidentiality; and the convenience of school-based care (Millstein, 1988).

FAMILIES. Families clearly play a critical role in the development and maintenance of health-related behaviors, both through their influence as role models and through the provision of opportunities to promote health. Despite the popular view of adolescents as rejecting all parental values, parents are viewed by adolescents as important resources regarding health issues, both as sources of information (Levenson et al., 1986; Parcel et al., 1977) and as sources of support (Metropolitan Life Foundation, 1988). Parents are the preferred sources when concerns about the family exist (Feldman et al., 1986; Parcel et al., 1977). An exception occurs in sensitive topic areas, when peers (ASHA, 1989) or other adults may be favored (Windle, Miller-Tutzauer, Barnes, & Welte, 1991). An exception may be emotional issues, for which parents may be the preferred source of information (Feldman et al., 1986).

Differences in the configuration of family structure may influence how the family is viewed. For example, black families are often characterized by the presence of extended family members within the domicile of the nuclear family (Chapter 4). These extended family members, such as grandparents, may provide additional resources for the adolescent. Family structure differences may help explain why nonwhite adolescents recognize parents and other adults as major sources of help in substance use problems (Windle et al., 1991), while significantly fewer white adolescents do so.

PEERS. Peers are a major source of health information for adolescents, with their importance increasing as the mid-adolescent years begin (Metropolitan Life Foundation, 1988). Although adolescents view health care providers as giving the most reliable information, they often find it difficult to disclose sensitive information spontaneously to them (Marks et al., 1983). They therefore often look to their peers as the primary source of information about health issues (ASHA, 1989). Friends, along with family, appear to be preferred sources of support for emotional issues (Feldman et al., 1986), although some issues may be sensitive enough to not be discussed with anyone. An example is sexual abuse, which is frequently not discussed with anyone (University of Minnesota, 1989).

MEDIA. In addition to interpersonal sources for information about health, adolescents report receiving a great deal of their health information from the mass media, including television, radio, and magazines (Price et al., 1988). Brown and Fritz (1988) found that television was the most frequently mentioned source of information about AIDS for youth and also the source to which the most information was attributed. The potential for using mass media, particularly television and radio, for adolescent health promotion has been discussed (Chapter 5). Research on adolescents' views of health promotion via the mass media would be useful, since this may give us important information about how to best use these sources for positive results.

Adolescents' Views of the Future

Western society generally views adolescence as a period of preparation for the future. The vision of one's future is likely to serve as an important motivator for adolescents, who are expected to work toward that vision, often delaying gratification in the meantime. Adolescents' future visions include hopes for academic success, a successful marriage, a pleasant home, employment and financial security, good health, happiness, and peace (Gillies, 1989). And for many adolescents, these visions are accompanied by significant optimism. A recent survey found that most adolescents expected to attend college and to have a satisfying, enjoyable job in the future (AHEA, 1988). In the Minnesota sample, a majority of youth felt that life was full of interesting opportunities.

But these samples probably fail to reflect the expectations of many adolescents, particularly those who are being raised in poverty, with limited opportunities for future economic and personal success. A survey of over 500 adolescents (AHEA, 1988) found that financial issues were a major concern, especially for black and Hispanic youth, who were more likely to be concerned about being able to pay for an education, the economic status of the country, and being able to live as well as their parents do. Overall, 60% of their sample believed that their lives would be more difficult than those of their parents (AHEA, 1988). The effects of negative economic conditions are also likely to influence associated belief systems, such as beliefs about work and work ethics. Pautler and Lewko (1987) found that adolescents who lived in economically depressed areas showed more negative attitudes about work than adolescents in economically thriving areas.

Summary and Future Directions

Health: A Salient Issue for Adolescents?

Although some authors have suggested that health is a nonsalient issue to adolescents (Gochman, 1986), their well-defined concepts of health, the frequency with which they think about health, and their interest in the topic argue against such a conception. As this chapter has pointed out, judgments about the salience of health to adolescents depends in part on whether one asks the adolescent or an adult.

Perhaps the question is not so much whether health is salient to adolescents, but how health concerns rank relative to other concerns in adolescents' lives. Clearly, this depends on how broadly one chooses to define the concept. Using a broad enough definition of health, almost any concern could be considered a health concern. If we limit the definition of health concerns to reflect diagnosable conditions, injuries, and illnesses, then we are likely to see less salience among younger people, who have had less experience with these negative health effects. More immediate concerns are likely to predominate, concerns relating to appearance, interpersonal relations, independence, and future work opportunities (Eme et al., 1979). Still, the AHEA survey (1988) found that out of a list of 32 concerns health ranked third, with 24% of the sample expressing a great deal of concern about health.

The concerns that predominate in adolescents' lives may also vary over generations as a function of social and economic factors that members of different cohorts experience. In an analysis of adolescent concerns from 1935 to 1970, Porteus

(1979) notes that there has been a growing emphasis on personal qualities, moral issues, and home and interpersonal relationships. Health concerns have shown increasing importance. Porteus's analysis is consistent with Natapoff and Essoka's (1989) comparison of adolescents' concepts of health in 1976, 1985 and 1988, which revealed much greater emphasis on physical fitness and personal health behavior as elements of the health concept in later years. As the larger culture has shown increasing attention to health and fitness, the emphasis on this theme in young people's definitions of health has also increased.

The Need for Qualitative Studies of the Adolescent Experience

Most of the research conducted on adolescents' beliefs and perceptions has relied on survey methodology, principally because it is an efficient method of getting a great deal of information relatively quickly from a large number of subjects. Surveys using representative samples allow for great generalizability of their results, and with low rates of sampling error, fairly reliable conclusions can be reached. Of course, the nature of the questions asked often precludes any in-depth appreciation of the participants' belief patterns, and the conclusions, while reliable and valid, may be relatively trivial.

Alternatives to the large-scale survey for capturing the adolescent experience do exist, although they are more commonly used in disciplines such as anthropology and sociology. These disciplines, which encourage the study of phenomenological experience, have developed methods for qualitative analysis that deserve to take their rightful place as acceptable methods of scientific inquiry. Research on adolescents has focused primarily on the quantitative research traditions of psychology and medicine. The few exceptions to this have provided rich and detailed descriptions of the adolescent experience (Porteus, 1979; Savin-Williams, 1987). Research using a combination of qualitative and quantitative approaches would be especially useful at this point (Savin-Williams, 1987).

Whatever the approach used, when researchers elicit information about adolescents' concerns, hopes, or fears, the situational context will significantly affect the responses. One such situational context has to do with the varying salience of particular issues at particular times. Asking adolescents about sources of stress during examination time, for example, is likely to generate far more responses targeting school as a source of stress (Porteus, 1979). Adolescents' concerns also show daily rhythms and patterns, as demonstrated by the innovative "beeper studies" of Csikszentmihaly and Larson (1984). The situational context is also reflected by the specific cohort in which the adolescent lives, along with its attendant fads and fashions. For example, issues regarding the salience of personal responsibility over health, which are more common among older adolescents, need to be examined within the context of real changes in viewpoints about preventive health that have taken place in our society.

An additional set of contextual variables includes those pertaining to the adolescent's social, cultural, and economic situations. Adolescents living in poverty are more likely to have health concerns that reflect their environmental circumstances, including concerns about jobs, crime, and safety. Adolescents from racial and ethnic minority groups are more likely to have concerns about discrimination than white adolescents (Sobal et al., 1988). The role of these contextual variables in adolescents' interpretations of the world requires far more investigation.

Using Adolescents' Perspectives to Inform Health Promotion Efforts

Although the knowledge base on adolescents' perspectives is clearly limited, it does provide some information that can be useful in thinking about health promotion efforts in this age group. Perhaps most obvious is the need to consider the developmental level of the adolescent when developing health promotion programs. The adolescent period is a decade of substantial growth physically, psychologically, and socially. Thus, while sexual behavior is a topic of interest for most adolescents, salient issues for 16-year-olds are unlikely to focus on reproductive physiology or the mechanics of sexual activity, issues that are prevalent in younger adolescents. Questions about sexual attraction and how to negotiate sexual relationships are far more pressing, suggesting that interventions tap into these areas for educating youth about sexuality and promoting their development at this stage. Furthermore, differences in the timing of physical maturation for males and females, which are accompanied by qualitatively different interests and concerns suggest that some health promotion efforts should be gender-segregated to ensure that they are developmentally appropriate.

This review also suggests that adults may have certain misperceptions about adolescents that may interfere with health promotion efforts. Some adolescent health concerns, such as oral health, seem to be virtually ignored by health educators. This represents a missed opportunity to educate youth about a topic of interest to them that has the potential to teach about more generic health issues as well (Chapter 11). To the degree that adults fail to understand adolescents' desires and motivations, they also fail to recognize potentially important means of providing adolescents with alternatives to health-damaging behaviors (Chapter 12). This is not to suggest that adolescents' views should be considered the definitive gold standard from which we ought to develop and implement health promotion programs. Rather, it suggests that programs developed without understanding the target population may be less likely to succeed, particularly when the goals and objectives of the programs and those of the recipients clash.

In considering the goals of health promotion, it is also useful to distinguish between short-term and long-term goals. Health promotion efforts often concentrate on the longer-term goals of adults (e.g., preventing substance use) while failing to consider the shorter-term goals of the adolescent (e.g., becoming one of the group). The degree to which we will be successful in promoting adolescent health is probably a function of how well we can *utilize adolescents' short-term goals* to reach adults' long-term goals. This is consistent with the views of numerous authors who suggest that in adolescence, health promotion efforts should focus on the short-term effects of health behaviors. It also echoes the view of many who believe that we should be shifting our long-term goals from altering behaviors such as substance use to intervening with the underlying generic causes of these health-damaging behaviors, such as inadequate life skills or personal support (Hamburg, 1990; Price, Cioci, Penner, & Trautlein, 1990).

With increasing recognition of the importance of evaluating the quality of *implementation* of interventions (Chapter 15), we also need to learn more about the translation of information from adults to adolescents. As mentioned earlier, programs assume that the message they intend to convey is the message that the adolescent receives. Yet few programs assess whether that is indeed the case. Adolescents' views about various information sources can also be used to improve program implementation by capitalizing on the strengths of particular sources and minimizing their limitations. For example, in educational settings, the use of health professionals to provide information about sensitive, health-related topics may be an appropriate adjunct to teachers. Teachers, who have more time to work with adolescents, may be more productively used to teach more generic life skills. Each of the sources described in this chapter has the potential to play an important role in adolescent health promotion. However, using these sources to their best advantage will require that we know more about adolescents' perspectives.

Attending to adolescents' viewpoints does more, however, than simply provide us with interesting data or information for use in improving interventions. More importantly, it supports the underlying philosophy that the beliefs and attitudes of youth are inherently important and worthy of consideration. Such a philosophy suggests that we not only ask but also listen to adolescents, include them in discussions relevant to their lives, and allow them to participate in decision-making forums. In doing so, we unequivocally demonstrate to adolescents that they are valuable participants in their social environment. These messages may be among the most crucial ones we communicate to youth in order to promote their healthy development.

References

Adler, N. E., Millstein, S. G., Irwin, C. E., Jr., & Kegeles, S. M. (1986, March). *Risk factors and health behaviors in adolescents.* Paper presented to the Annual Meeting of the Society for Behavioral Medicine, San Francisco.

Alexander, C. S. (1989). Gender differences in adolescent health concerns and self-assessed health. *Journal of Early Adolescence, 9,* 467–479.

Altman, D. G., & Revenson, T. A. (1985). Children's understanding of health and illness concepts: A preventive health perspective. *Journal of Primary Prevention, 6,* 53–67.

American Cancer Society (1979). *A study of health-related awareness and concerns among 4th, 5th and 6th graders* (C.R.S. No. 5649). New York: American Cancer Society.

American Home Economics Association (1988). *Survey of American Teens.* Washington, DC: Guideline Research Corporation.

American School Health Association, Association for the Advancement of Health Education, and Society for Publication Health Education, Inc. (1989). *The national adolescent student health survey: A report on the health of America's youth.* Oakland, CA: Third Party Publishing Co.

Armacost, R. L. (1989). Perceptions of stressors by high school students. *Journal of Adolescent Research, 4,* 443–461.

Becker, M. H., & Maiman, L. A. (1983). Models of health-related behavior. In D. Mechanic (Ed.), *Handbook of health, health care and the health professions* (pp. 539–568). New York: Free Press.

Benedict, V., Lundeen, K. W., & Morr, B. D. (1981). Self-assessment by adolescents of their health status and perceived health needs. *Health Values: Achieving High Level Wellness, 5,* 239–245.

Bloom-Feshbach, S., Bloom-Feshbach, J., & Heller, K. A. (1982). Work, family, and children's perceptions of the world. In S. B. Kamerman & C. D. Hayes (Eds.), *Families that work: Children in a changing world* (pp. 268–307). Washington, DC: National Academy Press.

Brown, L. K., & Fritz, G. K. (1988). Children's knowledge and attitudes about AIDS. *Journal of the American Academy of Child and Adolescent Psychiatry, 27,* 504–508.

Brunswick, A. F. (1969). Health needs of adolescence: How the adolescent sees them. *American Journal of Public Health, 59,* 1730–1745.

Brunswick, A. F., & Josephson, E. (1972). Adolescent health in Harlem. *American Journal of Public Health, 62* (Suppl), 7–62.

Burbach, D. J., & Peterson, L. (1986). Children's concepts of physical illness: A review and critique of the cognitive-developmental literature. *Health Psychology, 5,* 307–325.

Burke, R. J., & Weir, T. (1978). Sex differences in adolescent life stress, social support, and well-being. *Journal of Psychology, 98,* 277–288.

Byler, R. V., Lewis, G. M., & Totman, R. J. (1969). *Teach us what we want to know.* New York: Mental Health Materials Center.

Campbell, J. D. (1975). Illness is a point of view: The development of children's concepts of illness. *Child Development, 46,* 92–100.

Centers for Disease Control (1988). HIV-related beliefs, knowledge and behaviors among high school students. *Morbidity and Mortality Weekly Reports, 37,* 717–721.

Cleary, P. D. (1987). Why people take precautions against health risks. In N. D. Weinstein (Ed.), *Taking care: Understanding and encouraging self-protective behavior* (pp. 119–149). New York: Cambridge University Press.

Cohn, L., Macfarlane, S., & Yanez, C. (1991). *Unrealistic optimism in children and adolescents.* Paper presented at the Annual Meeting of the American Psychological Association. San Francisco.

Csikszentmihaly, M., & Larson, R. (1984) *Being adolescent.* New York: Basic Books.

DiClemente, R., Boyer, C., & Morales, E. (1988). Minorities and AIDS: Knowledge, attitudes and misconceptions among black and Latino adolescents. *American Journal of Public Health, 78,* 55–57.

DiClemente, R. J., Zorn, J., & Temoshok, L. (1986) Adolescents and AIDS: A survey of knowledge, attitudes and beliefs about AIDS in San Francisco. *American Journal of Public Health 76,* 1443–1445.

DiNicola, D. D., & DiMatteo, M. R. (1984). Practitioners, patients, and compliance with medical regimens: A social psychological perspective. In A. Baum, S. E. Taylor, & J. E. Singer (Eds.), *Handbook of Psychology and health. Volume IV: Social psychological aspects of health* (pp. 55–84). Hillsdale, NJ: Lawrence Erlbaum Associates.

Eisen, M., Zellman, G. L., & McAlister, A. L. (1985). A health belief model approach to adolescents' fertility control: Some pilot program findings. *Health Education Quarterly, 12,* 185–210.

Eiser, C., Patterson, D., & Eiser, J. R. (1983). Children's knowledge of health and illness: Implications for health education. *Child Care, Health and Development, 9,* 285–292.

Eme, R., Maisiak, R., & Goodale, W. (1979). Seriousness of adolescent problems. *Adolescence, 14,* 93–99.

Feldman, W., Hodgson, C., Corber, S., & Quinn, A. (1986). Health concerns and health-related behaviors of adolescents. *Canadian Medical Association Journal, 134,* 489–495.

Furby, L., & Beyth-Marom, R. (1990). *Risk taking in adolescence: A decision-making perspective.* Washington, DC: Carnegie Council on Adolescent Development.

Giblin, P., & Poland, M. (1985). Health needs of high school students in Detroit. *Journal of School Health, 55,* 407–410.

Gillies, P. (1989). A longitudinal study of the hopes and worries of adolescents. *Journal of Adolescence, 12,* 69–81.

Gochman, D. S. (1985). Family determinants of children's concepts of health and illness. In D. C. Turk & R. D. Kerns (Eds.), *Health, illness and families* (pp. 23–50). New York: Wiley.

Gochman, D. S. (1986). *Youngsters' health cognitions: Cross-sectional and longitudinal analyses.* Louisville, KY: Health Behavior Systems.

Gochman, D. S., & Saucier, J. (1982). Perceived vulnerability in children and adolescents. *Health Education Quarterly, 9,* 46–59.

Greene, A. L. (1988). Early adolescents' perceptions of stress. *Journal of Early Adolescence, 8,* 391–403.

Hamburg, B. A. (1990). *Life skills training: Preventive interventions for young adolescents.* Washington, DC: Carnegie Council on Adolescent Development.

Hodgson, C., Feldman, W., Corber, S., & Quinn, A. (1986). Adolescent health needs. II: Utilization of health care by adolescents. *Adolescence, 21,* 383–390.

Institute for Health Policy Studies, Center for Reproductive Health Policy, University of California, San Francisco. (1987). *A proposal to foster school-based comprehensive health services for secondary schools in the San Francisco Bay area.* New York: Carnegie Corporation of New York.

Kirscht, J. P. (1983). Preventive health behavior: A review of research and issues. *Health Psychology, 2,* 277–301.

Korbin, J. E., & Kahorik, P. (1985). Childhood, health, and illness: Beliefs and behaviors of urban American schoolchildren. *Medical Anthropology,* Fall, 337–353.

Levenson, P. M., Morrow, J. R. & Pfefferbaum, B. J. (1984). Attitudes toward health and illness: A comparison of adolescent, physician, teacher and school nurse views. *Journal of Adolescent Health Care, 5,* 254–260.

Levenson, P. M., Morrow, J. R., Gregory, E. K., & Pfefferbaum, B.J. (1984). A comparison of views of school nurses, teachers, and middle-school students regarding health information interests and concerns. *Public Health Nursing, 1,* 141–151.

Levenson, P. M., Morrow, J. R., Johnson, S. A., & Pfefferbaum, B. J. (1983). Assessing adolescent health needs: A factor analytic approach. *Patient Education and Counseling, 5,* 23–29.

Levenson, P. M., Morrow, J. R., & Morgan, W. C. (1986). Health information sources and preferences as perceived by adolescents, pediatricians, teachers and school nurses. *Journal of Early Adolescence, 6,* 183–195.

Levenson, P. M., Pfefferbaum, B., & Morrow, J. R. (1987). Disparities in adolescent–physician views of teen health information concerns. *Journal of Adolescent Health Care, 8,* 171–176.

Manning, D. T., & Balson, P. M. (1989). Teenagers' beliefs about AIDS education and physicians' perceptions about them. *Journal of Family Practice, 29,* 173–177.

Marks, A., Malizio, J., Hoch, J., Brody, R., & Fisher, M. (1983). Assessment of health needs and willingness to utilize health care resources of adolescents in a suburban population. *Journal of Pediatrics, 102,* 456–460.

Mechanic, D. (1983). Adolescent health and illness behavior: Review of the literature and a new hypothesis for the study of stress. *Journal of Human Stress, 9,* 4–13.

Melton, G. B. (1988). Adolescents and prevention of AIDS. *American Psychologist, 19,* 403–408.

Metropolitan Life Foundation (1988). *Health: You've got to be taught. An evaluation of comprehensive health education in American public schools.* Study No. 874024. New York: Louis Harris and Associates.

Michielutte, R., & Diseker, R. A. (1982). Children's perceptions of cancer in comparison to other chronic illnesses. *Journal of Chronic Diseases, 35,* 843–852.

Millstein, S. G. (1988). *The potential of school-linked centers to promote adolescent health and development.* Washington, DC: Carnegie Council on Adolescent Development.

Millstein, S. G. (in press). Perceptual, attributional and affective processes in perceptions of vulnerability through the life span. *Current issues and new directions in risk taking research and intervention,* Lubbock, TX: Texas Tech University Press.

Millstein, S. G., Adler, N. E., & Irwin, C. E. (1981). Conceptions of illness in young adolescents. *Pediatrics, 68,* 834–839.

Millstein, S. G., & Irwin, C. E., Jr. (1985). Adolescents' assessments of behavioral risk: Sex differences and maturation effects. *Pediatric Research, 19,* 112A.

Millstein, S. G., & Irwin, C. E. (1986). *Health protective and health risk behaviors in adolescents.* Unpublished manuscript. San Francisco: University of California at San Francisco.

Millstein, S. G., & Irwin, C. E. (1987). Concepts of health and illness: Different constructs or variations on a theme? *Health Psychology, 6,* 515–524.

Millstein, S. G., Irwin, C. E., Adler, N. E., Cohn, L. D., Kegeles, S. M., & Dolcini, M. M. (1992). Health risk behaviors and health concerns among young adolescents. *Pediatrics, 89,* 422–428.

Millstein, S. G., & Litt, I. (1990). Adolescent health and health behaviors. In S. S. Feldman and G. Elliott (Eds.), *At the threshold: The developing adolescent* (pp. 431–456). Cambridge, MA: Harvard University Press.

Morrison, D. M. (1985). Adolescent contraceptive behavior: A review. *Psychological Bulletin, 98,* 538–568.

Natapoff, J. N. (1978). Children's views of health: A developmental study. *American Journal of Public Health, 68,* 995–1000.

Natapoff, J. N., & Essoka, G. C. (1989). Handicapped and able-bodied children's ideas of health. *Journal of School Health, 59,* 436–440.

National Center for Health Statistics, U.S. Department of Health, Education, and Welfare, Public Health Service (1977). *The association of health attitudes and perceptions of youths 12–17 years of age with those of their parents: United States, 1966–1970.* DHEW Publication No. (HRA) 77-1643. Rockville, MD: Health Resources Administration.

Parcel, G. S., Nader, P. R., & Meyer, M. P. (1977). Adolescent health concerns, problems and patterns of utilization in a triethnic urban population. *Pediatrics, 60,* 157–164.

Pautler, K. J., & Lewko, J. H. (1987). Children's and adolescent's views of the work world in times of economic uncertainty. In J. H. Lewko (Ed.), *How children and adolescents view the world of work* (pp. 21–31). New Directions for Child Development, No. 35. San Francisco: Jossey-Bass.

Perry, C. L., & Jessor, R. (1985). The concept of health promotion and the prevention of adolescent drug abuse. *Health Education Quarterly, 12,* 169–184.

Porteus, M. A. (1979). A survey of the problems of normal 15-year-olds. *Journal of Adolescence, 2,* 307–323.

Price, R. H., Cioci, M., Penner, W., & Trautlein, B. (1990). *School and community support programs that enhance adolescent health and education.* Washington, DC: Carnegie Council on Adolescent Development.

Price, J. H., Desmond, S. M., Wallace, M., Smith, D., & Stewart, P. M. (1988). Differences in black and white adolescents' perceptions about cancer. *Journal of School Health, 58,* 66–70.

Radius, S. M., Dillman, T. E., Becker, M. H., Rosenstock, I. M., & Horvath, W. J. (1980). Adolescent perspectives on health and illness. *Adolescence, 15,* 375–384.

Resnick, M., Blum, R. W., & Hedin, D. (1980). The appropriateness of health services for adolescents. *Journal of Adolescent Health Care, 1,* 137–141.

Riggs, S., & Cheng, T. (1988). Adolescents' willingness to use a school-based clinic in view of expressed health concerns. *Journal of Adolescent Health Care, 9,* 208–213.

Ryan, S., Millstein, S. G., & Irwin, C. E., Jr. (1988). Pubertal concerns in young adolescents. *Journal of Adolescent Health Care, 9,* 267.

Savin-Williams, R. C. (1987). *Adolescence: An ethological perspective.* New York: Springer-Verlag.

Siddique, C. M., & D'Arcy, C. D. (1984). Adolescence, stress, and psychological well-being. *Journal of Youth and Adolescence, 13,* 459–473.

Sobal, J., Klein, H., Graham, D., & Black, J. (1988). Health concerns of high school students and teachers' beliefs about student health concerns. *Pediatrics, 81,* 218–223.

Sternlieb, J. J., & Munan, L. (1972). A survey of health problems, practices, and needs of youth. *Pediatrics, 49,* 177–186.

Strunin, L., & Hingson, R. (1987). Acquired immunodeficiency syndrome and adolescents' knowledge, beliefs, attitudes and behaviors. *Pediatrics, 79,* 825–828.

University of Minnesota (1989). *The state of adolescent health in Minnesota.* Minneapolis: University of Minnesota Press.

Violato, C., & Holden, W. B. (1988). A confirmatory factor analysis of a four-factor model of adolescent concerns. *Journal of Youth and Adolescence, 17,* 101–113.

Wagner, B. M., & Compas, B. E. (1990). Gender, instrumentality and expressivity: Moderators of adjustment to stress during adolescence. *American Journal of Community Psychology, 18,* 383–406.

Wallston, B. S., & Wallston, K. A. (1984). Social psychological models of health behavior: An examination and integration. In A. Baum, S. E. Taylor, & J. E. Singer (Eds.), *Handbook of psychology and health. Volume 4: Social psychological aspects of health* (pp. 23–53). Hillsdale, NJ: Erlbaum.

Weidman, H. H. (1988). A transcultural perspective on health behavior. In D. Gochman (Ed.), *Health behavior: Emerging research perspectives* (pp. 261–280). New York: Plenum Press.

Windle, M., Miller-Tutzauer, C., Barnes, G. M., & Welte (1991). Adolescent perceptions of help-seeking resources for substance abuse. *Child Development, 62,* 179–189.

7

Health-Enhancing
and Health-Compromising Lifestyles

Delbert S. Elliott

Health has typically been defined as the absence of disease. By this definition of health, the adolescent population in the United States is relatively healthy; adolescence could even be viewed as the peak period of health during the life span for persons living in developed countries. Why then is there a concern over adolescent health?

As the editors note in Chapter 1, our conceptualization of disease, illness, and health, and our understanding of the etiology and epidemiology of mortality and morbidity, have changed dramatically during the past decade. In developed countries, we now face a serious health crisis involving new sources of mortality and morbidity (O'Neill, 1983; World Health Organization [WHO], 1981). Of particular relevance to adolescents are diseases of lifestyle, the health consequences resulting from poverty and unemployment, and premature deaths resulting from risky behavior and accidents generally (Noack, 1987, p. 5). Indeed, the vast majority of all adolescent deaths and a substantial proportion of all adolescent morbidity can be attributed to one or more of these causes (Chapter 1). The prevalence rates for accidents, homicide, and suicide, the three major causes of death among adolescents, have been increasing over the past two decades (National Center for Health Statistics, 1980). Since risky behavior is a major contributing factor to the accident rate among adolescents and appears to be a characteristic of a particular lifestyle, it would appear that the major sources of adolescent mortality and morbidity in the United States can be linked to two general factors: (1) certain personal lifestyles and (2) social environments that involve high health risks.

This chapter focuses on adolescent lifestyles and the social contexts in which they emerge and are maintained. More specifically, our interest is in the health-promoting or health-compromising behaviors that are characteristic of particular lifestyles and those personality attributes and features of social environments that contribute to the emergence and maintenance of these lifestyles or increase the risks of mortality and morbidity directly. The general questions being addressed are how adolescents organize their lives and pattern their behavior in ways that put them at higher or lower risk for serious health problems, and how these patterns of behavior develop and persist.

119

We begin with a discussion of several theoretical issues to provide a clear conceptualization of *lifestyle*. The evidence for distinct lifestyles and the set or cluster of behaviors that comprise them are then reviewed, and the social environments that foster these lifestyles are described. We then turn to the developmental progression of health-compromising and health-enhancing lifestyles and an explanation of why these behaviors cluster into a coherent lifestyle. Finally, the implications of a lifestyle perspective for adolescent health promotion and intervention programs are discussed.

The Conceptualization of Lifestyle: Theoretical Issues

Sobel (1981, p. 2), in his classic work *Lifestyle and Social Structure,* notes that "there is almost no agreement either empirically or conceptually as to what constitutes a lifestyle." The literature is characterized by ambiguity in the way social scientists have defined and measured lifestyle. More specifically, there is a failure to separate determinants from definitional criteria, the frequent confounding of lifestyle and social class, an emphasis on particular components of lifestyle to the exclusion of others, and the frequent use of circumvention in the measurement of lifestyle. "This explains why researchers typically define lifestyle as a mode of living, a seemingly innocuous tautology, and then proceed directly to an eclectic and/or ad hoc set of measures" (Sobel, 1981, p. 16).

This criticism applies directly to the conceptualization and measurement of lifestyle in the adolescent health research literature to date. For example, many researchers who use the concept never define it (Newcomb & Bentler, 1988; Rajala, Honkala, Rimpela, & Lammi, 1980), and those who do define it very generally as a "way of life," "day-to-day habits and behavior patterns," the "ways people cope" with life conditions, or a "mode of living" (e.g., Breslow, 1990; Chassin, Presson, & Sherman, 1987; Henderson, Hall, & Lipton, 1979; Kulbok, Earls, & Montgomery, 1988), with little attention to explicating its essential properties as a guide to measurement and as a means of distinguishing lifestyle from its causes and effects. There is some agreement in both the health and criminology literatures that the definition and measurement of lifestyle should be restricted to observable behaviors (e.g., Jessor, 1987; Kulbok et al., 1988; Sampson & Lauritsen, 1990), but beyond this, there is little discussion of the essential properties of a lifestyle. As a means of bringing some consensus to the research in this area, a general definition of lifestyle and its essential properties is proposed, building upon and extending the earlier work of Sobel.

Sobel (1981, p. 28) notes that there is general agreement among sociologists that lifestyle refers to "a distinctive, hence recognizable, mode of living." It follows, he argues, that lifestyle is essentially behavioral. Further, these behaviors are recognizable, that is, observable. Attitudes, values, and motivations are thus excluded from this conceptual domain. They may be correlates of lifestyles or even causes or consequences of lifestyles, but they are not in themselves properties of a lifestyle.

Sobel further restricts the domain of content by adding the condition of expressiveness. Lifestyle refers to observable *expressive* behaviors, that is, behaviors over which the individual has considerable discretion or choice. This criterion implies that the individual has some choice between alternative behaviors that serve the same function or need, and it is the pattern of these individual voluntary choices that characterizes the lifestyle. For Sobel, then, lifestyle refers to observable, expressive behaviors that establish a distinctive mode of living.

To this set of criteria I would add several others. First, minimum involvement in a particular type of behavior over a minimum time period is essential to its being considered part of a lifestyle. If an individual uses marijuana twice over the course of a week and then stops using it, is it reasonable to include the use of this drug as a behavior in his or her lifestyle? I think not. Conceptually, a lifestyle denotes some continuity of involvement in an observable, expressive behavior, as implied in a "mode of living" or "day-to-day habits and patterns of behavior." It identifies a routine or established way of dealing with personal needs and the demands and expectations of others in one's environment, an established *pattern* of involvement in a particular type of behavior. Exploratory involvement with tobacco, alcohol, or illicit drugs (i.e., on one or two occasions) should not be considered evidence of a health-compromising lifestyle any more than sporadic use of physical exercise, an occasional well-balanced meal, or a few good nights' rest every month should be considered evidence of a health-enhancing lifestyle. This is not a trivial issue, as much of the research attempting to identify clusters of health-enhancing or health-compromising behavior has employed simple prevalence measures of behavior, that is, one or more reported acts of a given type. Further, for many forms of problem behavior, a large proportion of those initiating the behavior never become involved beyond an exploratory level. While there are as yet no clear, generally accepted rules for establishing what the minimum frequency and duration should be for classifying a behavior as *patterned* behavior, I propose that we not use simple prevalence measures to define lifestyles.

A further property of lifestyle is that it denotes combinations of behavior or behavioral domains that occur consistently. Conceptually, viewing a lifestyle as a way of life denotes a broad range of behaviors that are organized into a coherent way of responding to different life situations and different persons and environments. This *consistency* criterion, which requires that multiple types of behavior covary in a coherent pattern, has been explicitly or implicitly employed by several researchers (Chassin et al., 1987; Jessor, 1987).[1] The consistency criterion also implies that these diverse behaviors occur jointly or together in time (i.e., that the periods of active involvement in these behaviors overlap). Accordingly, persons who smoked two packs of cigarettes a day over several years would not, by virtue of their use of tobacco alone, be classified as having a health-compromising lifestyle. This would be patterned expressive behavior that might contribute to a lifestyle, but it would not by itself constitute a lifestyle. Further, the use of "ever" or lifetime prevalence measures to define a lifestyle would be inappropriate, since the joint occurrence of multiple, patterned behaviors at a particular time is not guaranteed with such measures.

Finally, the conceptualization of lifestyle implies that this set of patterned behaviors occurs with some consistency in individuals. Sobel (1981, p. 28) notes that while lifestyle might be seen as a property of groups or even cultures, it typically has been used by researchers as a property of individuals.

In summary, a lifestyle has been defined as a distinctive mode of living that is defined by a set of expressive, patterned behaviors of individuals occurring with some consistency over a period of time. The lifestyle construct is not intended to capture the totality of a person's behavior, but rather to reflect that complex subset of diverse behaviors that is relatively stable and predictable. This conceptualization of lifestyle also bears some similarity to the notion of a behavioral *syndrome*, which has been proposed by Jessor and his colleagues to describe the clustering of health-compromising (or problem) behaviors (Donovan & Jessor, 1985; Jessor, 1987; Jessor & Jessor, 1977). Both concepts reflect the consistency in covariation among multiple types of patterned behavior, but the lifestyle concept does not imply a common etiology for all of the individual types of behavior included in the lifestyle, whereas this *is* implied by the syndrome concept. Some commonality in causes is certainly expected, but it is not required by definition.

Our interest in this chapter is to identify lifestyles that incorporate specific types of patterned behavior that are either health-enhancing or health-compromising. In some cases there may be clear and immediate health consequences of lifestyle behaviors, while in others the effects may be indirect or delayed. This distinction may be important for health promotion programs, as it is more difficult to motivate persons to terminate health-compromising behaviors or initiate health-enhancing behaviors when the observable health consequences are not likely to appear for 20 to 30 years.

Given our conceptualization, a particular lifestyle may include *both* health-compromising and health-enhancing behaviors. Such an outcome might suggest that health considerations were not the primary factor (or perhaps not even a relevant factor) in the individual's selection of behaviors (Chassin et al., 1987). This possibility again raises the question of what ties the behaviors in a lifestyle together, what constitutes the common link for diverse, patterned, health-enhancing or health-compromising behaviors. We will return to this issue after we have considered the empirical evidence for health-enhancing and health-compromising lifestyles.

Health-Enhancing Lifestyles

In the search for empirical evidence of healthy lifestyles, there is a very uneven body of research. Relatively few general population studies focus on a range of health-promoting behaviors in adolescents. The few general population studies that have considered the clustering of multiple positive behaviors focus primarily upon seat belt use while driving, driving within the posted speed limits, eating nutritious foods, limiting the caloric fat content in food, sleep habits, dental hygiene habits, physical exercise, preventive physical exams, and seeking medical treatment when appropriate.

Some research suggests a clustering of behaviors that reflect preventive health care. Kulbok et al. (1988), using multidimensional scaling and factor analysis with a general set of health-related behaviors (e.g., physical exams, dental exams, brushing teeth, regularity of meals, adequate sleep, and seat belt use), substance use (tobacco, alcohol, and illicit drugs), and a variety of social activities (e.g., reading, hobbies, and chores), found that taking preventive health exams was correlated with seat belt use, good grades, brushing teeth, and reading and hobby activities. Covariation among preventive health measures has also been reported by Haefner, Kegeles, Kirscht, and Rosenstock (1967).

The most promising evidence of a health-promoting lifestyle comes from Donovan, Jessor, and Costa (1990), who found significant correlations among five of six measures in a general index of health (exercise, sleep, safety belt use, healthy diet, healthy food preferences, dental care) for a middle-school sample and among three of the six measures in a high school sample. Further, a confirmatory factor analysis indicated that a single underlying factor could account for the observed correlations among these health-promoting behaviors, and this single underlying factor was replicated for subsamples of males, females, Anglos, Hispanics, and blacks at each school level.

Some caution is necessary in interpreting these findings. The form of this analysis does not demonstrate that a single-factor model is the only or best model accounting for this set of correlations; the factor loadings are quite low for specific behaviors; and the zero-order correlations for half of the relationships between measures were weak (<.15) or nonsignificant. Clearly, there is some evidence for a clustering of these health-promoting behaviors in this study, but it is weak, particularly in the high school sample.

There is also some evidence that involvement in certain health-compromising behaviors (e.g., drug, tobacco, and alcohol use) involves a low likelihood of involvement in particular health-promoting behaviors. These behaviors include seat belt use (Kulbok et al., 1988; Mechanic, 1979), preventive exams or screenings (Kulbok et al., 1988; Mechanic, 1979) and perhaps regular teeth brushing (Kulbok et al., 1988; Nutbeam, Aar, & Calford, 1989). However, conflicting results have also been reported (Balding & Macgregor, 1987; Kulbok et al., 1988; Robinson et al., 1987; Sievers, Koskelalnen, & Leppo, 1974) and remain to be resolved.

Overall, studies on health-promoting behaviors among adolescents present a very confusing and sometimes contradictory set of findings. For example, regular exercise was associated with other health-enhancing behaviors in some studies (Nutbeam et al., Sievers et al., 1974) but not in others (Rajala et al., 1980; Rimpela, Eskola, & Paronen, 1978; Robinson et al., 1987) and with some health-promoting behaviors (seat belt use) but not others (preventive health behavior) in the study reported by Mechanic (1979). Other behaviors that make sense as part of a health-enhancing lifestyle fail to show expected relationships to other health-promoting behaviors. Adequate sleep, for example, was not related to preventive behaviors, exercise, or eating regular meals; nor was it negatively related to substance use (Hays, Stacy, & DiMatteo, 1984; Kulbok et al., 1988). Finally, nearly all of the general population studies reporting on relationships among positive health behaviors involve very weak relationships (Hays et al., 1984; Mechanic, 1979; Robinson et al., 1987).

In part, the contradictions and confusion stem from analyses involving different measures of particular behaviors, different sets of health-promoting and health-compromising behaviors (mostly limited to alcohol and tobacco use), different samples, and different methods for determining relationships. Donovan et al. (1990) are correct in noting that there are some potentially serious methodological problems with this body of research, particularly with the factor analyses reported. Still, there is considerable disagreement among researchers over whether there is or is not a coherent health-promoting lifestyle, and at present, the research base for making this judgment is simply inadequate.

Health-Compromising Lifestyles

The primary body of research on health-compromising lifestyles is found in the literature on adolescent problem behavior and deviance. Much of this work has focused on covariation between different forms of behavior within a single conceptual domain, such as different types of substance use (tobacco, alcohol, and illicit substances) or delinquent behaviors (violence, theft, public disorder, and vandalism).

The literature reviewed here is not exhaustive. It focuses on studies using probability samples from the general population rather than clinical or institutional samples, since findings from the latter cannot be generalized with any known degree of accuracy. In addition, it relies primarily on studies using similar definitions of problem behaviors; most involve self-reported measures of behavior, whose reliability and validity are generally acceptable (Hindelang, Hirschi, & Weis, 1981; Huizinga & Elliott, 1986).

The Cluster of Health-Compromising Lifestyle Behaviors

There is considerable empirical evidence that problem behaviors do indeed cluster in a way consistent with our definition of a lifestyle—that is, multiple forms of patterned, expressive problem behaviors that covary systematically. The core behaviors in this cluster involve two general domains: substance use/abuse and delinquent behavior (Donovan & Jessor, 1985; Elliott, Huizinga, & Menard, 1989; Osgood, 1991), but the general cluster also includes several other types of problem behavior. Because no single study to date has considered an extensive set of problem behavior domains, the full breadth of this health-compromising lifestyle may not be known, and much of what is known depends on inferences from observed covariation between overlapping pairs of behaviors considered in different studies.

The Core Behavioral Domains:
Substance Use/Abuse and Delinquent Behavior

Virtually all general population studies that have considered the relationship between minor forms of delinquency and the use of tobacco, alcohol, marijuana, and other illicit drugs have found a positive correlation between these behaviors (Dryfoos, 1990; Fagan, Cheng, & Weis, 1990; Grube & Morgan, 1989; Jessor & Jessor, 1977; Johnston, O'Malley, & Eveland, 1978; White, Labourie, & Bates, 1985). There is also evidence that high use levels or problem use of licit and illicit drugs covaries with involvement in serious forms of delinquency generally (Elliott et al., 1989; Fagan et al., 1990), and more specifically with serious violent offenses against persons (Ensminger, 1989; Johnston et al., 1978; Kandel, Simcha-Fagan, & Davies, 1986). Violent behavior is also clearly associated with drug smuggling and selling (Elliott et al., 1989; Johnson, Wish, Schmeidler, & Huizinga, 1986; White, 1990).

In sum, there is great consistency in studies of general populations that patterned forms of behavior from these two behavioral domains covary, that is, those involved in one of these types of behavior are also likely to be involved in the other. The pattern of positive correlations holds across the full range of behaviors in each domain. It thus appears that delinquency and drug use may be part of a more general deviant lifestyle, a lifestyle that includes behaviors that clearly put youth at risk for serious health problems.

Other Behaviors in the Deviant Lifestyle

It is well established that adolescents involved in delinquency and substance use are more likely to be sexually active (Dryfoos, 1990; Donovan & Jessor, 1985; Elliott & Morse, 1989; Mott & Haurin, 1988; Zabin, Hardy, Smith, & Hirsch, 1986). There is also limited evidence that contraceptive use may fit into this cluster, although studies reporting covariation between contraceptive use and delinquency or drug use have relied upon nonrepresentative samples (Kulbok et al., 1988; Zabin, 1984).

Research has also demonstrated that adolescents who use tobacco, become drunk, or use illicit drugs are less likely to use seat belts (Jonah, 1986; Lawson, Arora, & Jonah, 1982; Maron et al., 1986). Problem use of alcohol and/or use of illicit drugs is associated with other dangerous driving practices, as measured by traffic citations and accidents (Chapter 14). The relationship between risky driving behavior and delinquent or sexual behavior is less well studied, although Elliott (1987) has linked driving while under the influence (DUI) and the likelihood of an alcohol- or drug-related driving accident to involvement in serious delinquent behavior; and Jessor (1987) has reported that males who were involved in risky driving had higher frequencies of sexual intercourse.

While a number of researchers (DiFranza, Winters, Goldberg, Cirillo, & Biliouris, 1986; Jonah, 1986) claim that the high vehicle accident rate among adolescents is primarily a result of high rates of risky driving behavior (e.g., driving too fast and too close to vehicles in front, using gaps that are too narrow, driving without seat belts, and driving while impaired by alcohol or drugs), these risk-taking driving behaviors have *not* been linked directly to each other or to delinquency, substance use, and precocious sexual behavior. For example, speeding is not related to seat belt use (Jonah, 1986); nor are some other forms of risky driving related to seat belt use (Mechanic, 1979). Still, the available evidence suggests that DUI, nonuse of seat belts, and a higher risk for accidents are part of a general deviant behavior lifestyle.

School failure, truancy, and dropping out are also implicated in this deviant lifestyle; students who are invovled in delinquent behavior and substance use are more likely to do poorly in school (Elliott & Voss, 1974; Hawkins & Lam, 1987; Rutter & Giller, 1983). While research on the relationship between dropping out and substance use or any of the other behaviors identified above as deviant lifestyle behaviors is more limited (Wehlage & Rutter, 1987), it suggests that dropouts are involved in more serious and more frequent drug use but are less likely to be involved in drug selling than students still in school (Fagan & Pabon, 1990); that dropouts typically initiate sexual intercourse at an earlier age and are more likely to become pregnant (Mensch & Kandel, 1988; Yamaguchi & Kandel, 1985); and that those who are sexually active receive lower grades (Donovan, Jessor, & Costa, 1988; Hundleby, 1987).

The above review of research findings suggests that many types of patterned delinquent behavior and substance use, together with precocious sexual behavior, risky driving, and school-related problems, can be viewed as a coherent lifestyle. While it is possible that there are other problem behaviors that also cluster with this set of behaviors, such as suicide (Osgood, 1991), use of pornography (Zillman & Bryant, 1988), and sleeping disorders (Kosky, Sibburn, & Zubrick, 1990), the evidence for these behaviors is either very weak or conflicting.

The Strength of Relationships: Health-Compromising Lifestyle Behaviors

While it is true that youth with a patterned involvement in any one of the above health-compromising lifestyle behaviors are likely to be involved in others as well, is the risk of simultaneous, multiple health-compromising behaviors in individuals substantial? What proportion of youth can be said to have a health-compromising lifestyle? Given one of these behaviors, what is the increase in risk for the others? These are very difficult questions, both conceptually and empirically.

In most studies, the strength of these relationships is assessed in terms of correlations or other measures of association. To facilitate this discussion of the strength of relationships between lifestyle behaviors, Table 7.1 presents the correlations between lifestyle behaviors obtained from the National Youth Survey, a 14-year longitudinal study of a national sample of adolescents aged 11–17 in 1976 (Elliott et al., 1989). The correlations above the diagonal in the table are for the prevalence of patterned problem behavior, that is, the proportion of the sample who are involved in four or more behaviors of each type.[2] The correlations below the diagonal are those between frequency measures of these problem behaviors.

As expected, significant correlations between patterned involvement in these problem behaviors are all positive. The strength of the associations is slightly greater within particular domains than between them.[3] There are two important exceptions to this generalization. First, it appears that the less serious forms of delinquent behavior have a stronger relationship with alcohol, tobacco, and marijuana use, and with drunkenness, than with more serious forms of delinquent behavior. Second, the relationships between hard drug use, problem use of alcohol or drugs, and patterned delinquent behaviors are as strong as those within the delinquency or drug-use domains.

The strength of the associations between patterned behaviors in the delinquent and substance use domains with those in the sexual behavior domain are typically very weak. An exception is precocious intercourse, which appears to be moderately associated with substance use and nonserious forms of delinquency. Sexual deviance (see note d, Table 7.1), on the other hand, is only weakly associated with any of the other lifestyle behaviors in Table 7.1.[4]

In summary, using a correlation approach to estimate the strength of the relationship between health-compromising lifestyle behaviors, it would appear that the relationships between patterned involvement in delinquency, substance use, and problem use, DUI, and precocious sexual intercourse are weak to moderate, with involvement in one behavior typically accounting for 10% or less of the variance in the other. The strongest relationships identified (between hard drug use and drug sales, DUI, and marijuana use/drunkenness, marijuana use and status offenses, and theft and violent offenses) accounted for 25–35% of the variance. The relationships between sexual deviance, school failure, and other behaviors in the lifestyle were uniformly weak.[5]

A few studies provide a direct estimate of the proportion of youth who might be classified as having a health-compromising lifestyle, that is, simultaneous patterned involvement in two or more behavioral domains represented in the lifestyle. Mott and Haurin (1988) focused on substance use and sexual activity, and found that only modest percentages of youth were involved in more than one of these behaviors before their 17th birthday. For example, they report that 16% of males and 8% of females had become involved in patterned (monthly) alcohol use, marijuana use, and sexual intercourse before age 17. Approximately 30% of males and 45% of females reported no involvement in *any* of these behaviors prior to age 17.[6]

Elliott et al. (1989) focused on delinquent behavior and substance use, and found that 18% of youth (aged 11–17) were involved in both patterned alcohol use and patterned minor delinquent behavior. Nine percent were involved in patterned marijuana use and minor delinquency. Over 50% reported no patterned involvement in either delinquent behavior or substance use (alcohol, marijuana, or other illicit drugs). While the prevalence of joint delinquency and substance use was low, the overlap among those involved in one or the other behavior was quite high. Approximately 70% of patterned minor offenders were also using alcohol or some illicit substance (mostly alcohol), and 77% of patterned alcohol users were also patterned minor offenders. This overlap was much less for the more serious types of patterned behavior within these two domains: only 16% of serious offenders were also polydrug users, whereas 40% of polydrug users were also serious delinquents. This asymmetry in the overlap between serious delinquency and poly-

Table 7.1.   Correlations Between Types of Problem Behavior: Annual Prevalence and Frequency[a] Rates: National Youth Survey—1979[b]

Problem[c] Behavior Scales	No. of Items	Status	Public Disorder	Property Damage	Minor Theft	Minor Violence	Drug Sales	Serious Theft	Serious Violence	Tobacco
Status offenses	3	1.00	.47	.23	.26	.26	.30	.22	.21	.27
Public disorder	5	.34	1.00	.26	.27	.24	.25	.21	.21	.25
Property damage	3	.31	.28	1.00	.37	.34	.24	.33	.32	.12
Minor theft	3	.41	.35	.27	1.00	.29	.26	.42	.29	.13
Minor violence	3	.09	.04	.09	.04	1.00	.26	.29	.36	.11
Drug sales	3	.24	.21	.16	.23	.04	1.00	.35	.34	.19
Serious theft	4	.31	.15	.24	.55	.03[e]	.57	1.00	.43	.11
Serious violence	6	.20	.13	.32	.54	.08	.28	.53	1.00	.10
Tobacco	1	—	—	—	—	—	—	—	—	1.00
Alcohol	1	.42	.42	.15	.19	.01[e]	.28	.20	.15	—
Marijuana	1	.42	.33	.15	.17	.05	.35	.16	.13	—
Hard drugs	5	.24	.22	.17	.25	.02[e]	.76	.51	.17	—
Problem use of alcohol	8	.20	.28	.23	.22	.05	.17	.21	.20	—
Problem use of drugs	8	.26	.37	.23	.24	.03[e]	.32	.24	.16	—
Drunkenness[d]	1	—	.32	.07	.11	.24	.07	.11	.13	—
DUI[b]	1	—	.18	.02[e]	.12	.13	.10	.10	.13	—
Sexual intercourse	1	.16	.19	.07	.05	.01[e]	.29	.08	.05	—
Sexual deviance[d]	6	—	.15	.02[e]	.10	.06	.03[e]	.02[e]	.02[e]	—
STD[d]	1	—	—	—	—	—	—	—	—	—

[a]Correlations for prevalence of patterned behavior (i.e., four or more times per year) are shown above the diagonal; correlations for frequency are shown below the diagonal.

[b]Wave 4 of the NYS data set refers to calendar year 1979, when the sample was aged 14–20.

[c]For a description of the delinquency and drug use scales, see Elliott, Huizinga, and Morse (1986) and Elliott and Ageton (1980). Test-retest reliabilities for all scales are in an acceptable range; see Huizinga and Elliott (1986). The sexual deviance scale includes six items, including voyeurism, pedophilia, exhibitionism; use of pornographic materials, sadism, and masochism. STD = sexually transmitted diseases and involved a single item: Have you ever had a venereal disease such as genital herpes or gonorrhea? No frequency data are available for tobacco or STD. For Status Offenses (runaway, truancy), no prevalence or frequency data are available for subjects aged 18 and older; correlations for this behavior thus involve about half of the sample in 1979 and none of the sample in 1983. School failure refers to GPA's of 1.5 or lower.

[d]Correlations for this set of items was based upon NYS wave 6 data (1983), when the sample was aged 18–24. Information on these behaviors was not available on earlier waves. Sexual intercourse for wave 6 includes extramarital as well as premarital intercourse.

[e]$p > .05$. All other values are significant at $p \leq .05$.

drug use is associated with differences in the age distributions of these two types of behavior, an issue we will discuss later.

In general, then, the evidence suggests that there is a subgroup of adolescents who can be classified as having a health-compromising lifestyle that involves multiple types of delinquent, substance use, and/or precocious sexual behavior. Life-

Alcohol	Marijuana	Hard Drugs	Problem Use of Alcohol	Problem Use of Drugs	Drunkenness	DUI	Sexual Intercourse	Sexual Deviance	STD	School Failure
.42	.50	.32	.25	.28	—	—	.30	—	—	.11
.33	.46	.35	.34	.29	.53	.49	.33	.11	.06	.04[e]
.11	.17	.18	.21	.24	.08	.07	.11	.02[e]	−.02[e]	.08
.15	.28	.30	.26	.29	.15	.20	.12	.18	.03[e]	.08
.12	.16	.18	.19	.29	.08	.10	.12	.01[e]	−.02[e]	.08
.19	.38	.51	.23	.36	.15	.31	.22	.20	.11	.15
.11	.21	.28	.28	.35	.12	.17	.14	.10	.08	.14
.11	.21	.31	.25	.33	.08	.10	.17	.03[e]	.02[e]	.16
.30	.37	.27	.17	.16	.23	.23	.27	.05	.03[e]	.24
1.00	.43	.24	.20	.15	.32	.26	.31	−.00[e]	.04[e]	.10
.40	1.00	.46	.26	.31	.37	.48	.41	.13	.11	.15
.30	.28	1.00	.26	.36	.28	.44	.32	.16	.10	.14
.35	.18	.16	1.00	.42	.26	.29	.25	.14	.01[e]	.13
.25	.32	.35	.45	1.00	.11	.11	.17	.08	.13	.11
.48	.37	.26	.32	.25	1.00	.50	.24	.07	.05	—
.25	.67	.31	.23	.37	.45	1.00	.01	.16	.07	—
.27	.26	.17	.13	.19	.14	.06	1.00	.08	.07	.11
.23	.16	.08	.17	.07	.18	.12	.11	1.00	.19	—
—	—	—	—	—	—	—	—	—	1.00	—

styles limited to licit substances and minor delinquency involved approximately one in five adolescents in the 11–17 age range; for 15- 21-year-olds, one in four were involved in this kind of lifestyle. For those involved in either minor delinquent behavior or alcohol use, a large majority were also involved in the other form of behavior. However, lifestyles characterized by the more serious forms of behavior within these domains involved very few adolescents and lower levels of overlap. Even looking over time at the concomitance of these types of behavior by the end of adolescence (age 17), the percentages of adolescents that could be classified as having a health-compromising lifestyle involving multiple illicit drugs and premarital sexual behavior or serious/violent delinquent behavior are small. Still, from a health perspective, a lifestyle involving patterned use of tobacco, alcohol, and minor forms of delinquent behavior may have quite serious long-term consequences (Newcomb & Bentler, 1988), and substantial proportions of adolescents appear to be involved in these lifestyles.

Healthy and Unhealthy Environments

Deviant lifestyles tend to be concentrated in particular social contexts and are, at least in part, a patterned response to these environments (Chapter 13). Our concern in this chapter is with the social structural features of environments as they define specific neighborhood, school, and family contexts that operate to foster or inhibit the emergence of health-compromising lifestyles. Stated simply, neighborhoods differ substantially with respect to their social, cultural, and financial capital (Tienda, 1990), that is, the level of consensus about values and norms, the effectiveness of informal social networks and relationships, and the types and amounts of community resources available to residents. Together, these structural characteristics determine the level of social cohesion and the effectiveness of socialization and social control processes by providing exposure to particular behaviors and not to others (i.e., selected learning structures); by providing many opportunities to engage in particular behaviors and few or no opportunities to engage in functionally equivalent alternative behaviors that might have very different health implications (i.e., selected performance structures); and by the presence or absence of effective controls on illegal or dysfunctional behavior.

There is clear evidence that neighborhoods differ with respect to their official aggregated rates of predatory crime and violence, alcoholism, illicit drug use, and teenage sexual behavior and pregnancy (Bursik & Webb, 1982; Johnstone, 1978, 1983; Sampson, 1985; Taylor & Covington, 1988). The evidence linking neighborhood and school contextual effects to individual self-reported involvement in lifestyle behaviors (compared to aggregated official rates) is much more limited and indicates relatively weak neighborhood and school contextual effects when family backgrounds and relationships are controlled (Jencks & Mayer, 1987; Simcha-Fagan & Schwartz, 1986). There is general agreement, however, that there are serious conceptual and methodological problems with this body of research; and the observation that the effects of neighborhood structure and organization work primarily through the family, school, and peer group rather than independently (Simcha-Fagan & Schwartz, 1986) does not negate the significance of the neighborhood setting as a generating milieu for deviant, health-compromising lifestyles. Further, there may be significant interactions or conditional relationships between neighborhood contextual effects and family, school, and peer group effects. For example, Johnstone (1983) found that male involvement in delinquent gangs reflected the joint effects of a youth's self-identity; attachments to family, school, and friends; and the presence or absence of established gangs in the neighborhood.

At the family level, the relationship between characteristics such as economic status, race, family structure (both parents, single parent, stepparent), and the prevalence of delinquency and substance use during adolescence is very weak or nonexistent (Chapter 3; Kandel, 1978; Smith & Remington, 1989). Race and economic status are more strongly associated with dropping out, early sexual intercourse, teenage pregnancy, and risky driving behavior, with the more disadvantaged having higher rates of dropping out, intercourse, and pregnancy but lower rates of DUI (Elliott, 1987; Elliott & Morse, 1989; Fagan & Pabon, 1990; Mott & Haurin, 1988).

There is also some evidence that health-promoting behavior is positively related to the social class of parents (Nutbeam et al., 1989).

The Developmental Dynamics of Lifestyle Behavior

Our ability to describe the developmental dynamics of lifestyle behaviors is largely limited to health-compromising behaviors, given the inadequate research base on health-promoting behaviors during adolescence. Most of the available data on the developmental progression of lifestyle behaviors involves the sequencing of behaviors *within* particular behavioral domains. For example, drug substances are linked to one another in a developmental progression or series of stages that begins with the licit substances (tobacco and/or alcohol use) and escalates to include marijuana and then other illicit drugs (Johnston et al., 1978; Kandel & Faust, 1975; Kandel & Yamaguchi, 1985). These stages are hierarchical and cumulative; the behavior characteristic of lower stages is retained and actually increases in frequency with the escalation to a new stage and its characteristic behavior (Elliott et al., 1989; Kandel, 1988). The progression involves an add-on pattern rather than a replacement pattern, a movement toward diversification rather than specialization.

While there is a progression in drug use, the likelihood of escalation from one substance use stage to another is not high. For example, Elliott et al. (1989) report that, on average, one in five make the transition to the next advanced stage in any given year during adolescence. In late adolescence and early adulthood, progression to a more advanced stage is no more likely than regression to an earlier stage. As a result, the proportion of active, patterned polydrug users at any given age during the adolescent years is relatively small (10% or less). The cumulative proportion of adolescents who become patterned, multiple illicit drug users during their adolescent years is larger, but still less than 20% by age 17 (Elliott et al., 1989).[7] Entry into a particular stage is thus a necessary but not a sufficient prerequisite for entry into the next higher stage (Kandel, 1985, p. 5).

Although not as well established as for stages of substance use, there also appears to be a developmental progression from status offenses to misdemeanors to serious property crimes to serious violent crimes against persons (Elliott et al., 1989; Loeber, 1985). Again, the annual transition rates from stage to stage are low, and relatively few adolescents reach the last stage, but those reaching more advanced stages of patterned delinquent behavior are quite likely to be involved at high frequencies in earlier stage behavior.

Across domains, Elliott and his colleagues (Elliott et al., 1989; Elliott & Morse, 1989) reported on the temporal sequencing of delinquent behavior, sexual intercourse, and substance use for youth in the National Youth Survey. The most consistent ordering involved the onset of minor offending, followed by alcohol use, marijuana use, sexual intercourse, serious delinquent offending, and polydrug use. The progression was hierarchical, with an add-on pattern of involvement in these behaviors (see also Kandel, 1988). Given these data on temporal order, drug use cannot be a cause of the *onset* of delinquency. The onset of illicit drug use is associated with a higher frequency of delinquent behavior by those previously involved in delinquency, and the addition of illicit drug use to the behavioral repertoire is associated with a longer criminal career (Elliott et al., 1989). The addition of illicit drugs to the lifestyle thus has implications for both the rate and the continuity of other lifestyle behaviors.

The substance use, delinquent behavior, and sexual intercourse sequences appear to reflect increasingly serious violations of social and legal norms, and progression through these stages may well reflect an increasing commitment to a deviant lifestyle. However, this claim with respect to patterned use of tobacco and alcohol and sexual intercourse must be qualified by age, since these behaviors are normative in late adolescence and early adulthood and cease to be a characteristic of a deviant lifestyle (Newcomb & Bentler, 1988; Osgood, Johnston, O'Malley, & Bachman, 1988).

Age Dynamics in Lifestyle Behaviors

There are important differences in the developmental timing of different types of problem behavior included in the health-compromising lifestyle. To illustrate these differences, Figure 7.1 presents age-specific annual prevalence rates for the major

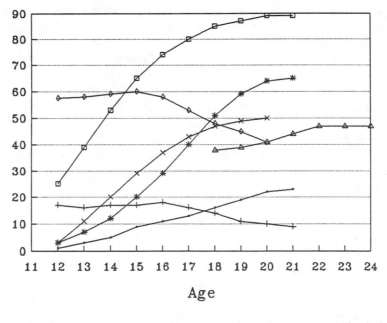

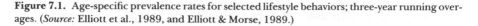

Figure 7.1. Age-specific prevalence rates for selected lifestyle behaviors; three-year running overages. (*Source:* Elliott et al., 1989, and Elliott & Morse, 1989.)

types of problem behavior included in the lifestyle. Several general observations can be made about the timing of involvement in these behaviors. First, 50% or more of all adolescents who will (by age 21) engage in delinquent behavior do so by age 12; for alcohol use, half of all adolescent users begin using by age 14; for marijuana use, by age 16; for sexual involvement and hard drug use, by age 17; and for DUI, by age 18 (or earlier). The onset of involvement in delinquency and alcohol use is thus quite early in adolescence, whereas it is later for sexual intercourse, illicit substance use, and serious delinquency.

Second, neither serious delinquent behavior nor the use of illicit drugs other than marijuana ever becomes normative (statistically) in the adolescent population, that is, the age-specific prevalence rates never reach 50% or more. The highest prevalence rate for serious delinquent behavior (18%) occurs at age 16 and for hard drug use (23%) at age 21 (or later).

Third, two behaviors do become statistically normative during adolescence: alcohol use in midadolescence and sexual intercourse in late adolescence. The link between these two behaviors and other lifestyle behaviors diminishes substantially as these behaviors become normative (Kandel, 1978; Newcomb & Bentler, 1988; Osgood et al., 1988; White et al., 1985). It appears that it is only *early* involvement in alcohol use and sexual intercourse that covaries with other forms of problem behavior or with a general tendency toward problem behavior as a lifestyle; initiation of these behaviors in late adolescence does not put youth at risk for other forms of deviant lifestyle behavior or appear to be a characteristic of a deviant lifestyle. Although the evidence is more limited, it appears that late onset of illicit drug use is also less likely to be associated with delinquency or crime (Elliott et al., 1989).

White (1990) notes that levels of covariation between delinquent behavior and substance use are highest in midadolescence (age 15) and are relatively low at ages 12 and 18. The particular spacing of these behaviors over the life span may reflect nothing more than changing opportunities in the social environment, social definitions about age-appropriate behaviors, and changing social roles in which adolescents and young adults are involved (Bachman 1987; Osgood et al., 1988), but some researchers argue that certain forms of lifestyle behavior (in particular, marijuana use) play a causal role in the onset of later behaviors in the sequence (Kandel, 1978; Osgood et al., 1988). In any event, timing is a phenomenon with great significance for interventions that target lifestyle behaviors, an issue that will be explored later.

Continuity and Discontinuity in Lifestyle Behaviors

There is greater continuity in substance use and sexual behavior than in delinquent behavior (Bachman, O'Malley & Johnston, 1984; Mechanic, 1979). For example, 8 out of 10 youth involved in serious, patterned delinquency and half of those involved in any patterned delinquency terminate their involvement by age 17. In comparison, only 13% of patterned alcohol users and 30% of patterned marijuana users terminate this behavior by age 17. The termination of polydrug use prior to adulthood is much higher (45%). However, a substantial proportion of polydrug users initiate this behavior after age 17, whereas initiation rates for criminal behavior after 17 are very low (Elliott et al., 1989).

Discontinuity in some lifestyle behaviors appears to be related to general demographic characteristics of youth. Females are more likely than males to terminate involvement in delinquent behavior (both minor and serious), marijuana use, and polydrug use during adolescence; blacks are more likely than whites to terminate minor offending but less likely to terminate serious delinquency; middle-class youth are more likely to terminate serious delinquency than lower-class youth; and urban youth are more likely to terminate alcohol and marijuana use but less likely to terminate serious delinquency than are rural youth (Elliott et al., 1989). These differences in termination rates suggest that those in disadvantaged social environments are less likely to mature out of these lifestyle behaviors than are adolescents from more advantaged social contexts, an outcome that may reflect the differences in access to jobs and other conventional roles associated with the transition from adolescence to adulthood.

Explanations for the Clustering of Behaviors into Lifestyles

A number of explanations have been proposed to account for the clustering of particular behaviors into lifestyles: (1) they have a common cause (e.g., personality trait, clinical disorder, social orientation, developmental process), (2) they are generally linked in social experience and learned as a set (e.g., drinking and smoking are typically linked with sexual intercourse in media presentations of this behavior), (3) they are alternative means of achieving personal goals, (4) they are linked in the normative expectations of particular groups or cultures, (5) they are causally linked to each other, and (6) the apparent clustering is purely coincidental.

The Clustering of Health-Compromising Behaviors

The most frequently cited and tested explanation for the clustering of problem behaviors is that they are all manifestations of a single underlying general propensity to deviance. This approach is most fully developed in problem behavior theory (Donovan & Jessor, 1985; Jessor, Donovan, & Witmer, 1980; Jessor & Jessor, 1977), and there is an extensive body of research examining Jessor's proposed explanation. According to this view, problem behaviors cluster because they have a common etiology; they are each a manifestation of a general predisposition to unconventionality. Variations of this approach are offered by others, such as general dispositions to hedonism (Hirschi, 1984), risk taking (Irwin & Millstein, 1986), or sensation seeking (Zuckerman, Eysenck, & Eysenck, 1978). The argument that problem behaviors cluster because they have a common etiology is compelling. However, it raises several critical questions.

First, is the observed level of clustering strong enough and consistent enough to support the claim that these behaviors are all manifestations of a single underlying general trait such as unconventionality (or hedonism, sensation seeking, or risk taking)? As Osgood (1991) notes, if this argument is pushed to its limit, the specific types of behavior in which an individual engages at any time would be strictly random, in which case the correlation between types of behavior should be perfect, limited only by the reliability of the measures employed. Clearly, this is not the case. As reported earlier, the level of covariation between problem behaviors is relatively modest, even when adjustments for reliability are made. Further, the strength of the covariation between behaviors appears to vary with the stage of the life span, increasing from late childhood to midadolescence and then declining with the transition to early adulthood (Gilmore et al., 1990; Newcomb & Bentler, 1988; Osgood et al., 1988; White, 1990). This life span pattern suggests that something in addition to a general stable propensity to unconventionality is operating, since presumably the individual propensity has not changed.

While Jessor et al. (1980) propose a general proneness to unconventionality as the key element in problem behavior theory, they note that when this proneness is present, the specific behavior selected is determined by exposure, social support, and modeling of specific behaviors in the immediate environment. This is an important addition, since the dynamics of clustering and sequencing in problem behavior would appear to be primarily the result of environmental influences rather than an individual predisposition to unconventionality.

Whether one views the causal structure as including only individual predispositions or both predispositions and environmental factors, the second issue in the common etiology argument concerns the claim that the same *set* of causes accounts for *each* of the forms of behavior in the lifestyle. While the available evidence clearly indicates that there is a common set of causal variables implicated in delinquent behavior, alcohol and illicit substance use, and adolescent sexual activity (Donovan & Jessor, 1985; Elliott et al., 1989; Kaplan, Martin, & Johnson, 1986; Newcomb & Bentler, 1988), there is also evidence for some unique causal variables involved in the explanation of specific types of problem behavior (Elliott et al., 1989; Ensminger & Kane, 1985; Fagan et al., 1987; Kandel et al., 1986; Mott & Haurin, 1988; Osgood, 1991). The evidence also indicates that the variables causally implicated in the onset of a particular type (domain) of behavior are not necessarily the same as those that lead to more serious forms of that behavior (Kandel, 1988; Kandel et al., 1978; Smith, Fisher, & Jarjoura, 1989).

Kandel (1988) argues that this common etiology explanation is too opportunistic to account for the highly structured sequences and progression observed both within and across behavioral domains. Illicit drug use, even when the drugs are generally available in the social environment, does not occur independently of alcohol or marijuana use, solely as a function of availability or opportunity. Further, the cumulative add-on pattern guarantees that those involved in all types of delinquency and users of all the different substances will share certain *initial* characteristics, since they all passed through the same initial stage of involvement. In addition to the common causes associated with the initial entry into problem behavior, Kandel argues that specific (unique) factors are necessary to explain why some persons are more likely to proceed further along the developmental path than others. The evidence reviewed above does suggest that there are indeed unique individual and environmental factors associated with progression to more serious or advanced stages of problem behavior.

The issues surrounding the common etiology explanation are far from being resolved. However, I believe the evidence reviewed above does indicate that the more simplistic common etiology arguments that involve a single personality trait or predisposition cannot account for the changing patterns of covariation or the observed sequencing of these behaviors over time. Some combination of individual characteristics and environmental conditions is necessary to explain the observed clustering of problem behaviors.

A second major explanation for the clustering of problem behaviors is that they are causally linked to one another. The popular view that involvement in drugs leads to involvement in delinquency as a means of sustaining one's drug habit is an example of this argument. While the evidence is mixed, there is more consistency when a distinction is made between the onset of a particular behavior and the continuity or discontinuity of involvement in that behavior, that is, initiation compared to annual prevalence or rate of offending/use. Most evidence on initiation indicates that there is no causal connection between delinquency, alcohol or illicit drug use, or sexual activity among adolescents (Carpenter, Glassner, Johnson, & Loughlin, 1988; Huizinga & Elliott, 1986; Johnson et al., 1986; Johnston et al., 1978; Kandel, 1978). One exception to this general conclusion is fairly well established: marijuana use does appear to be causally related to the initiation of later hard drug use (Kandel & Yamaguchi, 1985; Osgood, O'Malley, Bachman, & Johnston, 1989).

The evidence pertaining to the frequency or continuity of offending or use is more limited but suggests that the onset of substance use has a significant effect on the rate of delinquent offending (Elliott et al., 1989; Fagan et al., 1990). The evidence for this relationship is more compelling for adult samples. Among active drug users who have previously initiated criminal behavior, increasing or decreasing the frequency of substance use produces a corresponding increase or decrease in the frequency of (nondrug) criminal behavior (Anglin & Speckart, 1988; Clayton & Tuchfeld, 1982; Nurco, Schaeffer, Ball, & Kinlock, 1984).

In sum, while the size and consistency of the covariation between problem behaviors are too great to allow a pure coincidence explanation (cf. White, 1990), the level of covariation is too weak to support a single etiology explanation. In light of the evidence reviewed above, the most plausible explanation involves a partial commonality in etiology and some unique causal factors linked to specific types of problem behaviors, specifically those constituting more serious or later stages of the developmental progression. This position accounts for the consistent but moderate level of covariation and allows for the possibility that involvement in earlier developmental forms of problem behavior may have some causal influence on later forms. This position is sure to be controversial. Yet it provides at least one way to integrate the complex set of findings concerning the clustering of problem behaviors into a health-compromising lifestyle.

The Clustering of Health-Promoting Behaviors

Problem behavior theory (Costa, Jessor, & Donovan, 1989; Donovan & Jessor, 1985; Jessor, 1984) is the only theoretical perspective known to the author that attempts to explain both a problem behavior syndrome (lifestyle) and a health-promoting lifestyle. Just as problem behavior is a result of a proneness to unconventionality in the personality, perceived environment, and behavior systems of the individual, health-promoting behaviors are seen as a result of a proneness to conventionality in these systems. From this perspective, maintaining good health is a value that is endorsed and reinforced by conventional social institutions such as the family and school, and the adherence to this value should lead to involvement in health-promoting behaviors and avoidance of health-compromising behaviors. Problem behavior theory thus postulates that health-promoting behaviors should cluster as a result of a common etiology, in this case a proneness to conventionality. Further, a health-promoting lifestyle should be negatively related to a health-compromising lifestyle.

The empirical support for this perspective is weak. As noted earlier, the evidence for a cluster of health-promoting behaviors was limited and mixed; positive health behavior appears to be a multidimensional phenomenon. The relationship between health-promoting and health-compromising behaviors is inconsistent. There is some evidence that concerns about health tend to diminish relative to other personal concerns with the transition into adolescence (Chapter 6; Chassin et al., 1987; Eiser, Eiser, Gammage, & Morgan, 1989). The increasing influence of the peer group relative to that of the family and school may well encourage health-compromising behaviors rather than health-promoting behaviors (Elliott et al., 1989; Fagan, Weis, Cheng, & Watters, 1987; Kandel et al., 1986; Nutbeam et al., 1989; Osgood, 1991). These developmental variations in the salience of health and other concerns during adolescence argue against a coherent, stable "value on health." Finally, adolescents do not relate their involvement in many types of problem behavior, in particular alcohol use, to negative health outcomes (Radius, Dillman, Becker, Rosenstock, & Horvath, 1980).

Implications for Health Promotion and Treatment

In light of the evidence for a problem behavior lifestyle, how might our understanding of the content and dynamics of this lifestyle and its concentration in particular ecological and social environments inform our prevention and treatment efforts? First, the fact that most youth involved in the deviant lifestyle will terminate this behavior during late adolescence or early adulthood should make us cautious about implementing general interventions without *demonstrated* effectiveness and compelling evidence of immediate or short-term health consequences. In a sense, adolescent involvement in a deviant lifestyle is often self-limiting, and there is a danger that untested or undemonstrated interventions may make matters worse rather than better, particularly when the immediate consequences for health or quality of life are minimal. For example, some evidence indicates that official justice system interventions in the lives of minor juvenile offenders have iatrogenic effects, increasing rates of offending and lengthening delinquent careers (Gold & Williams, 1969; West and Farrington, 1977; Wolfgang, Figlio, & Sellin, 1972). This is not an argument for abandoning effective prevention and treatment programs, but rather an effort to put these objectives in perspective, given the evidence for maturational reform in lifestyle behaviors.

Second, the variety of behavioral domains and the developmental stage within a domain are indicators of the strength of an individual's underlying commitment to deviance. Most adolescents experiment with minor forms of delinquent behavior, tobacco and alcohol use, and sexual behavior; few become involved in these behaviors as a lifestyle; and the number who progress to serious delinquent behavior, problem use of alcohol, frequent DUI, and illicit substance use/problem use is quite small. Unfortunately, relatively little is known about the etiology of transitions, the variables and conditions that differentiate between those who will remain at a particular developmental stage (or return to an earlier one) and those who will escalate to more serious stages. Several researchers have studied the causes of transitions across drug stages (Kandel et al., 1978; Kandel & Yamaguchi, 1985; Kaplan, Martin, & Robbins, 1985), but to my knowledge no one has addressed the etiology of transitions across the multiple domains implicated in a deviant lifestyle.

Using a slightly different approach to this question, Chassin et al. (1989) proposed that there are two distinct types of youth who become involved in deviant lifestyles: (1) youth who are striving for independence and whose behavior can be understood as precocious involvement in conventional adult behaviors (constructive deviance) and (2) youth whose involvement represents a genuine alienation from society and a commitment to an unconventional lifestyle (destructive deviance). The former would be unlikely to escalate their involvement with tobacco, alcohol, and sex to serious delinquency or illicit drug use, as these are not conventional adult behaviors and reflect a strong commitment to a deviant lifestyle. Those with a genuine commitment to deviant forms of behavior would be much more likely to escalate their level of deviance or unconventionality. Should this distinction prove valid, there are obvious differences in approaches to treatment for these two groups. A better understanding of stage transitions would clearly facilitate our ability to target youth at risk for the more serious levels of lifestyle behavior.

Third, it must be acknowledged that from a health perspective, it is not only the more serious forms of deviant lifestyle behavior that pose significant health risks, but the more minor ones as well. While society views the use of crack cocaine as a more serious violation of social norms than the use of tobacco or alcohol, there are equally serious health problems associated with the latter; and the relative proportions of adolescents involved in these substances and the early onset and stability of these behaviors are such that many more persons will suffer serious illness and death from tobacco and alcohol use than from cocaine use. The arguments made above concerning the maturation effect and more serious forms of lifestyle behaviors must thus be qualified for selected lifestyle behaviors that occur relatively early in the developmental progression, in particular frequent or heavy tobacco and alcohol use and risky driving.

Fourth, the developmental progression findings suggest some particular intervention strategies and target behaviors. A program successful in preventing the onset of minor delinquency might well have a profound prevention effect on all of the other deviant lifestyle behaviors, as this behavior appears to be the first step in the developmental progression to deviant lifestyle behaviors. This argument also holds for the initiation of alcohol use, as the probability of ever using illicit drugs is extremely low (3% or less), and the risk of serious delinquency is reduced by a factor of 4 if an individual has never used alcohol (Elliott et al., 1989). A less demanding prevention objective would be to delay the onset of tobacco and alcohol use until late adolescence. There is substantial evidence that the later onset of use of these substances is not associated with other lifestyle behaviors and is less likely to result in problem use of substances. The argument for targeting these specific behaviors depends upon the claim that early stages in the progression are *necessary* conditions for later stages, and the evidence in support of this claim is not conclusive.

The developmental progression findings also suggest that the first official contact and possible intervention for those adopting a deviant lifestyle is likely to be the juvenile justice system, since delinquent behaviors are the predominant lifestyle behaviors during early adolescence. An effective intervention at this point should have a significant impact on the full set of problem behaviors and should reduce the likelihood of escalation to more advanced stages of the deviant lifestyle. Perhaps a greater allocation of resources ought to be made at this point, while many youth are still at early stages of lifestyle development.

Researchers generally agree that there are common causes for the set of behaviors included in the lifestyle, such as weak integration and bonding to the family and school; poor internal controls and an attenuated commitment to moral norms; and exposure, opportunities, and reinforcements for these behaviors in the peer group and family settings. If so, interventions aimed at these causes should impact broadly on the full set of lifestyle behaviors, affording a more parsimonious approach to designing interventions. By the same token, interventions focused on a particular behavior that emphasize only health risks are unlikely to be successful in changing the general underlying commitment to deviance or the social reinforcements for these behaviors found in certain social contexts. There is little evidence that health concerns play a direct role in the etiology of problem behaviors during adolescence (Castro, Newcomb, McCreary, & Baezconde-Garbanati, 1989; Chassin et al., 1987; Kulbok et al., 1988; Radius et al., 1980). Even if there is some success in reducing a particular problem behavior, it is likely to be replaced by another if there has been no change in the underlying commitment to deviance and social environment that supports this lifestyle.

Given the concentration of persons with deviant lifestyles in particular neighborhoods and communities, solutions that focus on neighborhood revitalization and reorganization might be more productive than those that focus on the rehabilitation of individuals (Chapter 13; Tienda, 1990). The emergence of gangs and drug distribution systems in particular neighborhoods reflects a more general declining resource base, a loss of normative consensus, and a failure of social control processes in the neighborhood; the chances of changing the lifestyles of adolescents in such neighborhoods through individually oriented treatment programs are small. Although paradoxical, such lifestyles are in some respects functional for survival in these settings, and efforts to change individual lifestyles without attending to neighborhood conditions may actually be dysfunctional.

Finally, the fact that separate, expressive, patterned problem behaviors cluster into a single lifestyle calls for a reexamination of the existing organization of prevention, treatment, and research organizations. The present system, which focuses narrowly on particular behavioral domains, is poorly equipped to address the lifestyle as a coherent set of interrelated behaviors. Our youth are the ultimate victims of this inappropriate and inefficient organizational structure.

Notes

1. This criterion is labeled *stylistic unity* by Sobel (1981, pp. 118–119), who does not consider it an essential property of lifestyle. He does consider it an important empirical feature of lifestyles, one that he documents in his analysis.
2. For the Problem Use Scales (Alcohol and Drug), the range of scores was 6 to 30, and patterned problem use was defined as a score of 9 or more. This score reflects six or more occasions of reported problems associated with alcohol or drug use in the past year, such as trouble with spouse/boyfriend/girlfriend; with friends; with family; with police; personal health problems; or fights. For the STD measure, prevalence reflects any reported sexually transmitted disease. Technically, the Problem Use Scales and the STD measure are not measures of behavior, although some of the items in the Problem Use Scales are behavior items. They are more properly conceptualized as outcomes related to problem behavior.

    The range of scores on the Sexual Deviance measure was from 0 to 6. Patterned prevalence was defined as a score of 2 or more, which reflected involvement in two or more of the six types of deviant sexual behavior included in this scale.
3. Throughout this discussion, I will refer to correlations below .20 that indicate 4% or less explained variation as weak; those between .2 and .5 that explain between 4 and 25% of the variance as moderate; and those above .5 that explain more than 25% of the variance as strong.
4. All correlations for drunkenness, sexual deviance, and STD involve the NYS sample at a slightly older age (18–24). This may partially account for the weaker associations (Newcomb & Bentler, 1988, pp. 112–114).
5. Osgood (1991) reports stronger relationships between GPA and delinquent behavior, substance use, and sexual intercourse (using a continuous measure of GPA) than are presented in Table 7.1, but he also concludes that school failure is not a "core" behavior in the cluster of health-compromising behaviors.
6. The estimates in this study involved a patterned use of alcohol measure, but the measures of illicit drug use and sexual intercourse involved *any* use or involvement in these behaviors. It is thus reasonable to assume that these estimates of the joint occurrence of these behaviors will be higher than would be expected with patterned measures of all three behavioral domains.
7. Several national studies report even lower cumulative prevalence rates for polydrug use by age 18; for example, Mott and Haurin (1988) report a rate of 16% for males and 13% for females. However, these estimates are based on a long retrospective recall period and are thus suspect.

References

Anglin, M. D., & Speckart, G. (1988). Narcotics use and crime: A multisample, multimethod analysis. *Criminology, 26,* 197–233.
Bachman, J. (1987). *Changes in deviant behavior during late adolescence and early adulthood.* Paper

presented at the Ninth Biennial Meetings of the International Society for the Study of Behavioral Development, Tokyo.

Bachman, J. G., Johnston, L. D., & O'Malley, P. M. (1981). Smoking, drinking and drug use among American high school students: Correlates and trends, 1975–1979. *American Journal of Public Health, 71,* 59–69.

Bachman, J. G., O'Malley, P. M., & Johnston, L. D. (1984). Drug use among young adults: The impacts of role status and social environments. *Journal of Personality and Social Psychology, 47,* 629–645.

Balding, V., & Macgregor, I. (1987). Health related behavior and smoking in young adolescents. *Public Health, 101,* 277–282.

Breslow, L. (1990). A health promotion primer for the 1990's. *Health Affairs, 9,* 6–21.

Bursik, R. J., & Webb, J. (1982). Community change and patterns of delinquency. *American Journal of Sociology, 88,* 24–42.

Carpenter, C., Glassner, B., Johnson, B., & Loughlin, J. (1988). *Kids, drugs and crime.* Lexington, MA: Lexington Books.

Castro, F., Newcomb, M., McCreary, C., & Baezconde-Garbanati, L. (1989). Cigarette smokers do more than just smoke cigarettes. *Health Psychology, 8,* 107–129.

Chassin, L., Presson, C. L., & Sherman, S. (1987). Applications of social developmental psychology to adolescent health behavior. In N. Eisenberg (Ed.), *Contemporary topics in developmental psychology* (pp. 353–374). New York: Wiley.

Chassin, L., Presson, C., & Sherman, S. (1989). Constructive vs. destructive deviance in adolescent health-related behaviors. *Journal of Youth and Adolescence, 18,* 170–177.

Clayton, R. R., & Tuchfeld, B. S. (1982). The drug–crime debate: Obstacles to understanding the relationship. *Journal of Drug Issues, 12,* 153–166.

Costa, F. M., Jessor, R., & Donovan, J. E. (1989). Value on health and adolescent conventionality: A construct validation of a new measure in problem behavior theory. *Journal of Applied Social Psychology, 19,* 841–861.

DiFranza, J., Winters, T., Goldberg, R., Cirillo L., & Biliouris, T. (1986). The relationship of smoking to motor vehicle accidents and traffic violations. *New York State Journal of Medicine, 86,* 464–467.

Donovan, J., & Jessor, R. (1985). Structure of problem behavior in adolescence and young adulthood. *Journal of Consulting and Clinical Psychology, 53,* 890–904.

Donovan, J., Jessor, R., & Costa, F. (1988). Syndrome of problem behavior in adolescence: A replication. *Journal of Consulting and Clinical Psychology, 56,* 762–765.

Donovan, J., Jessor, R., & Costa, F. (1990). *Structure of health-related behavior in adolescence: A latent variable approach.* Unpublished manuscript, University of Colorado, Institute of Behavioral Science, Boulder.

Dryfoos, J. G. (1990). *Adolescents at risk.* New York: Oxford University Press.

Eiser, J. R., Eiser, C., Gammage, P., & Morgan, M. (1989). Health locus of control and health beliefs in relation to adolescent smoking. *British Journal of Addiction, 84,* 1059–1065.

Elliott, D. S. (1987). Self-reported driving while under the influence of alcohol/drugs and the risks of alcohol/drug-related accidents. *Alcohol, Drugs and Driving, 3,* 31–44.

Elliott, D. S. & Ageton, S. S. (1980). Reconciling race and class differences in self-reported and official estimates of delinquency. *American Sociological Review, 45,* 95–110.

Elliott, D. S., Huizinga, D., & Menard, S. (1989). *Multiple problem youth: Delinquency, substance use and mental health problems.* New York: Springer-Verlag.

Elliott, D. S., & Morse, B. J. (1989). Delinquency and drug use as risk factors in teenage sexual activity. *Youth and Society, 21,* 21–60.

Elliott, D. S., & Voss, H. L. (1974). *Delinquency and dropout.* Lexington, MA: Lexington Books.

Ensminger, M. (1989, April). *Drug use and other problem behaviors among black urban adolescents.* Presentation to the Delta Omega Honorary, Public Health Society.

Ensminger, M. E., & Kane, L. P. (1985, March). *Adolescent drug and alcohol use, delinquency and sexual activity: Patterns of occurrence and risk factors.* Paper presented at the National Institute for Drug Abuse Technical Review on Drug Abuse and Adolescent Sexual Activity, Pregnancy and Parenthood. Rockville, MD.

Fagan, J., Cheng, Y. T., & Weis, J. G. (1990). Drug use and delinquency among inner-city youths. *Journal of Drug Issues, 20,* 349–400.

Fagan, J., & Pabon, E. (1990). Contribution of delinquency and substance use to school dropout among inner-city youth. *Youth and Society, 21,* 306–354.

Fagan, J., Weis, J. G., Cheng, Y. T., & Watters, J. K. (1987). *Drug and alcohol use, violent delinquency, and social bonding: Implications for intervention theory and policy.* San Francisco: URSA Institute.

Gold, M., & Williams, J. R. (1969). National study of the aftermath of apprehension. *Prospectus, 3,* 3–12.

Grube, J. W., & Morgan, M. (1989). The structure of problem behaviors among Irish adolescents. *British Journal of the Addictions, 85,* 667–675.

Haefner, D., Kegeles, S., Kirscht, J., & Rosenstock, I. (1967). Preventive actions in dental disease, tuberculosis and cancer. *Public Health Reports, 82,* 451–459.

Hawkins, J. D., & Lam, T. (1987). Teacher practices, social development and delinquency. In J. Burchard & S. Burchard (Eds.), *Prevention of delinquent behavior* (pp. 241–274). Newbury Park, CA: Sage.

Hays, R., Stacy, A., & DiMatteo, M. (1984). Covariation among health-related behavior. *Addictive Behaviors, 9,* 315–318.

Henderson, J. B., Hall, S. M., & Lipton, H. L. (1979). Changing self-destructive behaviors. In G. Stone, F. Cohen, & N. Adler (Eds.), *Health psychology: A handbook* (pp. 141–160). San Francisco: Jossey-Bass.

Hindelang, M., Hirschi T., & Weis, J. (1981). *Measuring delinquency.* Beverly Hills, CA: Sage.

Hirschi, T. (1984). A brief commentary on Aker's delinquent behavior, drugs and alcohol: What is the relationship? *Today's Delinquent, 3,* 49–52.

Huizinga, D., & Elliott, D. S. (1986). Reassessing the reliability and validity of self-report delinquency measures. *Journal of Quantitative Criminology, 2,* 293–327.

Hundleby, J. (1987). Adolescent drug use in a behavioral matrix: A confirmation and comparison of the sexes. *Addictive Behaviors, 12,* 103–112.

Irwin, C., & Millstein, S. (1986). Biopsychosocial correlates of risk-taking behaviors during adolescence. *Journal of Adolescent Health Care, 7,* 82S–96S.

Jencks, C., & Mayer, S. (1987). *The social consequences of growing up in a poor neighborhood: A review.* Unpublished manuscript, Northwestern University, Center for Urban Affairs and Policy Research, Evanston, IL.

Jessor, R. (1984). Adolescent development and behavioral health. In J. D. Matarozzo, S. M. Weiss, J. A. Herd, & N. E. Miller (Eds.), *Behavioral health: A handbook of health enhancement and disease prevention* (pp. 69–90). New York: Wiley.

Jessor, R. (1987). Risky driving and adolescent problem behavior: An extension of problem behavior theory. *Alcohol, Drugs and Driving, 3,* 1–11.

Jessor, R., & Jessor, S. (1977). *Problem behavior and psychosocial development: A longitudinal study of youth.* New York: Academic Press.

Jessor, R., Donovan, J., & Witmer, K. (1980). *Psychosocial factors in adolescent alcohol and drug use: The 1978 national sample study and the 1974–78 panel study.* Boulder: University of Colorado, Institute of Behavioral Science.

Johnson, B., Wish, E., Schmeidler, J., & Huizinga, D. (1986). The concentration of delinquent offending: Serious drug involvement and high delinquency rates. In B. D. Johnson & E. Wish (Eds.), *Crime rates among drug abusing offenders* (pp. 106–143). New York: Interdisciplinary Research Center, Narcotic and Drug Research.

Johnston, L., O'Malley, P., & Eveland, L. (1978). Drugs and delinquency: A search for causal connections. In D. B. Kandel (Ed.), *Longitudinal research on drug use: Empirical findings and methodological issues* (pp. 137–156). Washington, DC: Hemisphere.

Johnstone, J.W.C. (1978). Social class, social areas and delinquency. *Sociology and Social Research, 63,* 49–72.

Johnstone, J.W.C. (1983). Recruitment to a youth gang. *Youth and Society, 14*, 281–300.

Jonah, B. (1986). Accident risk and risk-taking behavior among young drivers. *Accident Analysis and Prevention, 18*, 255–271.

Kandel, D. (1978). Convergences in prospective longitudinal surveys of drug use in normal populations. In D. Kandel (Ed.), *Longitudinal research on drug use: Empirical findings and methodological issues* (pp. 3–38). Washington, DC: Hemisphere.

Kandel, D. (1988). Issues of sequencing of adolescent drug use and other problem behaviors. *Drugs and Society, 3*, 55–76.

Kandel, D., & Faust, R. (1975). Sequences and stages in adolescent patterns of drug use. *Archives of General Psychiatry, 32*, 923–975.

Kandel, D., Kessler, R., & Marguilies, R. (1978). Antecedents of adolescent initiation into stages of drug use: A developmental analysis. In D. Kandel (Ed.), *Longitudinal research on drug use: Empirical findings and methological issues* (pp. 73–100). Washington, DC: Hemisphere.

Kandel, D., Simcha-Fagan, O., & Davies, M. (1986). Risk factors for delinquency and illicit drug use from adolescence to young adulthood. *Journal of Drug Issues, 16*, 7–90.

Kandel, D., & Yamaguchi, F. (1985). *Developmental patterns of the use of legal, illegal and medically prescribed psychotropic drugs from adolescence to young adulthood.* Etiology of Drug Abuse: Implications for Prevention. NIDA Research Monograph 56 (pp. 193–235). DHHS Publication No. (ADM) 85-1335. Washington, DC: U.S. Government Printing Office.

Kaplan, H., Martin, S., & Johnson, R. (1986). Self-rejection and the explanation of deviance: Specification of the structure among latent constructs. *American Journal of Sociology, 92*, 384–411.

Kaplan, H., Martin, S., & Robbins, L. (1985). Toward an explanation of increased involvement in illicit drug use: Application of a general theory of deviant behavior. *Research in Community and Mental Health, 5*, 205–252.

Kosky, R., Sibburn, S., & Zubrick, S. (1990). Are children and adolescents who have suicidal thoughts different from those who attempt suicide? *Journal of Nervous and Mental Disease, 178*, 38–43.

Kulbok, P., Earls, F., & Montgomery, A. (1988). Lifestyle and patterns of health and social behavior in high-risk adolescents. *Advances in Nursing Science, 11*, 22–35.

Lawson, L. L., Arora, H., & Jonah, B. A. (1982). As cited by Jonah, B. (1986). Accident risk and risk-taking behavior among young drivers. *Accident Analysis and Prevention, 18*, 255–271.

Loeber, R. (1985). Patterns and development of antisocial child behavior. *Annals of Child Development, 2*, 77–116.

Maron, D., Telch, M., Killen, J., Vranizan, K., Saylor, K., & Robinson, T. (1986). Correlates of seat belt use by adolescents: Implications for health promotion. *Preventive Medicine, 15*, 614–623.

Mechanic, D. (1979). The stability of health and illness behavior: Results from a 16-year follow-up. *American Journal of Public Health, 69*, 1142–1145.

Mensch, B., & Kandel, D. (1988). Dropping out of high school and drug involvement. *Sociology of Education, 61*, 95–113.

Mott, F., & Haurin, R. J. (1988). Linkages between sexual activity and alcohol and drug use among American adolescents. *Family Planning Perspectives, 20*, 128–136.

National Center for Health Statistics. (1980). *Vital statistics, 86*, 10.

Newcomb, M. D., & Bentler, P. M. (1988). *Consequences of adolescent drug use: Impact on the lives of young adults.* Newbury Park, CA: Sage.

Noack, H. (1987). *Concepts of health and health promotion.* In T. Abelin (Ed.), *Measurement in health Promotion and protection* (pp. 5–28). World Health Organization (European Series). Copenhagen, Denmark: World Health Organization.

Nurco, D. C., Schaeffer, J. W., Ball, J. C., & Kinlock, T. W. (1984). Trends in the commission of crime among narcotic addicts over successive periods of addiction. *Journal of Drug and Alcohol Abuse, 10*, 481–489.

Nutbeam, D., Aar, L., & Calford, J. (1989). Understanding children's health behavior: The implications for health promotion for young people. *Social Science and Medicine, 29*, 317–325.

O'Neill, P. (1983). *Health crisis 2000*. London: Heinemann Medical Books.

Osgood, D. W. (1991). *Covariation among adolescent health problems*. Background paper for U.S. Congress Office of Technology Assessment's Adolescent Health Project. Washington, DC: U.S. Government Printing Office.

Osgood, D. W., Johnston, L., O'Malley P., & Bachman, J. (1988). The generality of deviance in late adolescence and early adulthood. *American Sociological Review, 53*, 81–93.

Osgood, D. W., O'Malley, P., Bachman, J., & Johnston, L. (1989). Time trends and age trends in arrests and self-reported illegal behavior. *Criminology, 27*, 389–417.

Radius, S., Dillman, T. E., Becker, M., Rosenstock, I., & Horvath, W. (1980). Adolescent perspectives on health and illness. *Adolescence, 15*, 375–384.

Rajala, M., Honkala, E., Rimpela, M., & Lammi, S. (1980). Toothbrushing in relation to other health habits in Finland. *Community Dental and Oral Epidemiology, 8*, 391–395.

Rimpela, M., Eskola, A., & Paronen, O. (1978). As cited in Kannas, L. (1981). The dimensions of health behavior among young men in Finland. *International Journal of Health Education, 24*, 146–155.

Robinson, T., Killen, J., Taylor, B., Telch, M., Bryson, S., Saylor, K., Maron, D., Macoby, N., & Farquhar, J. (1987). Perspectives on adolescent substance use. *Journal of the American Medical Association, 258*, 2072–2076.

Rutter, M., & Giller, H. (1983). *Juvenile delinquency: Trends and perspectives*. New York: Penguin Books.

Sampson, R. (1985). Neighborhood and crime: The structural determinants of personal victimization. *Journal of Research in Crime and Delinquency, 22*, 7–40.

Sampson, R. J., & Lauritsen, J. L. (1990). Deviant lifestyles, proximity to crime, and the offender–victim link in personal violence. *Journal of Research in Crime and Delinquency, 27*, 110–139.

Sievers, K., Koskelalnen, O., & Leppo, K. (1974). As cited in Kannas, L. (1981). The dimensions of health behavior among young men in Finland. *International Journal of Health Education, 24*, 146–155.

Simcha-Fagan, O., & Schwartz, J. E. (1986). Neighborhood and delinquency: An assessment of contextual effects. *Criminology, 24*, 667–703.

Smith, D. A., Fisher, C. A., & Jarjoura, R. G. (1989). *Dimensions of delinquency: Estimating the correlates of participation, frequency and persistence of delinquent behavior*. Unpublished manuscript, University of Maryland: Institute of Criminal Justice and Criminology.

Smith, P. F., & Remington, P. L. (1989). The epidemiology of drinking and driving: Results from the Behavioral Risk Factor Surveillance System (1986). *Health Education Quarterly, 16*, 345–358.

Sobel, M. E. (1981). *Lifestyle and social structure: Concepts, definitions, analysis*. New York: Academic Press.

Taylor, R. B., & Covington, J. (1988). Neighborhood changes in ecology and violence. *Criminology, 26*, 553–589.

Tienda, M. (1990). *Poor people and poor places: Deciphering neighborhood effects on poverty outcomes*. Presented at the 98th Annual Meeting of the American Psychological Association, San Francisco.

Wehlage, G., & Rutter, R. (1987). Dropping out: How much do schools contribute to the problem? In G. Natriello (Ed.), *School dropouts: Patterns and policies* (pp. 70–88). New York: Teachers College Press.

West, D. J., & Farrington, D. P. (1977). *The delinquent way of life*. New York: Crane Russak.

White, H. (1990). The drug use–delinquency connection in adolescence. In R. Weisheit (Ed.), *Drugs, crime and the criminal justice system* (pp. 215–256). Cincinnati: Anderson.

White, H., Labourie, E., & Bates, M. (1985). The relationship between sensation seeking and delinquency: A longitudinal analysis. *Journal of Research in Crime and Delinquency, 22*, 197–211.

Wolfgang, M. E., Figlio, R. M., & Sellin, T. (1972). *Delinquency in a birth cohort*. Chicago: University of Chicago Press.

World Health Organization. (1981). *Global strategy for health by the year 2000*. Geneva: World Health Organization.

Yamaguchi, K., & Kandel, D. (1985). Drug use and other determinants of premarital pregnancy and its outcome: A dynamic analysis of competing life events. *Journal of Marriage and the Family, 49,* 257–270.

Zabin, L. (1984). The association between smoking and sexual behavior among teens in U.S. contraceptive clinics. *American Journal of Public Health, 74,* 261–263.

Zabin, L., Hardy, J., Smith, E., & Hirsch, M. (1986). Substance use and its relation to sexual activity among inner-city adolescents. *Journal of Adolescent Health Care, 7,* 320–331.

Zillman, D., & Bryant, J. (1988). Effects of prolonged consumption of pornography on family values. *Journal of Family Issues, 9,* 518–544.

Zuckerman, M., Eysenck, S., & Eysenck, H. I. (1978). Sensation-seeking in England and America: Cross-cultural, age, and sex comparisons. *Journal of Consulting and Clinical Psychology, 46,* 139–149.

COMMENTARY ON PART I

The Adolescent, Health, and Society: From the Perspective of the Physician

Charles E. Irwin, Jr.

During the past two decades, researchers and practitioners have focused much of their efforts on understanding the initiation of adolescent risk behaviors, their prevalence patterns within specific groups, and the mechanisms by which the behaviors are maintained (Baumrind, 1991; Irwin & Millstein, 1986; Jessor & Jessor, 1977; Chapter 7). These efforts were fueled by the recognition that behaviors such as substance use, early sexual behavior, and recreational and vehicular use were increasingly responsible for the majority of deaths and disabling conditions through the fourth decade of life, and that most of the behaviors were initiated during adolescence (Report of the U.S. Preventive Services Task Force, 1989). However, the attention to risk factors and health-compromising behaviors has resulted in minimal emphasis being placed on identifying the mechanisms supportive of healthy development and health promotion.

Chapters 2 through 7 of this book provide the structural framework from which to begin to develop an integrated approach to health promotion during the second decade of life. More important, each chapter identifies what is missing in our knowledge base in order to increase our understanding of healthy development and effective health promotion programs for the adolescent population. All of these chapters call for the participation of multiple sectors of society in this effort, including health care professionals. What role might the physician play in these efforts?

The Role of the Physician

The majority of adolescents see a physician at least once a year. These visits represent opportunities for health promotion. Physicians, as well as other health care providers, are viewed by adolescents as credible sources of information (Chapter 6); for some sensitive topics, they may be the only adult with whom the adolescent discusses concerns.

The recent task force report on clinical preventive services highlighted six points that have direct relevance to the care of adolescents (Report of the U.S. Preventive Services Task Force, 1989). First, primary prevention of risk factors such as smoking, physical inactivity, poor nutrition, and alcohol/substance abuse generally holds greater promise for improving overall health than many secondary measures such as screening tests. Second, the need to be more selective in screening patients requires a greater emphasis on history taking and the evaluation of the personal health habits of patients. Third, counseling and patient education are within the purview of the clinician and should be developed around the specific age-appropriate risks of the patient. For example, during adolescence when a young person is often riding bicycles, a discussion of the utility of helmet use is critical. Fourth, at the same time that behavioral factors assume a larger role in health status, the individual is given greater responsibility in this area. Fifth, preventive services should be integrated into all clinical encounters. There is no need to wait for a physical examination for sports to discuss safety measures if an adolescent comes in with an acute injury (Cushman, James, & Waclawik, 1991; Runyan & Runyan, 1991). Finally, for most areas of health promotion and prevention, we have inadequate data on effectiveness to determine the optimal frequency of a preventive service (Lowenstein & Hunt, 1990). We do know that there are few immunizations for infectious diseases that give lifelong immunity; therefore, it would be naive for us to think that a single clinical encounter with a patient can provide lifelong immunity from the range of behavioral risks to which he or she is exposed.

Physicians working with adolescents also need to recognize some additional key points in order to be successful with this age cohort. Adolescents are in the process of making decisions regarding health habits, and the personal health habits of the clinician can be critical (Schwartz et al., 1991). Physicians who serve as positive role models through their own health-promoting behaviors may be more effective at health promotion with this group. In addition, physicians alone will have minimal impact on adolescent health promotion in the absence of efforts from the other sectors. As such, they will need to establish contacts with other health agencies and health professionals in the community in order to deliver a truly effective health promotion program. An appropriate method might be the development of an adolescent health advisory board for the community, which health professionals and educators would join to organize a community-based program for youth.

Adolescence as a Unique Developmental Period in the Life Cycle

Adolescence spans the decade between 10 and 21 years and encompasses the biological changes of puberty, as well as psychological, cognitive, and behavioral changes that take place within the organism and social, environmental, and legal transitions external to the organism. The 10-year-old is considerably different from the 15-year-old, yet both are considered adolescents. Just as pediatricians, educators, and social scientists utilize more than one term to describe all of childhood (*infancy, toddlers, preschoolers, school-age children*), we should disaggregate *adolescence*, since it is not a unified, undifferentiated stage of life. By using different terms, we create and permit different expectations for the individual child (Carnegie Council on Adolescent Development, 1989).

Health professionals often have a set of expectations for all adolescents rather than developing targeted services for the unique developmental needs of the different stages of adolescence (Carnegie Council on Adolescent Development, 1989; Hamburg, Nightingale, & Takanishi, 1987; Irwin & Vaughan, 1988). Although several investigators and organizations have attempted to define the stages of adolescence, little of this work has been translated into implications for clinical practice (Irwin, 1987). This may be due to the lack of communication among the disciplines caring for adolescents or the low priority given to this stage of the life cycle by developmentalists in the past (Hill, 1982; Petersen, 1988). We may need, however, to redefine adolescence into two or three distinct life stages to assist in our efforts for health promotion.

Furthermore, the continued emphasis on adolescence as a transitional period between childhood and adulthood encourages our society to view this unique and specific developmental period of the life cycle as a temporary perturbation. The major physiological and psychosocial changes occurring during adolescence are not inevitably associated with negative outcomes and instability; adolescence is not inherently turbulent (Irwin, 1987). By viewing adolescence as a temporary and negative stage, we miss opportunities for health promotion. For example, even though pubescence is one of the hallmarks of early adolescence, little effort is made to utilize this normal physiological process as a means of promoting health. In no other period of the life cycle (except infancy) is there such marked biological growth, and during puberty the young person has the emerging cognitive skills to understand the biological processes. Beyond these new cognitive skills, physicians can use the heightened self-consciousness of adolescents as a means of engaging young persons in the process of learning more about their developing bodies. This self-instruction about one's developing body should be one of the first steps in encouraging young people to assume more responsibility for themselves through health-enhancing behaviors. Since each phase of the life cycle (infancy, childhood, adolescence, young adulthood, middle age, old age) has specific biological events, the stage would be set for the individual to be more attuned to the physiological changes of later phases of life as well. Education about puberty could be taught in a variety of settings, including the home, schools, youth groups, and health clinics, with a slightly different focus in each setting. For example, in the clinical setting, the focus might be the individual's growth and development, whereas in a group setting the emphasis might be on gender differences and variations within the adolescent population.

Is Being Healthy Relevant to the Adolescent?

Most adolescents traverse the second decade of life with few illnesses and enter adulthood in excellent health by traditional standards (Irwin, 1990). In spite of the relatively steep increases in mortality rates from early to late adolescence, most adolescents will exit the second decade having incurred no major health problems (Irwin, Brindis, Brodt, Bennett, & Rodriguez, 1991). This will occur despite the fact that the majority of adolescents will have tried cigarette smoking, drunk alcohol, engaged in sexual intercourse, driven over the speed limit, not used a helmet while riding a bicycle, and ingested a considerable amount of junk food (Irwin, 1990). However, caution must be exercised in presenting such a scenario, since there are great variations within the adolescent population. In clinical settings, the patient population often represents a group at higher risk, who will experience more negative consequences from engaging in health-compromising behaviors (Neinstein, 1991). The degree of clustering of risk behaviors within adolescents will also vary, depending on the population; in clinical samples, the covariation appears to be greater (Moscicki, Millstein, Broering, & Irwin, 1988). Clinicians need to recognize the unique characteristics of their patient population in comparison with study populations while remembering that adolescents often participate in a number of health-damaging behaviors in an exploratory manner and do not experience any negative health outcomes.

Adolescence Does Not Occur in a Vacuum

To foster health promotion in adolescents, there needs to be a "prolongation of a supportive environment for adolescents with graded steps toward autonomy" (Irwin, 1987, p. 2). A supportive environment requires the participation of families, schools, the health care system, and communities that are responsive to the normative processes of adolescence, as well as the need to involve adolescents in a meaningful way with their own health and well-being and to have a role in the community, school, and family (Irwin & Vaughan, 1988). Sources of engagement for adolescents include community organizations, schools, parents, and voluntary organizations. Structured job experiences and volunteer activities may assist adolescents to realize that they have meaningful roles and can contribute productively to society (Greenberger, 1983). This engagement process may represent one of the most critical health-promoting activities for the adolescent.

Finally, in moving toward health promotion, perhaps adolescents themselves can teach us something. Clinicians tend to look for what is going wrong, and social scientists tend to seek out problems to solve. As an alternative, we might consider how adolescents conceptualize health. As Chapter 6 notes, adolescents view health quite broadly in terms of physical health, mental and emotional health, social health, and personal health. When a clinician asks an adolescent what he or she does to stay healthy, the young person often responds: "Do you mean my physical or mental health or how I am doing in school?" Adolescents clearly have a repertoire of behaviors to remain healthy. They are also capable of identifying the risks of most health-damaging behaviors (Irwin & Millstein, 1991). For health promotion to be effective, we need to listen to their voices.

References

Baumrind, D. (1991). The influence of parenting style on adolescent competence and substance use. *Journal of Early Adolescence, 11,* 56–95.

Carnegie Council on Adolescent Development (1989). *Turning points: Preparing American youth for the 21st century: The report of the Task Force on Education of Young Adolescents.* Washington DC: Carnegie Council on Adolescent Development.

Cushman, R., James, W., & Waclawik, H. (1991). Physicians promoting bicycle helmets for children: A randomized trial. *American Journal of Public Health, 81,* 1044–1046.

Greenberger, E. (1983). A researcher in the policy arena: The case of child labor. *American Psychologist, 38,* 104–111.

Hamburg, D., Nightingale, E. O., & Takanishi, R. (1987). Facilitating the transitions of adolescence. *Journal of the American Medical Association, 257,* 3405–3406.

Hill, J. (1982). Guest editorial [Special issue on early adolescence]. *Child Development, 53,* 1409–1412.

Irwin, C. E., Jr. (Ed.) (1987). Editor's Notes: Adolescent social behavior and health. In *New Directions for Child Development, Volume 37* (pp. 1–13). San Francisco: Jossey-Bass.

Irwin, C. E., Jr. (1990). The theoretical concept of at-risk adolescents. *Adolescent Medicine: State of the Art Reviews, 1,* 1–14.

Irwin, C. E., Jr., Brindis, C. D., Brodt, S. E., Bennett, T. A., & Rodriguez, R. Q. (1991). *The health of America's youth: Current trends in health status and utilization of health services.* San Francisco: University of California, San Francisco.

Irwin, C. E., Jr., & Millstein, S. G. (1986). Biopsychosocial correlates of risk-taking behaviors during adolescence. *Journal of Adolescent Health Care, 7*(Suppl), 82S–96S.

Irwin, C. E., Jr., & Millstein, S. G. (1991). Correlates and predictors of risk-taking behaviors during adolescence. In L. P. Lipsitt & L. L. Mitnick (Eds.), *Self-regulatory behavior and risk taking: Causes and consequences* (pp. 3–21). Norwood, NJ: Ablex Publishing Corporation.

Irwin, C. E., Jr., & Vaughan, E. (1988). Psychosocial context of adolescent development, research issues. *Journal of Adolescent Health Care, 9*(Suppl), 11S–19S.

Jessor, R., & Jessor, S. L. (1977). *Problem behavior and psychological development.* New York: Academic Press.

Lowenstein, S. R., & Hunt, D. (1990). Injury prevention in primary care. *Annals of Internal Medicine, 113,* 261–262.

Moscicki, B., Millstein, S. G., Broering, J., & Irwin, C. E., Jr. (1988). Adolescents' beliefs and behaviors concerning sexually transmitted diseases and AIDS. *Journal of Adolescent Health Care, 9,* 261.

Neinstein, L. S. (1991). *Adolescent health care, a practical guide* (2nd ed.). Baltimore: Urban and Schwarzenberg.

Petersen, A. C. (1988). Adolescent development. In M. R. Rozenzweig & L. W. Porter (Eds.), *Annual review of psychology, Volume 39* (pp. 583–607). Palo Alto, CA: Annual Reviews.

Report of the U.S. Preventive Services Task Force (1989). *Guide to clinical preventive services.* Baltimore: Williams and Wilkins.

Runyan, C. W., & Runyan, D. K. (1991). How can physicians get kids to wear bicycle helmets? A prototypic challenge in injury prevention. *American Journal of Public Health, 81,* 972–973.

Schwartz, J. S., Lewis, C. E., Clancy, C., Kinosian, M. S., Radany, M. H., & Koplan, J. P. (1991). Internists' practices in health promotion and disease prevention. *Annals of Internal Medicine, 114,* 46–53.

The Adolescent, Health, and Society: From the Perspective of The Nurse

Jeanette M. Broering

The research literature on adolescents and health promotion has exploded in the past 2 to 3 years, with representation from a variety of professional perspectives including psychology, sociology, medicine, nursing, and public health. The quantity of research illustrates the magnitude of concern about the future health of our youth. Attempts to define, explain, and codify the complex interaction between behaviors such as substance use and delinquency or factors such as poverty and health status appear to have marginal predictive ability when attempting to understand adolescent's choice of healthy lifestyle options (Chapter 7). And yet the question remains: have we generated enough research findings such that, armed with this knowledge, we find ourselves at a crossroad in establishing a new direction for the health of our youth? If so, then how does the profession of nursing further the improvement of the health status of adolescents? Are nurses adequately prepared for this task?

A Comprehensive Definition of Health: What Is the Relationship to Professional Nursing?

Contemporary trends in health care delivery have shifted from a strict medical model to a biopsychosocial model. Historically the emphasis has been on a simplistic, linear, causal model of one-cause, one-disease. Advances in social and behavioral science research have led to an understanding of the complex web of events, both biological and behavioral, that influence the health status of an individual (Lee, 1985). Utilizing the Perry and Jessor (1985) paradigm of health, the authors support the notion of the comprehensive dimensions of health (Chapters 2 and 6). From a philosophical perspective, the profession of nursing has always been committed to a wellness-oriented system of care that incorporates concepts of self-care and holistic care for the individual within the contexts of family, culture, and community. For nursing, health is defined as "a dynamic state of being in which the developmental and behavioral potential of an individual is realized to the fullest extent possible" (ANA *Social Policy Statement,* 1980, p. 5). This perspective is complementary to Bronfenbrenner's (1979) ecological perspective. Nursing can provide support for the attainment of optimal health status for adolescents in four domains: (1) direct service through clinical practice models such as schools or other primary care settings; (2) collaboration with other professionals who have contact with adolescents such as physicians, teachers, and administrators at a variety of levels, from local to national; (3) development of health policy and advocacy that positively affect health status; and (4) education for nurse researchers who support the overall adolescent health research agenda in domains like cross-cultural nursing, program evaluation of health care delivery by nurses, and implementation and evaluation of health promotion and disease prevention programs.

Are Nurses Adequately Prepared to Provide Health Care to Adolescents?

The expanded definition of health, which encompasses traditional indicators (e.g., sleep, nutrition, safety) as well as socially defined constructs (delinquency, school truancy and absenteeism, cultural context, and poverty), will place new demands on nursing education. Previously, nurses successfully provided comprehensive, school-based health care using a medical model that emphasized physical examinations; screening for vision, hearing, and scoliosis; and administration of immunizing vaccines. However, program evaluation revealed that the school-based nurses did little to affect the new morbidities such as mental health or learning problems. Until the discipline can incorporate these health problems in traditional training, it may be necessary to provide additional education for these nurses or possibly require a master's degree in order to sensitize the nurse to the relationship between school performance and the new morbidities on overall health status and health promotion (Meeker, De Angelis, Berman, Freeman, & Oda, 1986). This expanded scope of practice will demand that nurses be adequately prepared to screen and refer adolescents to appropriate colleagues from other professional disciplines.

Survey research from nurses in three different practice settings (public health, school health, and pediatric nursing) has concluded that all three groups felt they were inadequately prepared to address some of the most common health concerns of adolescents (Bearinger, Wildey, Gephardt, & Blum, 1991a+b). That over half of the nurses sampled had been educated at the graduate level (master's or doctorate) calls into question the gap between educational preparation and clinical practice demands. To prepare nurses and other practitoners of adolescent health promotion adequately to carry out meaningful health risk profiles, we must expand the nursing curriculum to include areas such as asynchrony between biological and psychological development; methods of assessing social functioning in the domains of academic performance, peers, family functioning, and acculturation issues; assessing mental health status; and evaluation of risk behaviors such as substance abuse, sexual activity, and involvement with the juvenile justice system. Yet the development of educational programs in adolescent health care and health promotion has been slow due to competing practice demands in other sectors and funding constraints (Panzarine et al., 1988; Ruszala-Herbst, 1985).

What Are the Current Trends in the Education of Professional Nurses?

Nurses comprise the largest group of health care providers in the United States, with approximately 1.5 million registered nurses (ANA *Facts About Nurses,* 1987). The profession of nursing is maturing, with the standardization of an academic track from the associate degree through the postdoctoral level in order to develop its own body of scientific literature. This consolidation has resulted in enhanced personal competency and increased scope of practice. This professional maturation has created new demands for nurses in the health care marketplace. The "graying" of America, the AIDS epidemic, and the health care needs of the homeless and poor create new demands for more providers in the areas of ambulatory care, home health care, and long term care (NLN, 1990a, 1990b). These practice demands in other sectors may detract from recruitment of adequate numbers of nurses who can provide services to adolescents in the area of health promotion. Already, 2,000 qualified applicants were squeezed out of baccalaureate programs of nursing in 1991 (McCarty, 1991). Development of the pool of baccalaurate-prepared nurses is essential for the education of the nurse generalist and recruitment into advanced specialty practice. Movement into advanced nursing practice, which allows for specialization in areas such as adolescent health promotion, currently occurs at the graduate level (NLN, 1990a, 1990b).

Board certification to document excellance in an area of specialty practice already exists through professional nursing organizations. Advanced practice nurses will demand access to more sophisticated continuing education. Conceptual models of adolescent health promotion will require a higher level of analysis in regard to the evolving social morbidities and their translation into changing models of health care delivery. The rate of change within the nursing profession requires those in positions of power and authority to engage in a continuing dialogue regarding the nature and scope of practice for adolescent health promotion. Participants in this dialogue would include faculty and administrators in schools of nursing, state boards of nursing, professional nursing organizations, health policy and financing agencies, and the National Center for Nursing Research.

What Do We Know About Health Promotion Services That Are Currently Being Rendered by Professional Nurses?

Because the delivery of nursing services is not directly linked to any data tracking mechanism such as financial reimbursement (office visits, hospital admission, or discharge data), it is difficult to quantify the impact of professional nursing care on health promotion. For example, hospital nursing costs are still merged with room charges on patient bills, and reimbursement mechanisms for primary health care by public health nurses or nurse practitioners are just now being developed. A review of surveys that describe practice characteristics does provide some insight into the level at which nurses participate in health promotion activities. For example, a nationwide survey of state boards of education regarding the role and function of school nurses revealed the most frequent activity mandated to be performed by school nurses was health appraisal such as physical care (i.e., emergency care, communicable disease control, health and developmental assessments, and problem management). Health education was mandated by 70% of the states that responded. Although the role of school nurses varied in this activity, 24% responded that school nurses serve as the primary disseminators of health education and 34% reported that nurses were used as primary consultants for resource materials and information. No minimal educational requirements by state boards of education exists on a national level. Responses by 38% of states revealed that the vast majority (95%) were prepared at the generalist level (BSN or below) in educational preparation (Thurber, Berry, & Cameron, 1991).

Survey data on nurse practitioners in traditional health care delivery systems provide additional information on nurses and primary care. Membership data from the National Association of Pediatric Nurse Associates and Practitioners revealed areas of specialty practice, with members spending 25.5% of their clinical time providing primary care to adolescents and an additional 8.5% providing gynecological or family planning care and 14.5% school health care. Practice characteristics of pediatric nurse practitioners revealed that 46% were employed in either public health departments, hospital clinics, or school health settings. These nurses see an average of 10–15 clients per day and spend 30 minutes for an initial visit and 20 minutes for follow-up visits. Their visits are equally divided between acute care and well care. They serve middle- to low-income families that are equally distributed between whites and blacks (Grey & Flint, 1989). A survey conducted by the American Academy of Nurse Practitioners does not describe the degree to which they provide health care/health promotion activities to adolescents. However, the majority of those practicing in freestanding clinics did respond that 78.4% of the families they cared for had incomes below $15,999 per year (Tower, 1991). In conclusion, it appears that nurse practitioners in primary care settings do devote a significant amount of time in the provision of primary health care to adolescents from diverse ethnic backgrounds and from poor families, some of which contain adolescents most at risk for deleterious health outcomes.

Conclusions

The authors in this volume have articulated a comprehensive definition of adolescent health encompassing the domains of biology, cognitive development, sociocultural context, and lifestyle. Parallel with this conceptual shift is the need to educate health professionals such as nurses to reframe their conceptual framework of practice to encompass these complex phenomena. The trend in nursing education is toward greater educational preparation for advanced clinical practice and research; however, the majority of nurses in school-based health delivery systems are not prepared at this level. Other practice demands and sociodemographic shifts in the population and chronic illness phenomena will tax the current supply of professional nurses. Educational and financial initiatives are needed to develop an adequate supply of professional nurses who are appropriately educated to participate in the promotion of optimal health for all adolescents utilizing this broader-based conceptual approach to health care.

Acknowledgments

During the preparation of this commentary the author was supported in part by a grant from the Bureau of Maternal and Child Health and Resources Development (MCJ 000978A).

References

American Nurses Association (1987). *Facts about nursing.* Kansas City, MO: American Nurses Association.

American Nurses Association (1980). *Nursing: A social policy statement.* Kansas City, MO: American Nurses Association.

Bearinger, L. H., Wildey, L., Gephardt, J., & Blum, R. W. (1992). Nursing competence in adolescent health: Anticipating the future needs of youth. *Journal of Professional Nursing, 8,* 80–86.

Bearinger, L. H., Wildey, L., Gephardt, J., & Blum, R. W. (1991a). *Self-assessed skills and knowledge in adolescent health nursing: A comparison of public health, school health and pediatric nurse practitioners.* Poster presentation to the annual meeting of the National League for Nursing.

Bearinger, L. H., Wildey, L., Gephardt, J., & Blum, R. W. (1991b). Nursing competence in adolescent health: Anticipating the future needs of youth. *Journal of Professional Nursing, 8,* 80–86.

Bronfenbrenner, A. (1979). *The ecology of human development: Experiments by nature and design.* Cambridge, MA: Harvard University Press.

Grey, M., & Flint, S. (1989). 1988 NAPNAP membership survey: Characteristics of members' practice. *Journal of Pediatric Health Care, 3,* 336–341.

Lee, P. R. (1985). Health promotion and disease prevention for children and the elderly. *Health Services Research, 19,* 783–792.

McCarty, P. (1991). Image campaign boosts student enrollments. *The American Nurse, Official Newspaper of the American Nurses' Assn.,* October, 1, 24.

Meeker, R. J., DeAngelis, C., Berman, B., Freeman, H. E., & Oda, D. (1986). A comprehensive school health initiative. *Image: Journal of Nursing scholarship, 18,* 86–91.

National League for Nursing (NLN). (1990a). *Nursing datasource 1990: A research report: Volume I: Trends in contemporary nursing education.* NLN Publication No. 19-2335. New York: Author.

National League for Nursing (NLN). (1990b). *Nursing student census, 1989.* NLN Publication No. 19-2291. New York: Author.

Panzarine, S., Broering, J., Gephart, J., Lucas, S., Minas, E., Savedra, M., St. Germaine, A., & Wildey, L. (1988). Adolescent health care: A challenge for nursing educators. *Journal of Nursing Education, 27,* 278–280.

Perry, C. L., & Jessor, R. (1985). The concept of health promotion and the prevention of adolescent drug abuse. *Health Education Quarterly, 12,* 169–184.

Ruszala-Herbst, J. (1985). Curriculum design for educating nurse practitioners in adolescent health care. *Journal of Nursing Education, 24,* 37–39.

Thurber, F., Berry, B., & Cameron, E. (1991). The role of school nursing in the United States. *Journal of Pediatric Health Care, 5,* 135–140.

Tower, J. (1991). Report of the national survey of the American Academy of Nurse Practitioners, part V: Comparison of nurse practitioners according to practice setting. *Journal of the American Academy of Nurse Practitioners, 3,* 42–45.

PART II

Topical Areas
for Promoting Health

8

Promoting Positive Mental Health during Adolescence

Bruce E. Compas

The promotion of positive mental health and the prevention of psychopathology are essential goals of a comprehensive model of mental health services for any age group. Efforts toward mental health promotion and the prevention of psychopathology are complementary to interventions to treat or remediate emotional and behavioral problems. However, the development and implementation of promotion and prevention programs require a fundamental shift in the paradigm that is typically used to guide most mental health services. Specifically, promotion and prevention programs require a model based on positive human development rather than pathology (Albee, 1982, 1986; Masterpasqua, 1989).

The importance of promoting positive mental health and preventing psychopathology may be especially pressing during adolescence, given the urgent needs and problems that arise during this developmental period (Hamburg & Takanishi, 1989). The purposes of this chapter are to discuss an approach to adolescent mental health based on a conceptualization of positive human development and to offer an agenda for future work in this area. This will include a discussion of the issues involved in defining positive development and positive mental health during adolescence, a description of programs that promote positive adolescent mental health, and an outline of future directions for research and program development.

Defining Positive Mental Health in Adolescence

Psychology's view of the adolescent has been sufficiently negative that, for much of the past, a discussion of the nature of positive mental health during adolescence would have constituted a contradiction in terms. Adolescence was viewed as period of stress and storm in which psychopathology, personal distress, and behavioral dysfunction were considered to be the norm. Adolescents were characterized as self-focused, depressed, rebellious, hostile toward the family, and likely to be involved in deviant peer groups activities (Erikson, 1968; Freud, 1958; Hall, 1904). The accumulation of considerable empirical data has led to substantial changes

159

such that we now characterize adolescence in more positive terms as a developmental stage offering tremendous opportunities for growth and positive outcomes[1] (Feldman & Elliott, 1990; Petersen, 1988; Powers, Hauser, & Kilner, 1989; Chapter 2).

In spite of the increasingly constructive view of adolescence, defining adolescent mental health remains a difficult task. It is unlikely that a single definition can be generated to satisfy the multiple, divergent perspectives that are needed to understand adolescent functioning. Rather, a multiaxial framework is needed to account for differences in positive mental health as a function of the views of adolescents and others in their lives (parents, teachers, peers, mental health professionals); developmental status; and sociocultural factors. Within this framework, the two primary dimensions of positive mental health involve (1) the development of skills to *protect* oneself from stress and (2) the development of skills to *involve* oneself in personally meaningful activities (cf. Noack, 1987).

Protection from Stress

The protective functions of positive adolescent mental health center on the ability and motivation to cope with stress and adversity adequately (Compas, 1987a; Garmezy & Rutter, 1983). Effective coping contributes to positive mental health by providing ways to deal with stressful life experiences of an acute or chronic nature. The multiple stresses associated with adolescence, especially early adolescence, make the attainment of effective coping skills an especially important developmental task during this period (Compas, 1987a, 1987b; Hamburg, 1974). Effective coping includes the development of skills and abilities that protect the well-being of the individual and involves processes that are primarily reactive in nature. That is, it includes the ability of the individual to react effectively to threats, challenges, and losses in the relationship between the self and the environment (Lazarus & Folkman, 1984).

Recent evidence has helped to clarify the nature of the coping processes used by adolescents in the face of stress (see Compas, 1987; Compas, Malcarne, & Banez, in press, for reviews). Effective coping may include the flexible use of strategies for problem solving and emotion management (Band & Weisz, 1988; Compas, Malcarne, & Fondacaro, 1988), the ability to match strategies to the demands of the specific situation (Compas et al., 1988), and the ability to draw on others as sources of social support (Cauce & Srebnik, 1989).

Involvement in Personally Meaningful Activities

The second dimension of positive mental health is characterized by generative functions that include the ability and motivation to involve oneself in personally meaningful instrumental and/or expressive activities that are goal-directed, experienced by the individual as autonomous, and initiated by the self. Personal commitments to meaningful activities and relationships have been central to a number of theories of human functioning, development, and adaptation (Bandura, 1986;

Deci & Ryan, 1985; Lazarus & Folkman, 1984). These various theories propose different mechanisms to explain how commitments are developed and maintained, including the presence of drives that are present from birth (Deci & Ryan, 1985), the effects of contingent rewards and perceptions of self-efficacy (Bandura, 1986), and emotions (Lazarus & Folkman, 1984). Regardless of the source of personal commitments, the involvement in personally meaningful activities and relationships and the pursuit of personally meaningful goals are central to mental health.

Research on this topic has been limited. A recent study by Maton (1990) provided evidence for the relation between meaningful involvement in instrumental activities and adolescents' feelings of subjective well-being. Meaningful instrumental activity was defined as "task or skill related activity which has positive significance or value to the individual involved" (Maton, 1990, p. 298). Maton found that adolescents' life satisfaction and self-esteem were predicted by their level of meaningful instrumental activity independent of social support received from friends and parents. Similarly, involvement in meaningful interpersonal relationships with family and peers has been found to relate to adjustment and well-being (Reisman, 1985).

Domains of Functioning

Adolescents can employ their skills at managing stress and involve themselves in ways that are personally meaningful in a variety of life domains. These different life domains offer various avenues for developing and achieving the central features of positive mental health. Several different systems have been developed to define the central domains of personal functioning. For example, in their descriptions of fundamental human needs, Connell and colleagues (Connell, in press; Connell & Wellbourn, in press; Deci & Ryan, 1985) have highlighted the significance of interpersonal relationships (relatedness), achievement in instrumental activities (competence), and feelings of self-determination (autonomy). In her elaboration of self-system processes, Harter (1985) has distinguished among the domains of academics, interpersonal relationships, athletics, personal appearance, and behavioral conduct.

Individuals differ in the degree to which they are engaged in and committed to different life domains. For a given individual, experiencing success is likely to be more important in some activities and domains than others (Bandura, 1986; Novacek & Lazarus, 1989). Adolescence represents an important developmental period during which personal commitments to different life domains are forged as youth are increasingly exposed to adult roles and opportunities. Further, there are likely to be a variety of commitment patterns that emerge during adolescence as a result of exposure to models, experiences of success and failure, and values that shape what is personally meaningful for the individual. For example, there appear to be gender differences during adolescence in the degree of commitment to instrumental and relationship-oriented domains (e.g., Maton, 1990; Wagner & Compas, 1990).

Positive development has been distinguished from maladaptive developmental paths based the level of individuals' engagement as opposed to disaffection in certain domains (Connell, in press). Not all adolescents develop high levels of involvement in and commitment to domains that they experience as meaningful in their lives. Further, there may be substantial differences in what are considered meaningful and appropriate domains for adolescent involvement as a function of the perspectives of different individuals (adolescents, parents, teachers), developmental level, and sociocultural factors (Chapter 6).

Perspectives of Different Informants

A fundamental problem in the assessment and evaluation of the behavior of any individual is that reports of the occurrence of a behavior and judgments about the acceptability of that behavior will depend on who has provided the information. When different informants are asked to provide their perspectives on what constitutes positive mental health and whether a particular adolescent is "well adjusted," there is likely to be considerable disagreement on both of these grounds. Of particular importance is the possibility of such disagreement between adolescents and adults in their social environments.

This point has been clearly illustrated in research examining reports of different informants on emotional/behavioral problems or psychopathology in adolescents and children. In their meta-analysis of studies in which multiple perspectives were obtained on child and adolescent maladjustment, Achenbach, McConaughy, and Howell (1987) found that the average correlations between reports by parents, teachers, mental health professionals, observers, and self-reports by children or adolescents were quite modest. For example, the correlation between parent and child reports was on average .25. This modest level of correspondence may be due to several factors, including situational differences in behavior and differences in judgments about the nature of problematic emotions and behaviors.

Along this line, Phares and Compas (1990) found that young adolescents made a distinction between emotions and behaviors that they experienced as personally distressing and those that they believed were distressing to their parents. Adolescents reported more personal distress over internalizing problems and perceived their parents to be more distressed by externalizing problems. For example, of those adolescents who reported strong feelings of guilt, 87% reported that this bothered them but only 65% felt that it bothered their mother and only 55% felt that it bothered their father. In contrast, of those adolescents who reported that they "hang around with kids who get in trouble", 54% reported that they were bothered by this, whereas 79% felt that this bothered their mother and 73% felt that it bothered their father. Similar research on the correspondence between the perspectives of adolescents and others on positive mental health has not been conducted. However, it is a reasonable hypothesis that disagreement will occur regarding the nature and occurrence of positive behaviors and emotions as well. For example, it would not be surprising to find that adolescents and their parents disagree about the value of a number of recreational activities that are common for many teens (e.g., playing video games, spending unsupervised time with peers).

Given the possibility or probability that adolescents, parents, and teachers will disagree on the nature and occurrence of various characteristics of positive mental health, how are we to reconcile these differences? Strupp and Hadley (1977) offer a useful framework for comparing divergent perspectives on mental health. They describe the definitions of mental health held by the individual, by society, and by mental health professionals. Individuals, in this case adolescents, define mental health in terms of their own *subjective well-being and feelings of happiness and contentment.* Society, which in the present analysis includes parents and teachers, defines mental health in terms of *behavioral stability, predictability, and conformity to social rules.* Finally, mental health professionals tend to view mental health from the vantage point of *a specified theory of personality or human behavior,* which may include criteria for maladjustment or psychopathology. As Strupp and Hadley note: "It follows from the preceding that the divergent vantage points described may result in different definitions of 'mental health' and consequently in discrepant evaluations of a given individual's functioning and performance" (1977, p. 189). One can go beyond this framework to include the diverse perspectives associated with sociocultural factors. The behaviors that are valued by society and mental health professionals may or may not be related to positive subjective states for adolescents. When we intervene with the goal of promoting positive mental health, considerable care must be taken to account for the potentially divergent goals of the interested parties and to employ measures that are sensitive to these multiple perspectives. Different intervention strategies may be needed to achieve successful outcomes according to these divergent perspectives, and these differences may not always be reconcilable.

Prior research and theory concerned with the concept of positive mental health has included both the *subjective* and *objective* components described above (Connell & Wellborn, in press; Jahoda, 1958; Offer & Sabshin, 1984; Powers et al., 1989; Seeman, 1989; Taylor & Brown, 1988). The subjective components of positive mental health identified by mental health professionals and behavioral scientists have centered on cognitive and affective factors, including an affective experience of subjective well-being or personal happiness, belief in one's personal competence or efficacy in achievement contexts (work and school), a sense of personal control or autonomy, a sense of relatedness to others, and motivation to direct behavior toward personally relevant goals. The relation between positive and negative affect is complex; at a given moment they are inversely related to one another, while over the course of longer periods of time they are essentially unrelated (Diener, 1984; Diener & Emmons, 1985). However, it appears that the predominance of positive affect over negative affect through time is a hallmark of a sense of subjective well-being.

The subjective component of positive mental health is not necessarily characterized by positive beliefs about the self or positive emotions in all domains of life or in all social contexts in which the individual functions. On the contrary, adolescence is marked by increasingly greater differentiation of various aspects of the self (Harter, 1990). The well-adjusted adolescent may feel relatively more competent or efficacious in some domains or social contexts than others. Further, the well-adjusted adolescent may be more or less invested in or committed to certain domains of functioning. As a whole, positive adolescent mental health is likely to be characterized by feelings of competence and positive affect in domains and contexts that are important or meaningful to the individual. Feelings of competence and well-being are achieved through a balance of accurate assessments of the reality of one's skills and life situations, and a set of positively biased self-perceptions or illusions (Taylor & Brown, 1988). That is, accurate assessment of the demands one faces in everyday life and one's personal capacity to handle them is a necessary ingredient of effective functioning in the face of daily problems and stress. However, a strong sense of optimism and the ability to create adaptive positive illusions may be important factors in the ability to cope effectively with more extreme levels of adversity and stress.

The most widely used external representation of positive mental health has been the construct of social competence. Dodge (1986) defines social competence as the degree to which significant others rate an individual as successful in solving and completing relevant social tasks. He outlines five sequential social information processing skills that may serve as the core of adaptive responding in a variety of social contexts: (1) decoding social cues in the environment; (2) interpreting these cues in a meaningful way; (3) accessing and generating potential behavioral responses to the interpreted cues; (4) evaluating the consequences of alternative responses and selecting an optimal choice; and (5) enacting the selected response with behavioral effectiveness and monitoring its effects.

The specific behaviors that characterize social competence will vary with the particular context or situation in which the individual is functioning. As a consequence, social competence requires a diverse repertoire of cognitive and behavioral skills that can be applied in requisite situations. For example, maintaining close ties with one's family will be adaptive for many adolescents but may prove highly maladaptive for youth whose families are characterized by high levels of dysfunction or psychopathology. Thus, observable characteristics of positive mental health cannot be identified independently of the environmental conditions in which the individual adolescent is functioning.

Developmental Factors in Adolescent Mental Health

A developmental perspective underscores the need to conceptualize mental health in dynamic rather than static terms. Emphasis is placed on the identification of adaptive paths or trajectories of development during adolescence rather than a specified endpoint or outcome (Powers et al., 1989). Failure to account for developmental processes during childhood will lead to a misinterpretation of the significance of events during adolescence. Although the facilitation of positive development during adolescence is a goal in its own right, it is equally important to consider the longer-range effects of adolescent experiences on adult development and functioning (see Chapter 2 for a description of the life span developmental perspective). A developmental perspective also highlights the importance of the sequence and the timing of developmental changes relative to peers during adolescence (e.g., the onset of puberty; Brooks-Gunn & Reiter, 1990; Chapters 2 and 9).

Life span developmentalists have emphasized the importance of understanding the effects of events that serve as shared experiences for various age groups or cohorts. These shared events define, to a degree, the experience of growing up for members of a cohort and may affect the developmental paths of many or all members of a group. Social change (or lack of change) at the local, national, or global level may have important effects on what is required for successful adaptation during adolescence. The possibility of mandatory military service in late adolescence, exposure to high rates of violent crime throughout adolescence, and the pressure to experiment with drugs during early adolescence are among the many experiences that distinguish various cohorts as they move through adolescence. Failure to account for such differences may result in inadequate definitions of positive mental health for a particular group.

Sociocultural Differences in Adolescent Mental Health

Perhaps the single most important contextual factor that needs to be considered in defining and promoting the development of positive mental health involves sociocultural differences in the nature of valued and adaptive personal characteristics and behavior (Angel & Thoits, 1987; Spencer & Dornbusch, 1990). Appropriate social norms within a majority culture may not be shared by those outside of that culture. To the extent that majority cultures fail to recognize this, minorities suffer (Chapter 4). The importance of sociocultural differences in the United States will certainly increase in coming years as the proportion of African-American, Hispanic-American, and Asian-American youth increases dramatically. Further, the types of mental health and behavioral problems faced by youth of different sociocultural groups may influence the basic needs of their communities. For example, the growing problems associated with violence and homelessness in urban areas present a different set of concerns than the difficulties faced in more rural communities. A pluralistic definition of mental health will be needed if we are to be responsive to the needs of our society's different groups of adolescents (Laosa, 1984).

Evidence indicates that sociocultural factors are related to the physical and mental health concerns and problems reported by adolescents. For example, Dubow, Lovko, and Kausch (1990) found differences in concerns about psychological and behavioral problems as a function of socioeconomic status and differences in concerns about sexual problems as a function of race. However, similar information about sociocultural differences in definitions of positive or optimal functioning during adolescence has not been reported.

A Multiaxial Framework of Adolescent Positive Mental Health

Integrating these multiple aspects of functioning and varied perspectives on adolescent mental health represents a formidable task. What is required is a multiaxial framework of positive mental health similar to the multiaxial taxonomy of developmental psychopathology proposed by Achenbach (1985; in press). As noted above, the two core axes of a framework for positive mental health involve (1) skills and motives for protecting the self from stress and (2) skills and motives for involving the self in meaningful activities. A third axis is needed to reflect the divergent perspectives and sources of information: adolescents, parents, teachers, and mental health professionals. A fourth axis must reflect developmental changes in the nature of mental health. And a fifth axis is required to represent sociocultural differences in the nature of positive mental health. These five axes are represented in Table 8.1.

Based on this framework, positive mental health during adolescence is defined as *a process characterized by development toward optimal current and future functioning in the capacity and motivation to cope with stress and to involve the self in personally mean-*

Table 8.1.   Multiaxial Framework of Positive Adolescent Mental Health

Axis I: Coping with Stress and Adversity

- Includes skills and motivation to manage acute, major life stressors and recurring daily stressors.
- Includes skills to solve problems (problem-focused coping) and skills for emotion management (emotion-focused coping).
- Effectiveness is characterized by flexibility and the ability to meet the demands of varying types of stress.

Axis II: Involvement in Personally Meaningful Activities

- Includes skills and motivation to engage in instrumental and/or expressive activities that are personally meaningful.
- Includes behaviors and activities that are experienced as autonomous and self-determined.

Axis III: Perspectives of Interested Parties

- Includes the perspectives of adolescents, parents, teachers, and mental health professionals.
- Adolescents emphasize subjective well-being.
- Societal agents (parents, teachers) emphasize behavioral stability, predictability, and conformity to social rules.
- Mental health professional emphasize specified theories of personality or human behavior.

Axis IV: Developmental Factors

- Adolescent development is viewed in light of previous development during childhood and subsequent development during adulthood.
- Developmental changes during adolescence in cognitive, affective, social and biological functioning.
- Cohort differences in events and social context affect the development of positive mental health.

Axis V: Sociocultural Factors

- Sociocultural differences in values regarding optimal development and functioning during adolescence.
- Sociocultural differences in perceived threats to positive mental health and the risk of maladjustment.

ingful instrumental activities and/or interpersonal relationships. Optimal functioning is relative and depends on the goals and values of the interested parties, appropriate developmental norms, and one's sociocultural group. Based on a multiaxial approach to positive mental health during adolescence, this construct cannot be characterized by a single profile or developmental trajectory (Powers et al., 1989). Rather, multiple different developmental paths during adolescence could represent adaptive functioning.

Promotion of Adolescent Mental Health: Examples of Programs That Work

Having outlined a framework to identify the characteristics of positive mental health during adolescence, it is now possible to consider efforts designed to foster systematically adolescent mental health. Existing programs will be discussed in terms of three mechanisms through which change is achieved: (1) programs that facilitate the development of skills for coping with stress and for involvement in personally meaningful activities, (2) programs that promote the development of healthy social environments, and (3) programs that promote positive mental health through public policy.[2]

Skill-Building Programs

TEACHING COPING AND PROBLEM - SOLVING SKILLS. The most widely used programs have been aimed at the enhancement of a set of positive outcomes variously labeled *social competence, life skills,* or *coping skills* (see Hamburg, 1990, for a comprehensive review of these programs). These programs share a common set of concerns centered on the development of the adaptive skills of the individual adolescent. One group of these programs is generic or broad-based in nature, typically delivered as part of the public school curriculum, and aimed at the development of a set of basic skills that enhance individuals' abilities to solve social problems and cope with life stress. A second group of programs has been designed to teach a similar set of skills with the goal of preventing specified problems such as substance abuse (Chapter 12), teen pregnancy (Chapter 9), or aggressive/antisocial behavior (Chapter 13).

The primary goals of generic programs center on the development of a set of attitudes and behaviors that foster positive feelings toward the self, mutually adaptive relations with others, and skills to solve life problems and stressors. These include but are not limited to a sense of self-efficacy; the ability to control one's emotions under stress; the ability to act assertively in changing one's environment in response to a problem; the ability to consider alternative solutions to a problem; the capacity to pursue goal-directed behavior; the capacity to resist pressure from others and, concomitantly, to experience a sense of autonomy and personal control over one's behavior; and the capacity to evaluate the effectiveness of one's actions and pursue alternative solutions if necessary. These goals are shared by several programs, including the Yale–New Haven Social Problem Solving Project (YNH-SPS; Weissberg, Caplan, & Bennetto, 1988) and the Comprehensive Stress Management Program for Children (CSMPC; Ledoux, 1985).

These basic skills are critical in the proactive process of developing a positive sense of oneself, a sense of subjective well-being, and a repertoire of behaviors that allows one to deal with the social environment in a manner that is perceived by others as socially skilled and acceptable. Further, these skills enable the individual to maintain these positive attributes in the face of major life crises and chronic or intermittent daily stress. The goal of these programs is the development of a diverse set of coping skills that can be applied to the variety of stressful events that adolescents are likely to encounter. These coping skills include both active responses to change the source of stress (problem-focused coping) and responses directed to the negative emotions that are experienced in the face of stress (emotion-focused coping). Effective coping is at least in part a function of the individual's ability to match these two forms of coping with controllable as opposed to uncontrollable stress (Folkman, Lazarus, Dunkel-Schetter, DeLongis, & Gruen, 1986; Forsythe & Compas, 1987).

A commonly used protocol involves teaching youth to identify sources of stress in their lives, to recognize the physical and emotional consequences of stress, and to implement adaptive coping responses in the face of stressful events. Specific skills include a six-step response sequence developed by Weissberg et al. (1988) based on an information-processing model of social competence: (1) stop, calm down, and think before you act; (2) state the problem and how you feel; (3) set a positive goal; (4) think of many solutions; (5) think ahead to the consequences; and (6) try the best plan.

Programs have been implemented in schools using formats varying from 8 to 20 sessions during the school year, typically delivered on a weekly basis as part of the regular school curriculum. The programs have usually been carried out by school personnel (teachers, counselors) who have received special training from mental health professionals. Many recent models have argued for a more explicitly developmental approach to the promotion of positive mental health through a series of developmentally appropriate interventions ranging from kindergarten through the twelfth grade (Long, 1986). The YNH-SPS program has shown sensitivity to sociocultural factors by focusing on those sources of stress that are of greatest concern to the inner-city population that has been served by the program. Both the YNH-SPS and CSMPC programs have addressed the developmental level of their participants by focusing on those stressors that are most salient to young adolescents.

Evaluation studies have focused on a variety of outcomes and have shown that these programs are quite promising in promoting various aspects of positive mental health and preventing emotional/behavioral problems. Relative to untrained controls, the YNH-SPS program participants improved their ability to solve social problems effectively; increased their peer involvement; experienced increased impulse control, sociability with peers, and improved academic performance as rated by teachers; and decreased self-reports of misbehavior, including fighting, stealing, and being sent out of the classroom (Weissberg & Caplan, 1989). Young adolescents who participated in the CSMPC, compared with controls, have shown increased ability to use emotion-focused coping skills, decreased perceptions of stress, increased perceptions of personal competence, and lower rates of externalizing emotional/behavioral problems (Compas et al., 1991).

A second set of interventions has been developed to address specific problems or types of psychopathology. An example is the Life Skills Training (LST) approach to the prevention of substance abuse (Botvin, 1983; Botvin & Dusenbury, 1989). The LST program consists of 15 to 20 class periods with seventh graders focusing on three broad areas: (1) information and social resistance skills targeted specifically at substance abuse prevention; (2) generic personal coping skills; and (3) generic social skills. These are addressed through five components of the program whereby participants learn (1) factual information concerning the negative consequences of substance abuse; (2) self-directed behavior change; (3) independent decision making; (4) skills to cope effectively with anxiety; and (5) interpersonal skills (Botvin & Dusenbury, 1989). Efforts have been made to make necessary changes in the program as it has been applied to inner-city minority youth. The Positive Youth Development Program (PYD; Caplan et al., 1992) follows a similar format and has been developed as a more focused adjunct to the generic skills taught in the YNH-SPS program described above.

Programs that target specific problems have documented considerable success. The LST program has proven successful in deterring substance abuse, as program participants have been found to be less likely than controls to begin smoking cigarettes (Botvin & Eng, 1982; Botvin, Eng, & Williams, 1980; Botvin, Renick, & Baker, 1983), to consume alcohol (Botvin, Baker, Botvin, Filazzola, & Millman, 1984), or to use marijuana (Botvin, Baker, Renick, Filazzola, & Botvin, 1984). Similar positive effects have been reported for the PYD program (Caplan et al., 1992).

ENHANCING INVOLVEMENT IN PERSONALLY MEANINGFUL ACTIVITIES. Other programs, in some instances in conjunction with teaching life skills, have focused on increasing adolescents' involvement in roles and activities that are personally meaningful. Most of these programs have developed a network of volunteer opportunities for youth in their local communities that offer youth the opportunity to: explore career roles that have relevance for their future; develop employment-relevant skills; make a contribution to their local communities; and experience a level of engagement and commitment that exceeds many other activities that are typically available to adolescents. Some of these programs are primarily school-based, while others are part of community organizations and structures, including youth service groups, religious groups, and community agencies.

The Teen Outreach Program of the Association of Junior Leagues is an example of an intervention that utilizes volunteer opportunities to prevent problems and promote positive development in adolescents in grades 7 through 12 (Allen, Philliber, & Hoggson, 1990). Volunteer activities include work as aides in hospitals and nursing homes, participation in walkathons, and volunteer work at school. These activities are coupled with classroom-based group discussions on issues related to self-awareness, social awareness, human development, and making life decisions. Program participants, compared to controls who were not exposed to the program, evidenced fewer behavior problems (i.e., pregnancy, school failure, and school suspension) at the end of the program. These changes were positively related to the amount of volunteer activity in which adolescents participated, such that greater volunteer activity was related to fewer behavior problems (Allen et al., 1990). Interestingly, this is one of the few programs that has shown different effects as a function of developmental level. Program participants who were in the higher grades were significantly more likely to have fewer behavior problems than those in the lower grades. Further, participation in more classroom discussions was related to fewer behavior problems in the younger but not the older students. Although the outcome of the program has been measured in terms of the reduction of behavior problems rather than the promotion of positive mental health, this intervention shows considerable promise as an approach to promoting positive development.

The Early Adolescent Helper Program is another program that attempts to create meaningful roles for adolescents through their involvement in volunteer work (developed by Schine and described by Hamburg, 1990). Adolescents serve as "interns, assistants, and helpers two or three times a week in early childhood and after-school child care programs, senior centers, community agencies, and other appropriate settings" (Hamburg, 1990, p. 44). The program has been implemented in over 16 New York City schools and has involved over 1,000 youth as participants. Although evaluative data on the program have not been reported, it represents another promising approach for fostering adolescents' involvement in personally meaningful activities and roles.

Promoting Healthy Social Environments

Relatively fewer programs to develop healthy social environments for adolescents have been the subject of controlled empirical evaluations. However, there are sufficient data available to highlight the promise of this approach as well.

Felner and colleagues (Felner & Adan, 1988; Felner & Felner, 1989) developed and evaluated a program designed to alter the social environment of schools to reduce problems associated with the transitions to junior and senior high school. The intervention included two major components: (1) changing the role of homeroom teachers to provide a link between students, parents, and the rest of the school and to increase support for students; and (2) establishing a stable peer support system by assigning students to all of their academic subjects with the same set of classmates. Participants in the program were absent less often, improved their grade point averages relative to controls, and maintained stable self-esteem, while controls reported lowered self-esteem over the same period of time.

The School Development Program of Comer and his colleagues (Cauce, Comer, & Schwartz, 1987; Comer, 1980, 1988) provides another important example of fostering positive development through the creation of more adaptive social environments in schools. This program is designed to facilitate positive interaction between parents and school staff. A governance and management team is formed, led by the school principal and made up of elected parents and teachers, a mental health specialist, and a member of the nonprofessional support staff. The team decides issues ranging from the school's academic and social programs to changes in school procedures that seem to engender behavior problems. The goal is to facilitate positive social and academic development in students by creating a stronger bond between schools and families. Considerable success has been achieved with the program in elementary schools, and the model is now being applied to junior and senior high schools.

Finally, the Rochester Schools Experiment is designed to increase student engagement (active involvement in tasks or activities) and decrease disaffection (uninterest and alienation) by restructuring the social and physical environments of public schools (Connell, in press). The program alters the social environment by increasing the degree of structure and involvement provided by teachers and by encouraging student initiative and autonomy. Based on the conceptual model described above (Connell, in press; Connell & Wellbourn, in press), the program is designed to increase students' feelings of competence, autonomy, and relatedness as a mechanism for increasing engagement and reducing disaffection. Evaluative data on this promising program are currently being collected.

Promoting Positive Mental Health Through Public Policy

The development and evaluation of interventions to build personal skills and create healthy social environments, and the development and implementation of public policy to promote positive mental health, are different but complementary processes, each requiring unique skills (Cowen, Hightower, Johnson, Sarno, & Weissberg, 1989). A number of efforts to develop public policy to promote healthy development in adolescence have been initiated to accompany the interventions described above; we will provide a brief discussion of their approach.

One function of policy and legislative action is to ensure the effective implementation, continuation, and dissemination of school- and community-based interventions (Cowen et al., 1989). Without adequate financial support for the training of professional and nonprofessional staff to carry out interventions, even programs of the highest quality will fail to make a meaningful contribution to the promotion of adolescent mental health. For programs to succeed, continual monitoring of legislative decision making regarding the allocation of funds will be needed.

Other policy decisions are designed to affect adolescents' behaviors, directly or indirectly, either by providing necessary supports to facilitate the development of adaptive behavior or by imposing limits to deter maladaptive behavior. For example, one major effort involves the restructuring of junior high and middle schools and the relationships among schools, families, communities, and health care settings (Carnegie Corporation of New York, 1989; Comer, 1988; Jackson & Hornbeck, 1989). Policy changes may affect significant risk factors for maladaptive development during adolescence, including laws regarding the purchase of alcohol and the availability of information and services regarding sexual functioning and pregnancy.

Future Directions in the Promotion of Positive Adolescent Mental Health

It is evident from the research reported above that considerable strides have been made in the effort to understand and promote positive mental health during adolescence. Returning to definitional issues discussed earlier, it is clear that (1) programs have achieved success in building both the skills to cope with stress and involvement in personally meaningful activities; (2) both the subjective and objective features of positive mental health have been addressed by these programs; (3) evaluations have included the perspectives of adolescents, parents, teachers, and mental health professionals in determining the effects of the programs; (4) some attention has been paid to the developmental level of the participants; and (5) programs have served diverse groups with socioeconomic backgrounds ranging from inner-city to suburban to rural youth. Building on these initial efforts, the following issues and concerns need to guide future research and intervention in the promotion of adolescent mental health.

Toward a Multiaxial Model of Positive Adolescent Mental Health

The foremost research need in this area is the further investigation of the characteristics of positive adolescent mental health from the perspectives of adolescents, their parents, and their teachers and from the perspectives of different sociocultural groups. What do these groups define as the characteristics of desirable adolescent functioning? How can these perspectives be reliably and validly assessed? These questions are essential to address because of their heuristic importance, and additionally because of their importance in identifying the goals of interventions (see below).

A number of existing instruments should prove useful in the investigation of adolescents', parents', and teachers' perspectives on mental health. For example, Harter (1985) has developed measures of children's and adolescents' self-perceptions of competence and behavior that reflect different domains of functioning (social relationships, academic achievement, athletics, behavior, physical appearance, and global self-worth), vary with developmental level, and can be completed by adolescents, teachers, or parents. Similarly, parallel ratings of social competence can be obtained from adolescents, parents, and teachers on the parent, teacher, and adolescent self-report versions of the Child Behavior Checklist (Achenbach & Edelbrock, 1983, 1986, 1987).

Although existing instruments may adequately assess the occurrence of behaviors and emotions that are central to divergent views of adolescent mental health, further work is needed to understand the significance of these variables for adolescents and others. By examining the value that adolescents, parents, and teachers place on various behaviors and emotions, we will better understand the similarities and differences among these groups in their notions of optimal adolescent functioning if we are to incorporate their perspectives to create meaningful contexts for health promotion. Further, the importance of various behaviors and emotions must be investigated with populations of varying developmental levels and from diverse sociocultural backgrounds. For example, there may be considerable agreement about the importance of desirable subjective states of happiness and contentment as components of good mental health, but greater disagreement between adolescents and adults about the behaviors that comprise adaptive functioning. It seems likely that adolescents will place greater importance on autonomous behaviors, while parents and teachers will put a higher premium on behavior that is responsive to social rules and norms (Strupp & Hadley, 1977). Such areas of potential agreement and disagreement need to documented.

Development and Evaluation of Intervention Programs

Researchers and practitioners concerned with the continued development and refinement of mental health promotion interventions for adolescents are faced with a number of conceptual and pragmatic tasks. These include (1) formulating goals for interventions that reflect the divergent perspectives and values of all interested parties, (2) integrating interventions during adolescence with interventions during childhood and adulthood, (3) identifying the most beneficial ways to sequence generic and problem-specific interventions, (4) ensuring that interventions facilitate change in both adolescents and their social environments, and (5) generating data that evaluate the implementation and effects of such programs.

The need for continued clarification of adolescents', parents', and teachers' views of adolescent mental health has been discussed above. The applied significance of this research lies in its importance for the formulation of goals for intervention programming. The initiation of any intervention should begin with an assessment of the different groups' perceptions of need. Given the high probability that adolescents, parents, and teachers will identify different needs, interventionists will be required to generate program goals that are mutually acceptable to these parties and/or to modify the programs.

For example, in attempting to help families cope with the stress of divorce, programs geared separately for children, for parents, and for parents and children together have been shown to have different effects (Stolberg & Garrison, 1985). Since adolescents, parents, and teachers may have quite different needs, all of which are related to the enhancement of adolescent mental health, separate but coordinated interventions may be required. Because of limited knowledge about the goals of adolescents, parents, and teachers, existing interventions have been skewed toward achieving outcomes that are valued by mental health professionals. As we increase our knowledge of more diverse views of positive mental health, we will be able to achieve outcomes that satisfy the interested parties.

Efforts to promote positive mental health must be sensitive to the developmental needs of the population that is being served. However, an intervention delivered at one point in development cannot be expected to produce effects that last throughout the life span (Weissberg, Caplan, & Harwood, 1991; Zigler & Berman, 1983). Instead, intervention will need to be developmentally sequenced and designed to address the important tasks for a specified period. For example, a case has been made for the need to develop social competence promotion programs that could be delivered in developmentally appropriate ways from preschool through high school (Long, 1986; Weissberg, Caplan, & Sivo, 1989). Future research needs to determine which types of interventions should be uniquely tied to adolescence as part of such a sequence.

In addition, for sequential mental health promotion interventions to be effective, the relation between generic, broad-focused programs and those designed to target specific problems or specific risk factors must be clarified. For example, Weissberg and colleagues found that a generic social competence promotion program did not affect substance abuse in young adolescents, while a program that taught skills and knowledge specific to substance abuse did affect attitudes and behaviors related to drug and alcohol use (Caplan et al., 1989). The timing and sequencing of broad and specific programs have not been determined.

Adaptive and maladaptive patterns of development are the result of ongoing transactions between the person and the environment. As a result, interventions need to be targeted to building adaptive emotions, cognitions, and behaviors in adolescents *and* creating social environments that can facilitate individual development. Interventions need to expand beyond a person-centered model to include a range of helping and socializing interventions. These efforts need to create environments that can accommodate and facilitate the development of varied adaptive patterns of individual adolescent development (Adelman & Taylor, 1988; Powers et al., 1989). This means that the attitudes and behaviors of teachers, parents, and others who interact with adolescents will need to be included as targets of interventions. Moreover, the very structure of educational settings and programs for young adolescents may require alteration to meet the needs of youth during the transition to adolescence (Jackson & Hornbeck, 1989).

Issues in Delivery of Services

Schools have been the primary context for the delivery of formal mental health promotion programs for adolescents. Because of our compulsory education system, the enormous contact between children and schools over the course of childhood and adolescence, and the mission of our educational system to foster adequate social development, schools are likely to remain the primary context for implementing prevention and promotion programs. However, we need to know more about the culture of schools if such programs are to become integrated parts of the school environment (Meyers, 1989).

There are a number of effective ways to establish prevention and promotion within the schools (Bond & Compas, 1989). A novel and potentially important avenue is through School Mental Health Centers (Adelman & Taylor, 1989). The UCLA School Mental Health Project is developing a model for providing mental health services in school-based health centers. Resources for carrying out mental health education programs would include adolescents as peer helpers, parents and other family members, community volunteers, regular school staff, special support staff, and mental health professionals in the community (Adelman & Taylor, 1989). This type of inclusive participation will be necessary if schools are to become an optimal setting for the promotion of positive mental health.

While the schools should remain a primary context for the promotion of positive adolescent mental health, we need to expand the focus of intervention efforts to include out-of-school youth and other settings and contexts, especially the family (Bond & Wagner, 1988). In spite of widespread recognition of the family as a primary resource for adaptive development and a major source of risk for psychopathology, systematic efforts to promote positive adolescent mental health through the family have been lacking. Although interventions for families can be delivered through the schools, alternative interventions are particularly important for reaching adolescents who drop out of high school.

Positive adolescent mental health can also be promoted through agencies and settings in the community, such as youth service organizations, religious institutions, and health care settings. Programs such as those offered by Girls' Clubs provide a means for inner-city youth to participate actively in the larger social environment; similarly, Project Spirit utilizes black churches to reach African-American youth (Price, Cioci, Penner, & Trautlein, 1990). As evidence for the connected roles of mental health and physical health has grown, so has recognition of the need to integrate mental and physical health promotion efforts (Taylor, 1990). As yet, however, health systems have not been well utilized for the promotion of adolescent mental health, either as a goal in itself or as a means to achieve more optimal physical health. Efforts to promote positive mental health should become a part of overall health promotion efforts to facilitate the physical and social development of adolescents (Millstein, 1989).

Summary

It is evident that substantial progress has been made in our understanding of the nature of positive mental health during adolescence and in our ability to promote the development of adaptive functioning in this developmental period. In spite of this outstanding work, formidable research and program development tasks remain. Our efforts to facilitate the development of good mental health during adolescence are likely to be successful only if it is guided by a pluralistic and inclusive model of mental health that represents the perspectives of adolescents and significant adults in their lives, as well as the diverse cultural and ethnic groups in our society. Active collaboration between mental health professionals, adolescents, parents, teachers, policymakaers, and other members of the community is essential to our efforts to define and promote positive and healthy psychological development.

Acknowledgments

Preparation of this chapter was supported in part by National Institute of Mental Health Grant MH43819. The author is grateful to Howard Adelman, members of our research group (especially Kathy Grant), Susan Millstein, and three anonymous reviewers for their comments.

Notes

1. Given our focus on positive mental health, we will not discuss psychopathology in adolescence. It should be noted, however, that rates of some types of psychopathology do increase during adolescence (e.g., delinquency, substance abuse, suicide), most likely as a result of the dramatic changes in biological and social development that occur during this developmental period (Petersen & Hamburg, 1987; Rutter, 1986).

2. It is necessary that this review be selective, as the literature on programs to promote positive mental health and prevent psychopathology in children and adolescents is vast and growing rapidly (for more extended discussion of this literature, see Bond & Compas, 1989; Bond & Wagner, 1988; Hamburg, 1990). The focus here will be on a few programs that exemplify the components of positive mental health outlined above and have specifically targeted adolescents.

References

Achenbach, T. M. (1985). *Assessment and taxonomy of child and adolescent psychopathology*. Beverly Hills, CA: Sage.

Achenbach, T. M. (in press). The derivation of taxonomic constructs: A necessary stage in the development of developmental psychopathology. In D. Cicchetti (Ed.), *Rochester symposium on developmental psychopathology (Vol. 3)*. Hillsdale, N. J: Erlbaum.

Achenbach, T. M., & Edelbrock, C. S. (1983). *Manual for the child behavior checklist and revised child behavior profile*. Burlington: University of Vermont, Department of Psychiatry.

Achenbach, T. M., & Edelbrock, C. S. (1986). *Manual for the teacher's report form and teacher version of the child behavior profile*. Burlington: University of Vermont, Department of Psychiatry.

Achenbach, T. M., & Edelbrock, C. S. (1987). *Manual for the youth self-report and profile*. Burlington: University of Vermont, Department of Psychiatry.

Achenbach, T. M., McConaughy, S. H., & Howell, C. T. (1987). Child/adolescent behavioral and emotional problems: Implications of cross-informant correlations for situational specificity. *Psychological Bulletin, 101*, 213–232.

Adelman, H. S., & Taylor, L. (1988). Clinical child psychology: Fundamental intervention questions and problems. *Clinical Psychology Review, 8*, 637–665.

Adelman, H. S., & Taylor, L. (1989). *Guidebook for a mental health focus*. Los Angeles: UCLA, Department of Psychology.

Albee, G. W. (1982). Preventing psychopathology and promoting human potential. *American Psychologist, 37*, 1043–1050.

Albee, G. W. (1986). Toward a just society: Lessons from observations on the primary prevention of psychopathology. *American Psychologist, 41*, 891–898.

Allen, J. P., Philliber, S., & Hoggson, N. (1990). School-based prevention of teenage pregnancy and school dropout: Process evaluation of the national replication of the Teen Outreach Program. *American Journal of Community Psychology, 18*, 505–524.

Angel, R., & Thoits, P. (1987). The impact of culture on the cognitive structure of illness. *Culture, Medicine, and Psychiatry, 11*, 465–494.

Band, E. B., & Weisz, J. R. (1988). How to feel better when it feels bad: Children's perspectives on coping with everyday stress. *Developmental Psychology, 24*, 247–253.

Bandura, A. (1986). *Social foundations of thought and action: A social cognitive theory*. Englewood Cliffs, NJ: Prentice-Hall.

Bond, L. A., & Compas, B. E. (1989). (Eds.). *Primary prevention and promotion in the schools*. Newbury Park, CA: Sage.

Bond, L. A., & Wagner, B. M. (Eds.). (1988). *Families in transition: Primary prevention programs that work*. Newbury Park, CA: Sage.

Botvin, G. J. (1983). *Life skills training: Teacher's manual (seventh grade curriculum)*. New York: Smithfield Press.

Botvin, G. J., Baker, E., Botvin, E. M., Filazzola, A. D., & Millman, R. B. (1984). Alcohol abuse prevention through the development of personal and social competence: A pilot study. *Journal of Studies on Alcohol, 45,* 550–552.

Botvin, G. J., Baker, E., Renick, N. L., Filazzola, A. D., & Botvin, E. M. (1984). A cognitive-behavioral approach to substance abuse prevention. *Addictive Behaviors, 9,* 137–147.

Botvin, G. J., & Dusenbury, L. (1989). Substance abuse prevention and the promotion of competence. In L. A. Bond & B. E. Compas (Eds.), *Primary prevention and promotion in the schools* (pp. 146–178). Newbury Park, CA: Sage.

Botvin, G. J., & Eng, A. (1982). The efficacy of a multicomponent approach to the prevention of cigarette smoking. *Preventive Medicine, 11,* 199–211.

Botvin, G. J., Eng, A., & Williams, C. L. (1980). Preventing the onset of cigarette smoking through Life Skills Training. *Preventive Medicine, 9,* 135–143.

Botvin, G. J., Renick, N. L., & Baker, E. (1983). The effects of scheduling format and booster sessions on a broad-spectrum psychosocial approach to smoking prevention. *Journal of Behavioral Medicine, 6,* 359–379.

Brooks-Gunn, J., & Reiter, E. O. (1990). The role of pubertal processes in the early adolescent transition. In S. S. Feldman & G. R. Elliott (Eds.), *At the threshold: The developing adolescent.* Cambridge, MA: Harvard University Press.

Caplan, M., Weissberg, R. P., Grober, J. S., Sivo, P. J., Grady, K., & Jacoby, C. (1992). Social competence promotion with inner-city and suburban young adolescents: Effects on social adjustment and alcohol use. *Journal of Consulting and Clinical Psychology, 60,* 56–63.

Carnegie Corporation of New York (1989). *Turning points: Preparing American youth for the 21st century.* Washington, DC: Carnegie Council on Adolescent Development.

Cauce, A. M., Comer, J. P., & Schwartz, D. (1987). Long term effects of a systems-oriented school prevention program. *American Journal of Orthopsychiatry, 57,* 127–131.

Cauce, A. M., & Srebnik, D. S. (1989). Peer networks and social support: A focus for preventive efforts with youths. In L. A. Bond & B. E. Compas (Eds.), *Primary prevention and promotion in the schools* (pp. 235–254). Newbury Park, CA: Sage.

Comer, J. P. (1980). *School power: Implications of an intervention project.* New York: Free Press.

Comer, J. P. (1988). Educating poor minority children. *Scientific American, 259,* 42–48.

Compas, B. E. (1987a). Coping with stress during childhood and adolescence. *Psychological Bulletin, 101,* 393–403.

Compas, B. E. (1987b). Stress and life events during childhood and adolescence. *Clinical Psychology Review, 7,* 275–302.

Compas, B. E., Ledoux, N., Howell, D. C., Phares, V., Williams, R. A., Giunta, C. T., & Banez, G. A. (1991). *Enhancing coping and stress management skills in children and adolescents: Evaluation of a school-based intervention.* Unpublished manuscript, University of Vermont.

Compas, B. E., Malcarne, V. L., & Banez, G. A. (in press). Coping with psychosocial stress: A developmental perspective. In B. Carpenter (Ed.), *Personal coping: Theory, research and application.* New York: Praeger.

Compas, B. E., Malcarne, V. L., & Fondacaro, K. M. (1988). Coping with stressful events in older children and young adolescents. *Journal of Consulting and Clinical Psychology, 56,* 405–411.

Connell, J. P. (in press). Context, self, and action: A motivational analysis of self-system processes across the life-span. In D. Cicchetti (Ed)., *The self in transition: From infancy to childhood.* Chicago: University of Chicago Press.

Connell, J. P., & Wellborn, J. G. (in press). Competence, autonomy, and relatedness: A motivational analysis of self-system proceses. In M. Gunnar & L. A. Sroufe (Eds.), *Minnesota symposium on child psychology (Vol. 23).* Hillsdale, NJ: Erlbaum.

Cowen, E. L., Hightower, A. D., Johnson, D. B., Sarno, M., & Weissberg, R. P. (1989). State-level dissemination of a program for early detection and prevention of school maladjustment. *Professional Psychology: Research and Practice, 20,* 309–314.

Deci, E. L., & Ryan, R. M. (1985). *Intrinsic motivation and self-determination in human behavior.* New York: Plenum.

Diener, E. (1984). Subjective well-being. *Psychological Bulletin, 95,* 542–575.

Diener, E., & Emmons, R. A. (1985). The independence of positive and negative affect. *Journal of Personality and Social Psychology, 47,* 1105–1117.

Dodge, K. A. (1986). A social information processing model of social competence in children. In M. Perlmutter (Ed.), *Minnesota symposium on child psychology (Vol. 18,* pp. 77–125). Hillsdale, NJ: Erlbaum.

Dubow, E. F., Lovko, K. R., & Kausch, D. F. (1990). Demographic differences in adolescents' health concerns and perceptions of helping agents. *Journal of Clinical Child Psychology, 19,* 44–54.

Erikson, E. H. (1968). *Identity: Youth and crisis.* New York: Norton.

Feldman, S. S., & Elliott, G. R. (1990). (Eds.). *At the threshold: The developing adolescent.* Cambridge, MA: Harvard University Press.

Felner, R. D., & Adan, A. M. (1988). The school transition environment project: An ecological intervention and evaluation. In R. H. Price, E. L. Cowen, R. P. Lorion, J. Ramos-McKay, & B. Hitchins (Eds.), *Fourteen ounces of prevention: A casebook of exemplary primary prevention programs.* Washington, DC: American Psychological Association.

Felner, R. D., & Felner, T. Y. (1989). Primary prevention programs in the educational context: A transactional-ecological framework and analysis. In L. A. Bond & B. E. Compas (Eds.), *Primary prevention and promotion in the schools* (pp. 13–49). Newbury Park, CA: Sage.

Folkman, S., Lazarus, R. S., Dunkel-Schetter, C., DeLongis, A., & Gruen, R. J. (1986). Dynamics of a stressful encounter: Cognitive appraisal, coping, and encounter outcomes. *Journal of Personality and Social Psychology, 50,* 992–1003.

Forsythe, C. J., & Compas, B. E. (1987). Interaction of cognitive appraisals of stressful events and coping: Testing the goodness of fit hypothesis. *Cognitive Therapy and Research, 11,* 473–485.

Freud, A. (1958). Adolescence. *Psychoanalytic Study of the Child (Vol. 13).* New York: International Universities Press.

Garmezy, N., & Rutter, M. (1983). (Eds.). *Stress, coping, and development in children.* New York: McGraw-Hill.

Hall, G. S. (1904). *Adolescence: Its psychology and its relations to physiology, anthropology, sociology, sex, crime, religion, and education (Vols. 1 and 2).* New York: Appleton.

Hamburg, B. A. (1974). Early adolescence: A specific and stressful stage of the life cycle. In G. Coelho, D. Hamburg, & J. Adams (Eds.), *Coping and adaptation* (pp. 102–124). New York: Basic Books.

Hamburg, B. A. (1990). *Life skills training: Preventive interventions for young adolescents.* Washington, DC: Carnegie Council on Adolescent Development.

Hamburg, D. A., & Takanishi, R. (1989). Preparing for life: The critical transition of adolescence. *American Psychologist, 44,* 825–827.

Harter, S. (1985). *Manual for the self-perception profile for children.* Denver: University of Denver.

Harter, S. (1990). Self and identity development. In S. S. Feldman & G. R. Elliott (Eds.), *At the threshold: The developing adolescent* (pp. 352–387). Cambridge, MA: Harvard University Press.

Jackson, A. W., & Hornbeck, D. W. (1989). Educating young adolescents: Why we must restructure middle grade schools. *American Psychologist, 44,* 831–836.

Jahoda, M. (1958). *Current concepts of positive mental health.* New York: Basic Books.

Laosa, L. M. (1984). Social competence in childhood: Toward a developmental, sociocultural relativistic paradigm. In J. M. Joffe, G. W. Albee, & L. D. Kelly (Eds.), *Readings in the primary prevention of psychopathology* (pp. 261–285). Hanover, NH: University Press of New England.

Lazarus, R. S., & Folkman, S. (1984). *Stress, appraisal, and coping.* New York: Springer.

Ledoux, N. (1985, November). *A comprehensive stress management program for elementary and secondary students and their families.* Paper presented at the Seventh National Conference on Child Abuse and Neglect, Chicago.

Long, B. B. (1986). The prevention of mental-emotional disabilities: A report from a National Mental Health Association Commission. *American Psychologist, 41,* 825–829.

Masterpasqua, F. (1989). A competence paradigm for psychological practice. *American Psychologist, 44,* 1366–1371.

Maton, K. I. (1990). Meaningful involvement in instrumental activity and well-being: Studies of older adolescents and at risk urban teen-agers. *American Journal of Community Psychology, 18,* 297–320.

Meyers, J. (1989). The practice of psychology in the schools for the primary prevention of learning and adjustment problems in children: A perspective from the field of education. In L. A. Bond & B. E. Compas (Eds.), *Primary prevention and promotion in the schools* (pp. 391–422). Newbury Park, CA: Sage.

Millstein, S. G. (1989). Adolescent health: Challenges for behavioral scientists. *American Psychologist, 44,* 837–842.

Noack, H. (1987). Concepts of health and health promotion. In *Measurement in health promotion and protection* (pp. 5–28). Geneva: World Health Organization.

Novacek, J., & Lazarus, R. S. (1989). *The structure and measurement of personal commitments.* Tulsa, OK: Tulsa Institute of Behavioral Sciences.

Offer, D., & Sabshin, M. (1984). *Normality and the life cycle.* New York: Basic Books.

Petersen, A. C. (1988). Adolescent development. *Annual Review of Psychology, 39,* 583–607.

Petersen, A. C., & Hamburg, B. A. (1987). Adolescence: A developmental approach to problems and psychopathology. *Behavior Therapy, 17,* 480–499.

Phares, V., & Compas, B. E. (1990). Adolescents' subjective distress over their emotional/behavioral problems. *Journal of Consulting and Clinical Psychology, 58,* 596–603.

Powers, S. I., Hauser, S. T., & Kilner, L. A. (1989). Adolescent mental health. *American Psychologist, 44,* 200–208.

Price, R. H., Cioci, M., Penner, W., & Trautlein, B. (1990). *School and community support programs that enhance adolescent health and education.* Washington, DC: Carnegie Council on Adolescent Development.

Reisman, J. M. (1985). Friendship and its implications for mental health or social competence. *Journal of Early Adolescence, 5,* 383–391.

Rutter, M. (1986). The developmental psychopathology of depression: Issues and perspectives. In M. Rutter, C. E. Izard, & P. B. Read (Eds.), *Depression in young people: Developmental and clinical perspectives* (pp. 3–30). New York: Guilford.

Seeman, J. (1989). Toward a model of positive health. *American Psychologist, 44,* 1099–1109.

Spencer, M. B., & Dornbusch, S. M. (1990). Challenges in Studying Minority Youth. In S. S. Feldman & G. R. Elliott (Eds.), *At the threshold: The developing adolescent* (pp. 123–146). Cambridge, MA: Harvard University Press.

Stolberg, A. L., & Garrison, K. M. (1985). Evaluating a primary prevention program for children of divorce: The Divorce Adjustment Project. *American Journal of Community Psychology, 13,* 111–124.

Strupp, H. H., & Hadley, S. W. (1977). A tripartite model of mental health and therapeutic outcomes: With special reference to negative effects in psychotherapy. *American Psychologist, 32,* 187–196.

Taylor, S. E. (1990). Health psychology: The science and the field. *American Psychologist, 45,* 40–50.

Taylor, S. E., & Brown, J. D. (1988). Illusion and well-being: A social psychological perspective on mental health. *Psychological Bulletin, 103,* 193–210.

Wagner, B. M., & Compas, B. E. (1990). Gender, instrumentality, and expressivity: Moderators of the relation between stress and psychological symptoms during adolescence. *American Journal of Community Psychology, 18,* 383–406.

Weissberg, R. P., Caplan, M., & Harwood, R. L. (1991). Promoting competent young people in competence-enhancing environments: A systems-based perspective on primary prevention. *Journal of Consulting and Clinical Psychology, 59,* 830–841.

Weissberg, R. P., Caplan, M. Z., & Bennetto, L. (1988). *The Yale-New Haven Social Problem-Solving Program for Young Adolescents.* New Haven, CT: Yale University, Department of Psychology.

Weissberg, R. P., Caplan, M. Z., & Sivo, P. J. (1989). A new conceptual framework for establishing school-based social competence promotion programs. In L. A. Bond & B. E. Compas (Eds.), *Primary prevention and promotion in the schools* (pp. 255–296). Newbury Park, CA: Sage.

Zigler, E., & Berman, W. (1983). Discerning the future of early childhood intervention. *American Psychologist, 38,* 894–906.

9

"Sex Is a Gamble, Kissing Is a Game": Adolescent Sexuality and Health Promotion

Jeanne Brooks-Gunn and Roberta L. Paikoff

Adolescence is characterized by a series of developmental tasks that need to be mastered. In the realm of sexual development, such tasks include learning to manage feelings of sexual arousal, developing new forms of intimacy and autonomy, experiencing interpersonal relationships with the opposite sex, and developing skills to control the consequences of sexual behavior.

The conceptual framework in which we study sexuality, or what we term *sexual well-being*, employs the constructs of vulnerability and resilience from developmental psychopathology. Vulnerability implies that a particular child or group of children who are at risk in a probabilistic sense for manifesting a certain behavior or set of behaviors are also susceptible to decrements in well-being. Risk factors are those biological, psychosocial, and environmental conditions, broadly defined, known to be associated with negative outcomes or decrements in well-being. The opposite of vulnerability and risk factors are resilience and protective factors. Protective factors and their links to resiliency have not been studied as extensively as risk factors and their links to vulnerability, yet they are critical to the promotion of well-being (Furstenberg, Brooks-Gunn, & Morgan, 1987; Garmezy & Rutter, 1988; Werner & Smith, 1982).

In this chapter, we focus on sexual well-being, first providing a working definition and describing variations in the sexual health of American youth today. Then we turn to a discussion of the risk and protective factors associated with decrements in sexual well-being. The possible factors that are antecedents of vulnerability or resilience include biological, cognitive, social cognitive, and emotional factors, as well as contextual factors (family, peer, school, community, and culture). The ways in which the developmental literature on each of the possible risk factors might be used to promote healthy sexuality are considered, and exemplars of interventions that have been implemented are given. Most of the interventions, while using principles of behavioral change in their design, have not been explicitly linked to the developmental literature on risk factors and vulnerability.

180

Sexual Well-Being: A Definition

What is adolescent sexual well-being? That this question is almost never raised speaks to the cultural construction of adolescent sexuality. We offer a working definition (see also Katchadourian, 1990) that includes four developmental challenges—positive feelings about one's body and the acquisition of secondary sexual characteristics; feelings of sexual arousal and desire; the engagement in sexual behaviors; and, for those teenagers who are engaging in sexual intercourse, the practice of safe sex. All of these occur in the context of the other social, emotional, and cognitive challenges facing the adolescent (Feldman & Elliott, 1990). (1) The transformation into a reproductively mature individual is a major part of the first half of adolescence. How the adolescent experiences these changes, as well as others' responses to the adolescent's emerging adult body, lay the groundwork for teenagers' feelings about their bodies. Healthy feelings include eventual comfort with pubertal changes, satisfaction with body shape and size, beliefs about physical attractiveness, and acceptance of sexual desirability. (2) The emergence of sexual arousal is a response to internal hormonal changes and external responses to the physical manifestations of the internal changes. The desired outcome is an acceptance of these feelings. (3) Sexual behaviors result from arousal and contextual factors. They may be expressed individually or with another person. Typically, individual responses focus on masturbation. Healthy sexuality includes feeling comfortable about choosing to engage in individual sexual behaviors or not to practice them. Sexual behaviors with a partner include kissing, genital and breast touching, vaginal intercourse, oral sex, and anal intercourse. These sexual behaviors may be voluntary or involuntary. Sexual well-being involves engaging in such behavior voluntarily with respect to one's partner.[1] (4) For those youth who are engaging in intercourse, healthy sexuality involves the practice of safe sex. Safe sex typically refers to practices to avoid pregnancy and/or sexually transmitted diseases (STDs). Both contraceptives and sexual practices other than intercourse may prevent pregnancy. While safe sex prevents STDs, including human immunodeficiency virus (HIV) infection, only one contraceptive method—condom use—is known to be effective in preventing STDs. Sexual practices other than intercourse also may reduce the likelihood of acquiring STDs.

Feelings About Pubertal Changes

Adolescent sexuality emerges as the child acquires a reproductively mature body via the process of puberty (Brooks-Gunn & Reiter, 1990). Puberty itself elicits a wide array of emotions—excitement and trepidation, pleasure and dismay—given the rapidity with which changes occur and the radical alterations in the body.

Research in the last decade suggests that puberty per se is not as upsetting as had been thought for both girls and boys. Most girls are not particularly upset by menarche or breast development, although they are sometimes reluctant to discuss these changes (Brooks-Gunn & Warren, 1988; Brooks-Gunn & Zahaykevich, 1989). Certain girls are more likely to have negative experiences, for instance, girls who are early maturers and who receive little or no information from their mothers

(Brooks-Gunn, 1988; Brooks-Gunn & Ruble, 1982). Less is known about boys' feelings about pubertal changes. In a small study of pubertal boys who had an ejaculation, their emotional reactions to it were comparable to girls' reactions to menarche—surprise and pride. Few boys were upset (Gaddis & Brooks-Gunn, 1985).

Boys and girls alike learn a great deal about cultural constructions of pubertal changes via the acceptability of discussing such changes. Information about menarche is obtained primarily through discussions with the mother and close girlfriends, almost never from boys or fathers (Brooks-Gunn, 1987). Even then, clear limits are placed on the range of acceptable topics; girls talk about menarche frequently but seldom discuss breast or pubic hair changes with others (Brooks-Gunn & Zahaykevich, 1989). Much less is known about boys' discussions, but boys seem to learn that pubertal changes are not to be discussed with most people in their lives and certainly not in mixed company. They have no adults to whom they turn for even rudimentary knowledge and no peers with whom they can discuss what these changes mean or how to cope with them (Gaddis & Brooks-Gunn, 1985). Of course, ejaculation, unlike menarche, is directly associated with masturbation, a topic not discussed by girls either.

Satisfaction with one's body shape and size is another aspect of the development of positive feelings about the pubertal body. Generally, girls are less happy with their bodies than are boys throughout the pubertal period (Blyth, Simmons, & Zakin, 1985; Petersen, Tobin-Richards, & Boxer, 1983; Richards, Boxer, Petersen, & Albrecht, 1990). Additionally, girls' dissatisfaction increases with pubertal development (as body fat increases), while boys' discontent decreases (as muscle mass increases; Gross, 1984). Girls are more likely to have poor body images, to diet and binge, and to exhibit frank eating disorders than are boys (Attie & Brooks-Gunn, 1989; Attie, Brooks-Gunn & Petersen, 1990; Chapter 2, Chapter 10).

Feelings of Sexual Arousal

Increases in sexual feelings and arousal follow pubertal changes. Unfortunately, discussing feelings of sexual desire is taboo. Girls' emerging feelings of sexual desire are treated as if they did not exist or, worse, as if they were not normal. In such an atmosphere, it is not surprising that relatively few teenage girls talk about desire or masturbation. Boys are allowed to acknowledge sexual arousal via jokes (although not to refer directly to their own feelings).

Girls respond less to erotic or provocative stimuli than boys. However, differences in sexual arousal are smaller than have been assumed, especially among sexually experienced adolescents and young adults. Many routine messages in the youth culture, such as advertisements, music, rock videos, movies, and fashion, have the potential to stimulate sexual arousal in both boys and girls. However, girls are more likely to respond to erotic stimuli in the context of a heterosexual relationship than are boys (Chilman, 1983).

Sexual Behavior

Almost all boys masturbate during the adolescent years. While fewer girls do so, and do so less frequently, it is believed that the incidence has increased over the last two decades, with a third of all girls having masturbated by the middle adolescent years (Chilman, 1983; Coles & Stokes, 1981).

Youth typically engage in a series of sexual behaviors with partners of the opposite sex prior to sexual intercourse. These include kissing and genital and breast touching. Such behaviors are often practiced in the late elementary school years (Westney, Jenkins, & Benjamin, 1983). We do know that the expected progression of behaviors for white youth goes from kissing to petting to intercourse; black youth are more likely to move directly from kissing to intercourse (Udry, 1988).

Over the past 25 years, youth have been having heterosexual intercourse at earlier and earlier ages.[2] In the 1940s, less than 10% of white girls had intercourse by age 16 (as estimated in select samples; Kinsey, Pomeroy, & Martin, 1948). In 1971, a third of all unmarried white girls 16 years of age had had intercourse, with an increase to almost half by 1988 (Hofferth & Hayes, 1987; Pratt, 1989). Ethnic differences exist, with higher prevalence rates in blacks compared to whites, although the gap is narrowing.

Historically, boys have been far more likely to have intercourse as teenagers than have girls (Hofferth & Hayes, 1987), although proportionally more girls than boys have become sexually active in the last decade. According to the National Survey of Adolescent Males, in 1988, one-half of 16-year-old boys and 86% of 19-year-old boys were sexually active (Sonenstein, Pleck, & Klu, 1989). Ethnic differences are particularly striking, since 69% of black boys had intercourse by age 15 or earlier compared to 26% of white boys. These differences do not diminish until age 18 (83% of black boys and 71% of white boys reported having had intercourse by age 18).[3]

While we know about age at first intercourse, our knowledge about the early sexual experiences of youth is scanty (Brooks-Gunn & Furstenberg, 1989; Hayes, 1987; Hofferth & Hayes, 1987; Paikoff & Brooks-Gunn, in press). We do not know how youth feel about their first experiences, with whom they share and from whom they withhold information, or how they decide to have sex the first time (although most recall not having planned for it). Information on the conversations between boys and girls that lead to intercourse or negotiations regarding the use of contraception is nonexistent.

The majority of teenagers believe that it is acceptable to have sex with a steady partner (53%), with more boys than girls agreeing (63% vs. 43%) and more tenth than eighth graders agreeing (63% vs. 43%; American School Health Association, 1988). At the same time, teenagers do not believe that it is acceptable to have sex with several different people (80%), with more girls subscribing to this belief than boys (91% vs. 69%). At the same time, even in 1979, about one-half of sexually active teenagers reported having one partner, the rest having two or more (Zelnik, 1983).

Safe Sex

As mentioned previously, safe sex is dependent on the use of contraception or sexual practices that do not expose the youth to pregnancy or STDs. The contraceptive literature has been reviewed elsewhere (Brooks-Gunn & Furstenberg, 1989).

Adolescence as an age group has the highest rate of STDs (U. S. Congress, 1991), excluding HIV infection and acquired immune deficiency syndrome (AIDS). However, concern is growing about the spread of HIV in adolescents via sexual behavior and drug use (Brooks-Gunn, Boyer, & Hein, 1988; Brooks-Gunn et al., 1989; Miller, Turner, & Moses, 1990).

Between two-thirds and four-fifths of teenagers know that using condoms reduces the risk of HIV infection (Brooks-Gunn & Furstenberg, 1990; DiClemente, Boyer, & Morales, 1988), and virtually all believe that sexually active people should use condoms (National Adolescent Student Health Survey, 1988). Have teenagers altered their sexual behavior since the HIV epidemic?[4] A significant number report using condoms more frequently (but not always) as a response to the risk of HIV (Sonenstein et al., 1989; Brooks-Gunn & Furstenberg, 1990). Looking at condom use over a 10-year period, condom use at last intercourse for 17- to 19-year-old metropolitan boys generally rose from 21% in 1979 to 58% in 1988. And, condom use at first intercourse increased 110% in 1987–1988 compared to a 1975–1982 base period (Sonenstein et al., 1989). However, teenagers do not use condoms every time they have sex. Individuals engaging in known risk behaviors for contracting HIV are the ones least likely to use condoms. Only about 29% of the adolescents in the 1988 National Adolescent Student Health Survey who had used intravenous drugs, who had sex with someone who had used drugs intravenously, or who had sex with a prostitute had used a condom at last intercourse, in comparison to 58% of the total sample of boys (Sonenstein et al., 1989).

Developmental Issues in the Study of Sexual Well-Being

At least three developmental issues need to be considered—the timing of behaviors associated with sexual well-being, the co-occurrence of sexual behaviors with other behaviors, and age trends in the expression of sexual behaviors.

TIMING OF BEHAVIORS ASSOCIATED WITH SEXUAL WELL-BEING. *Timing* refers to where an individual falls with respect to a certain behavior vis-à-vis her or his peer group (Brooks-Gunn, Petersen, & Eichorn, 1985). The peer group may be defined in terms of national norms, community norms, or school or subgroup norms (the most common subgroup classifications being racial, gender, and cultural; see Chapter 4).

Literature on the timing of puberty suggests that early development renders girls vulnerable to various behaviors—smoking, drinking, depressive symptomatology, negative body image, and dieting behavior (Brooks-Gunn, 1988; Brooks-Gunn et al., 1985). The early maturer probably experiences sexual arousal earlier, given the links between arousal and hormonal levels. The early-maturing girl requests (or demands) earlier independence from her parents and has older friends. Additionally, girls with mature bodies probably elicit responses from males that lead to earlier dating and earlier sexual experiences (Gargiulo, Attie, Brooks-Gunn, & Warren, 1987; Magnusson, Strattin, & Allen, 1985). Thus, timing of puberty has implications for the timing of other sexual events.

While the timing of sexual intercourse has been studied, little work has addressed the timing of other sexual behaviors (see Udry, 1988; Westney, Jenkins, & Benjamin, 1983, for exceptions). Sexual experience by late adolescence has become so common over the last two decades as to be normative. By the end of the 19th year today, three-quarters of white girls, four-fifths of black girls, four-fifths of white males, and almost all of black boys have had intercourse, based on data from four national surveys (Moore, Nord, & Peterson, 1989; Sonenstein et al., 1989). This state of affairs in part has shifted concern to the timing of onset during adolescence (rather than after adolescence) and to the practice of safe sex. Early onset of intercourse is defined here as intercourse at age 15 or earlier, and late onset is defined as first intercourse occurring after adolescence. Distinctions also may be made between onset at ages 16–17 and at ages 18–19. Unfortunately, different surveys have used various age classifications, making it difficult to use these classifications across studies. The same is true of studies focusing on risk factors associated with early sex.

The timing of the onset of sexual intercourse raises moral, legal, and developmental issues. Moral perspectives suggest that intercourse should be postponed until marriage, and few adolescents marry. Legal perspectives center on the rights and responsibilities of minors, as well as those of the parents of minors (with most of the legal concerns centering on access to contraceptive information and abortion; see Gardner, Scherer, & Tester, 1989; Melton, 1990). Developmental perspectives tend to sidestep moral and legal concerns, focusing instead on the abilities of different-aged youth to make informed decisions about engaging in sexual behavior and on the identification of antecedent factors that contribute to the timing of sexual behavior.

CO-OCCURRENCE OF OTHER BEHAVIORS. Another issue involves the co-occurrence of sexual behavior with other behaviors. The early onset of sexual behavior is associated with early onset of smoking and drinking, use of illegal substance, dropping out of school, and juvenile delinquency (Furstenberg, Brooks-Gunn, & Morgan, 1987; Jessor & Jessor, 1977). When such behaviors cluster together, youth are vulnerable to long-term problems. Little work exists on how such behavior patterns translate into later problems, that is, whether certain behaviors render youth more vulnerable to later problems than others (Chapter 7).

AGE TRENDS. It is believed that younger adolescents exhibit fewer health-promoting behaviors than do older adolescents or adults. Literature on the chronically ill supports this contention (see Brooks-Gunn, in press, for a discussion of this literature). With respect to sexual well-being, comparisons are usually made between the sexual behavior of younger and older sexually active adolescents, with differences in the antecedent factors contributing to sexual well-being, as discussed later.

Critical Cultural and Individual Factors Related to Sexual Well-Being

Earlier reviews have summarized the primarily sociological literature specifying risk factors for engaging in unprotected intercourse (see Brooks-Gunn & Furstenberg, 1989; Chilman, 1986, pp. 207–208; Morrison, 1985). We wish to discuss three sets of antecedent conditions in detail—the cultural context in which youth develop their sexuality, individual factors that may render teenagers vulnerable to decrements in sexual well-being (biological, emotional, and social cognitive factors), and the proximal environmental contexts in which adolescents find themselves (family, peer, and school). Developmental research is reviewed, and examples of intervention programs based on what is known about each factor are presented. A list of current programs targeting pregnancy prevention (Table 9.1) is presented. STD prevention programs are reviewed in Table 9.2 (taken from the U. S. Congress OTA Report, 1991). Each presents a description of the program evaluation results. Not all are presented in the text for brevity's sake.

Cultural Context

All societies have devised controls for adolescent sexuality because sexual desire emerges as the adolescent acquires a reproductively mature body rather than when a particular society deems it appropriate to begin producing offspring. Diverse strategies for controlling youthful sexuality have been developed, as historical and cross-cultural studies suggest (Paige & Paige, 1985).

MORALITY AND PROHIBITIONS AGAINST SEX DURING ADOLESCENCE. The moral standard states that sex outside marriage is bad for old and young alike. Yet media messages constantly bombard youth with sexual scenarios in which sex outside marriage is the norm. Because of the persistence of sexual prohibitions that are couched in moralistic and judgmental terms, youth are placed in a cultural double bind. If it is unacceptable to be sexually active, then contraceptive advice and planning become less salient and perhaps not even acceptable. At the same time that they are urged to avoid sex, youth are also told to act responsibly. But if intercourse is morally reprehensible, it is also wrong to plan for it. In fact, contraceptive use is lower in youth who have negative attitudes about having sex than among those who have positive attitudes (Fisher, Byrne, & White, 1983).

Mixed messages from adult society may deter adolescents from developing positive attitudes. While adolescents are told to act responsibly, birth control services are not effectively delivered to the teenage population (Jones et al., 1985). We believe that the contradiction between the increasing number of sexually active girls and the moral prohibitions against sexuality fuel many of the institutional, familial, and individual responses to contraceptive use in the United States. This contradiction may underlie our apparent failure to assist teenagers in responsible contraceptive use, a failure grimly reflected, in spite of similar rates of sexual activity, in our higher rates of teenage pregnancy compared to most Western European countries.

GENDER AND CULTURE. Societal constructions of youthful sexuality differ for boys and girls. Even as sexual behavior has increased in girls, as female sexual arousal has been acknowledged, and as reciprocity in sexual relationships is seen as a goal for adults, teenagers still receive gender-linked messages (Fine, 1988), as illustrated by the following rap song (author unknown).

Sex is a gamble/kissin is a game/boys do the action/girls get the blame.
One night of pleasure/nine months of pain/four nights in the hospital/and a baby to name.
They say you're pretty/they say you're fine/nine months later/they say it's not mine.
Think about it/sex is a *sensation*/to the *teenage* generation.

Sexual desire is seen as paramount for boys and is ignored for girls, as seen in the phrase "boys do the action." Girls' desires are almost never discussed, only the consequences of their sexuality, specifically pregnancy. By pretending that female desire does not exist, girls are given few strategies for incorporating it into their lives or for planning on how to handle it. Contrast this situation with that of males, for whom desire is a given. Males may even be socialized to emphasize demonstration of their potency as more important than acting responsibly, limiting their options as well.

Females, in being portrayed as having little desire and having to face the practical and moral consequences of sexuality, are characterized as victims. Girls must protect themselves against the desires of men outside of marriage, given that many societal controls to protect girls seem no longer to be in place (chaperonage, after-school parental supervision, community sanctions encouraging marriage when a pregnancy occurs, sex not being explicitly portrayed in the media) and that the majority of teenagers are having sex. Finally, although females are viewed as victims, males are also viewed as victims—of their hormonal drives. In this scenario, females become perpetrators (e.g., dressing provocatively, contributing to the males' drives). Again, girls must protect themselves, but they are expected to censor themselves as well or risk being blamed. Even in cases without direct physical coercion (perhaps one-fifth to as many as one-quarter of all young women have had sex against their will; see note 1), such a situation sets up males and females as antagonists, in that males are the perpetrators and females the victims of sexual desire. How sexuality is negotiated in such a situation is not clear.

These gender-linked messages about youthful sexuality have probably impeded discussions about sexual well-being and discouraged negotiation over responsible sex. The negative consequences of sexual behavior are emphasized, rather than the positive conditions that are associated with the delay of sexual activity and the practice of responsible sexual behavior. Additionally, males and females are seen as antagonists, and reciprocity is not emphasized. An example of miscommunication between males and females follows: In one study, girls believed that their boyfriends were not very likely to want to use condoms, while boys tended to believe that girls wanted them to use condoms (Kegeles, Adler, & Irwin, 1988). At the same time, boys were more likely to report their intention to use condoms than were girls.

MEDIA. Another window on the cultural milieu in which teenagers develop sexual well-being is the media. Youth, like adults, are bombarded with media messages about attractiveness and sexuality; at least a third of all prime time commercials are

Table 9.1. Teen Pregnancy Prevention Programs

Title	Population Served	Goals	Brief Description	Pregnancy Prevention Evaluation
Baltimore Project (Zabin et al., 1986)	Junior and senior high students, Baltimore public schools; inner city, low socioeconomic status.	Education regarding personal responsibility, goal setting, communication with parents.	Nurses and counselors in school plus an out-of-school clinic: reproductive, educational, group discussion services offered.	Reduced delay in clinic visit after initial sexual intercourse for females, substantial increases in contraceptive knowledge, positive attitudes, delays in sexual initiation, and decreases in sexual activity.
Health Belief Model Intervention Program (Eisen, Zellman, & McAllister, 1990).	13- to 17-year-old volunteers, Texas.	Provides increasing awareness of negative consequences of teen parenting, merits of delaying sexual activity, reducing perceived barriers to contraceptive use.	Sessions on factual information; group discussion of factual information; group discussion of values, feelings, and emotions; making decisions and taking personal responsibility for behavior.	For males, virgins more likely to maintain abstinence, nonvirgins more likely to use contraception.
Human Sexuality: Values & Choices (Donahue, 1987).	Public school seventh and eighth grades, at four sites (Midwest & Southwest).	Promotes values in approach to sexual issues; stress on communication with parents, techniques to resist peer pressure and postpone sexual initiation.	15-session course for adolescents, 3-session course for parents, teaching facts and promoting values.	Initial posttest showed participants to be more knowledgable about sex and to have talked to parents about it more than controls. Effects showed sizable decay, however, over the long term.

Program	Target Population	Goals	Intervention	Results
Postponing Sexual Involvement (Howard & McCabe, 1990)	Eighth graders in Atlanta public schools (within city limits)	Presents facts about sexual behavior and develop skills to assist teens in resisting social pressures that lead to early sexual involvement.	Ten classroom periods of education; five periods of education by adult health educator; five sessions of skill training by peer educators; reproductive health services available as well.	For preintervention virgins, long-term program effects on postponement of first intercourse, lower frequencies of first intercourse, and fewer pregnancies.
McMaster Team Project (Thomas et al., 1992)	Seventh and 8th graders in Hamilton, Ontario, randomly assigned.	Improves responsible decision making about sexual behavior and decrease the incidence of pregnancy in teens 16 years of age and under.	Ten-hour small group coed sessions focusing on problem solving and decision making.	None yet.
Mayor Frasers' Project on Adolescent Pregnancy and Parenting Information from Mayor's office, City of Minneapolis, MN. (no other ref. available)		A 20% reduction of pregnancy by 1990; a 20% increase in services to teenage mothers; educational attainment by teenage parents.	Broad-based community campaign through the media, schools, family planning clinics, and public health services.	Rates of pregnancy stabilized for 10- to 11-year-olds from 1986 to 1987; no final date.
School/Community Program for Sexual Risk Among Teens (Vincent et al., 1987)	Adolescents in a county of South Carolina.	To reduce the number of unintended pregnancies by unmarried adolescents.	Educational sessions in school, along with sessions for parents and clergy; media and public speaking on topic.	Dramatic decrease in teen birth rates when target county compared with other local counties and with prior years within the target county.
Youth Health Services (Pratt & Pollard, 1988)	Adolescents in the community of Elkins, West Virginia.	Provides assistance to youth in order to delay sexual initiations and pregnancy.	Depends on the client's risk status; ranges from media and civic groups to individual counseling on decision making.	At 1-year follow-up, only 1 of 146 adolescents at moderate risk of pregnancy reported initiation of sexual intercourse (no comparison group studied).

Table 9.1. Teen Pregnancy Prevention Programs (*continued*)

Title	Population Served	Goals	Brief Description	Pregnancy Prevention Evaluation
Girls' Club of America (Nicholson & Postrado, 1990)	Nine- to 18-year-old girls across the United States.	Improves communication with parents, provides assertiveness training, presents life options.	Group discussion sections that vary by age and access to community health clinics.	Significant effects in assertiveness training; joint participation effects for assertiveness training and parent communication sessions; however, parent communication program participants at less risk prior to intervention.
Teen Aid Family Life (Weed et al., 1988)	Junior high school males and females.	Promotes value of abstinence from sexual activity; value of individual life.	Three-week curriculum unit in schools.	Pre-post test impact on values, greater for females than for males.
Role-Playing Intervention (Gilchrist & Schinke, 1983)	High school males and females, suburban population.	Aids teens in role-playing and assertiveness training techniques.	Curricular sessions on human sexuality, modeling techniques, communication skills, problem solving.	Adolescents did better than controls in role playing assertiveness techniques.
Fertility Appreciation for Families (Kirby & Paradise, 1987)	Volunteer teenagers and parents; no controls.	Promotes parent–child communication, stressing value of delaying the onset of sexual activity.	Four sessions with parents and children.	Lowest pregnancy rates among participants than in general population, but participants were a volunteer (and hence nonrandom) subsample of the community.
Youth Incentive Entitlement Pilot Program (Olsen & Farkas, 1987)	Black urban teenagers aged 14–19; only females analyzed.	Promotes academic success and provides work.	Employment guaranteed to program participants if they continued in school. Youth worked part-time during the school year, full time in the summer.	Childbearing delayed by 10% when employment opportunities increased between 25% to 45% (but see Olsen & Farkas, 1987, for discussion of fixed vs. nonfixed effects models).

Program	Target population	Purpose	Intervention	Results
Teen Outreach (Philliber & Allen, 1992).	Eleven- to 19-year-old youth in 30 schools nationwide.	Promotes school continuation; aims to reduce pregnancy and delinquency rates.	Classroom instruction, group discussion, out-of-school volunteer work.	Participants had lower rates of school failure, suspension, dropping out, and pregnancy compared to both random and nonrandom controls.
Condom Mailing Program (Kirby et al., 1989)	National random sample of 16- to 17-year-old males.	Promotes knowledge and condom use among teenage males.	Mailing of pamphlet about condom use, order form for free condoms.	Telephone interview. The majority receiving the pamphlet remembered it; higher scores on knowledge about condoms test; no difference in condom use.
Summer Training and Education Program, STEP (Sipe, Grossman, & Milliner, 1988)	Aimed at 14- and 15-year-olds with academic problems.	Aids teenagers via remedial instruction and employment experience.	Fifteen-month program: two summers of half-time employment; 1 full year of school support.	Participants who were sexually active increased their knowledge of contraception; at 14- to 17-month follow-up, participants had greater knowledge about pregnancy prevention than controls, but sexual initiation, sexual activity, and pregnancy rates were unaffected.
"I Have a Future" Program Information available from: Dr. Lorraine Williams Greene The Mehany Medical College Box A90 1005 D.B. Todd Blvd. Nashville, TN 37208	Ten- to 17-year-old African-American youth in housing projects in Nashville, Tennessee.	Increase positive cultural association, delay onset of sexual activity and pregnancy.	Volunteer participation in a variety of group activities (e.g., sessions on substance abuse, job readiness, human sexuality).	None yet.

Table 9.2. Results of Primary Prevention Efforts for STDs and HIV Infection Among Adolescents

Reference	Goal	Intervention(s)/ Outcome Measure(s)	Research Design	Study Population/ Sample Size/Data Collection Year	Brief Description
Schools: Brown, et al. (1989)	Improve knowledge, attitudes toward future behaviors and tolerance for people with AIDS, and coping strategies.	*Intervention:* Two 45-minute classes on AIDS taught by health teachers. About half of each session was a film presentation; the remaining time was an open class discussion. *Outcome Measure:* Performance on knowledge, attitude, and coping survey.	Pretest/posttest design, no comparison group.	*Study Population:* Predominantly white, suburban, middle-class Rhode Island seventh and 10th graders. *Sample Size:* 7th grade: 174; 10th grade: 139 *Year Data Collected:* NA	Knowledge test scores increased significantly for both grades. Students in both grades reported a greater likelihood to engage in safer behaviors. The seventh graders changed their attitudes toward risk behaviors and tolerance of people with AIDS. Only the former changed significantly for tenth graders. Seventh-grade males and tenth-grade females reported being more tolerant. Seventh graders reported endorsing wishful thinking and self-criticism coping strategies less frequently, and tenth graders reported endorsing social withdrawal less frequently and problem-solving coping strategies more frequently.
DiClemente, et al. (1989)	Improve knowledge of AIDS, decrease misconceptions, and increase tolerance of individuals with AIDS.	*Intervention:* Three class period AIDS prevention curricula presented on consecutive days. *Outcome Measure:* Performance on knowledge questionnaire.	Pretest/posttest control group design. Comparison of the intervention and control groups.	*Study Population:* Middle and high school students in the San Francisco Unified School District. *Sample Size:* High school: 254 Middle School: 385 *Year Data Collected:* 1986 or 1987.	Intervention group showed statistically significant knowledge gains and fewer misconceptions. Middle school students demonstrated more knowledge gain (mean of 4.8) than high school students (mean of 3.5), and both groups had more knowledge than the nonintervention group. Students in the intervention group showed less fear of having a student with AIDS in the classroom.

Huszti et al. (1989)	Increase knowledge of AIDS and improve attitudes toward people with AIDS and practicing preventive behaviors.	*Intervention:* 45-minute AIDS educational program using either a lecture or a film. *Outcome Measure:* Performance on knowledge and attitude questionnaire.	Pretest/posttest and 1-month follow-up design. Volunteer subjects were randomly assigned to one of three conditions: lecture, film, or no program. *Study Population:* Tenth-grade students aged 14 to 17 attending two suburban Oklahoma City area public schools. *Sample Size:* 448 students completed the pretest, posttest, and follow-up. *Year Data Collected:* NA	Intervention groups' knowledge scores increased significantly from pretest to posttest and decreased significantly at 1-month follow-up, although scores were still higher than at the pretest. Students hearing the lecture had significantly higher knowledge scores than either the film or no-program group at both posttest and follow-up. Students watching the film had significantly higher scores than the no-program group. In addition, the intervention groups had significantly more positive attitudes toward people with AIDS and preventive behaviors than the no-program group. However, these attitudes decreased significantly 1 month later. Students' attitudes toward preventive behaviors were not significantly different than at pretest. Females had significantly higher levels of knowledge and more positive attitudes toward people with AIDS at all measurement times and more positive attitudes toward preventive behaviors than males at posttest and follow-up. *Remark:* Students' initially high positive attitudes toward preventive behaviors may have created a ceiling effect.
Miller and Downer (1987)	Improving knowledge of AIDS and attitudes.	*Intervention:* 50-minute multimedia AIDS program. *Outcome Measure:* Performance on knowledge and attitude survey.	Pretest/posttest design, no comparison group. *Study Population:* Seattle high school students. *Sample Size:* 114 students completed pretest 1 month prior to and 1 week after educational program; 53 students completed a posttest 8 weeks later. *Years Data Collected:* 1986–87.	Students' knowledge test scores increased from 78% to 90%. The percentage who thought they might get AIDS did not decrease significantly. The 8-week posttest showed retention of knowledge.

Table 9.2. Results of Primary Prevention Efforts for STDs and HIV Infection Among Adolescents (*continued*)

Reference	Goal	Intervention(s)/ Outcome Measure(s)	Research Design	Study Population/ Sample Size/Data Collection Year	Brief Description
Sroka (1986)	Improve knowledge and modify attitudes and behavioral intentions.	*Intervention:* 5 days of STD education. *Outcome Measure:* Performance on knowledge, attitudes, and behavioral intentions survey.	Pretest (1 week before)/posttest (1 week after) design involving a control group. Teachers were also asked to evaluate what they perceived to be significant gains in students' knowledge, attitudes, and behavioral intentions.	*Study Population:* Ninth-grade students in an urban inner-city area. *Sample Size: Intervention group:* 67 (completed pretest and posttests) *Control group:* 87 (completed pretest and posttests) *Year Data Collected:* 1986.	Knowledge, attitudes, and behavioral intentions improved in the intervention group compared with the control group (although significance was not determined). In general, a large proportion of teachers felt that significant gains had been made in students' knowledge (98%), attitudes (81%), and behavioral intentions (77%). *Remark:* Evaluation was not broad based. Teachers surveyed were located in only three states. Results are not generalizable to other populations.

NA = not available.

[a]This study reviews the following five school sex education programs: Dawson (1986), Furstenburg et al. (1986), Kirby (1984), Marsiglio and Mott (1986), and Zelnick and Kim (1982).

[b]The clinics are located in Gary, Indiana; Muskegon, Michigan; Jackson, Mississippi; Dallas, Texas; Quincy, Florida; and San Francisco, California.

Source: U.S. Congress, OTA

what have been termed *beauty* advertisements, the selling of products using young, attractive women (Tan, 1979), and the number and explicitness of sexual references have increased dramatically in the last decade. In 1985, the average teenage viewer saw almost 2,000 sexual references on television; in stark contrast, references to birth control or to STDs were almost nonexistent (Brown, Childers, & Waszak, 1990).

The media have the potential to reach almost all teenagers and their families. For media messages to be effective in changing attitudes or behavior, they must be repetitive, consistent, understandable, and receive community support (Flay, 1987; U. S. Congress, 1991).

Public health service messages on condom use to prevent HIV were aired starting in 1988. Mass mailing campaigns have been attempted by the Centers for Disease Control (CDC) with its brochure "Understanding AIDS," which describes modes of HIV transmission as well as methods of prevention. Such campaigns, however, rely on the communication of such material to adolescents either through discussion with parents or reading of the pamphlet, and it appears that a majority of parents who received the pamphlet did not discuss it with their 10- to 17-year-old children (Brooks-Gunn & Furstenberg, 1990; U. S. Congress, 1991). These findings suggest that the more local media efforts, in conjunction with other community efforts, also have been initiated (see Table 9.1, notably the Program for Sexual Risk Reduction Among Teens; Vincent, Clearie, & Schluchter, 1987).

Individual Factors

BIOLOGICAL FACTORS. Of the biological changes associated with puberty, hormonal factors are thought to account in part for the onset of sexual activity, either through effects occurring prenatally or via activation effects that change hormonal levels at puberty. Hormonal activation may influence behavior directly by increasing arousal or indirectly by the social stimulus associated with physical changes.

Additionally, contextual effects, if entered into the equation, might account for more of the variation in sexual activity than hormonal levels. Initiation of sexual behavior is highly associated with what is perceived as normative in one's peer group (Furstenberg, Moore, & Peterson, 1986), so it is likely that while very early sexual initiation may be in part hormonally mediated, by the time that behavior is normative, social factors may account for sexual initiation (see, Gargiulo et al., 1987, for a similar argument about dating behavior). Thus, even when hormonal effects are demonstrated, they must be evaluated relative to social factors before assuming direct or large hormonal–sexual behavior associations (Brooks-Gunn & Warren, 1988). Race differences in the initiation of intercourse prior to puberty also speak to the importance of social and contextual factors in sexual behavior (Clark, Zabin, & Hardy, 1984; Westney, et al., 1983).

SOCIAL COGNITIVE FACTORS. A number of social cognitive processes could influence adolescents' ability to manage their sexual well-being, including (1) understanding of intimate relationships, (2) understanding of the biological process of conception, (3) decision-making or problem-solving skills, and (4) perceptions of risk.

UNDERSTANDING OF INTIMATE RELATIONSHIPS. Social cognitive developmental models positing the development of social relational concepts have been applied to the study of peer relationships (Damon, 1977; Selman, 1980), to friendships (Savin-Williams & Berndt, 1990), and to sexual behavior (Gfellner, 1986). In general, these models find that with age, adolescents are increasingly able to take others' perspectives and to understand concepts of mutuality and reciprocity in relationships with age mates (however, see Gfellner, 1986, for a contradictory discussion of sexual behavior concepts through adulthood). As in other areas of social cognitive research, explicit links between social cognitive abilities and behavior in friendships and intimate relationships have not been assessed. However, it seems reasonable to posit that an individual who is capable of applying concepts of mutuality and reciprocity to a sexual relationship might also be more willing to communicate with a partner regarding sexual activity and contraception.

UNDERSTANDING THE BIOLOGICAL PROCESS OF CONCEPTION AND HIV TRANSMISSION. Several studies have applied neo-Piagetian models to the development of understanding the process of conception (Bernstein & Cowan, 1975; Goldman & Goldman, 1982). In most cultures, by late childhood (ages 10 or 11), children appear able to articulate a fairly accurate understanding of conception and pregnancy. U. S. youth are seen to lag a year or two behind those of other Western countries, perhaps due to the lack of early and nationally mandated sex education programs (Goldman & Goldman, 1982).

Virtually all teenagers know that HIV is transmitted via sexual intercourse and intravenous drug use, at least in urban areas such as San Francisco, New York City, Philadelphia, and the state of Massachusetts (over 90% by 1988; Brooks-Gunn & Furstenberg, 1990; Sonenstein et al., 1989). These percentages are comparable to those reported by adults in the National Health Interview Survey (Hardy & Dawson, 1989). At the same time, more misinformation is reported by teenagers than by adults (i.e., beliefs that casual contact and donating blood are transmittal modes; for example, in the Philadelphia sample, over a fifth of the teenage girls believed that the virus could be transmitted by giving blood).

DECISION- MAKING SKILLS. The possibility that decision-making or problem-solving abilities might influence adolescents' ability to manage sexual well-being has received particular interest in recent years (Fischhoff, 1989; Furby & Beyth-Marom, 1992; Luker, 1975; Paikoff, 1990). There is very little evidence to suggest that older adolescents (e.g., 15 years or above) differ substantially from adults in their decision processes and general abilities; however, little age-comparative research exists (Furby & Beyth-Marom, 1992). Although adults and older adolescents may be quite similar in the processes by which they make decisions, they may differentially weight both positive and negative consequences of decisions regarding sexuality and contraception. Such developmental differences might lead to extreme risk taking in adolescents when viewed through adult eyes (Furby & Beyth,-Marom, 1992, Gardner, 1990).

PERCEPTIONS OF RISK. Generally, health-related behavior is not altered unless the consequences are seen as serious (Janz & Becker, 1984). Therefore, all other things being equal, a teenager would have to believe that she was likely to become pregnant if engaging in unprotected intercourse and that becoming pregnant would have serious negative consequences in order to alter her behavior (e.g., use contraceptives or delay sexual activity). Teenagers often say that they had unprotected intercourse because they did not think they would conceive and/or were not anticipating having intercourse. Individuals tend to underestimate the personal risk of an undesirable outcome and to believe that they are at less risk than are their peers (Turner, Miller, & Moses, 1989; Weinstein, 1987).[5]

Many pregnant teenagers report that they took risks and procrastinated with respect to contraceptive use, suggesting that they have some awareness of the risk of pregnancy (Zabin & Clark, 1981). Poor insight, lack of future orientation, or lack of other high-level cognitive processes may explain in part such risk taking, but such notions have not been directly tested. At the same time, younger adolescents probably have a hard time calculating precise probabilities about risk, despite the general recognition that "they took a chance." Studies suggest that probability estimates are very inaccurate and that many teenagers are unable to complete a pregnancy probability task (Smith, Nenney, Weinman, & Mumford, 1982).

If an event has not yet occurred, the probability of risk is usually underestimated (Turner et al., 1989). Teenagers who become pregnant for the first time usually seem surprised; "It couldn't happen to me" (Brooks-Gunn & Furstenberg, 1989). Researchers have not yet investigated risk perception as a function of sexual experience, however.

Teenagers also are often misinformed or uninformed about the time of the month when one is most likely to get pregnant and the effectiveness of various types of contraceptives. Only one-third of all teenagers are able to identify the phase of the cycle in which the risk of pregnancy is greatest (Morrison, 1985; Zelnik & Kanter, 1977), with younger teenagers being less likely to do so (although some have suggested that this in itself does not increase teenagers' risk taking; see Kirby, 1988).

Finally, assessing personal risk may be difficult, given that teenagers' sexual identity is probably characterized by ambivalence, secretiveness, and negativity, reflecting the cultural backdrop. Whether and in what ways teenagers differ from adults and from each other with respect to these dimensions of risk assessment is not known.

Environmental Factors

PEERS. Teenagers depend on peers for much of their sexual information and may be influenced by peers' sexual behavior. Misinformation is probably communicated with great frequency throughout peer networks. For example, teenagers are likely to perceive their peers as having more permissive attitudes toward sex than they themselves hold. In a 1988 national survey of students, one-third believed that it is not acceptable to have sex, but believed that one-quarter of their peers would agree. Four-fifths felt that it is acceptable to say no to sex, but only three-fifths believed that their peers would agree (American School Health Association, 1988). We know little about how friends influence teenagers' sexual behavior. At the very least, teenagers act on what they believe their friends are doing (leaving aside the question of whether their perceptions are accurate; Newcomer, Gilbert, & Udry, 1980). Blacks may be less influenced by their peers than whites, boys less than girls, and older teens less than younger ones (Furstenberg et al., 1986; Smith & Udry, 1985; Udry & Billy, 1987). Perhaps peers are more salient when the behavior in question is less common or has acquired less normative status in a particular group. Several programs attempt to train adolescents in specific social skills germane to delaying the onset of sexual activity, often including role-playing situations (Eisen, Zellman, & McAlister, 1985; Gilchrist & Schinke, 1983; see Table 9.1).

FAMILIAL FACTORS. Discussions about sex and reproduction between parents and their adolescent children occur more frequently than is commonly thought. In a 1982 survey, approximately two-thirds of 15-year-old girls had talked about intercourse and one-half about contraception with their parents; similar percentages were reported by 18-year olds (Dawson, 1986). Large discrepancies exist between the perceptions of parents and their teenagers on their discussions regarding sex and birth control (Newcomer & Udry, 1985). Teenagers who rate perceived communication with their parents as poor are likely to initiate sex, as well as smoking and drinking, earlier than those who do not (Jessor & Jessor, 1977). While reported close relationships and communication with parents are associated with later age of intercourse and better contraceptive use, almost no process-oriented research has examined how parents may influence their teens' sexual behavior (Brooks-Gunn & Furstenberg, 1989; Morrison, 1985).

Many parents report discussing AIDS with their children. In 1990, 68% of parents had discussed AIDS with their 10- to 17-year-olds, with more mothers (78%) than fathers (56%) doing so (Dawson, 1990). However, little is known about the content of these discussions.

Familial discussions can be enhanced. A mass mailing of pamphlets on condoms resulted in a large number of boys reporting that they had discussions with their parents (Kirby, Harvey, Claussenius, & Novar, 1989). Parent–child programs have been used to enhance family discussions (Nicholson & Postrado, 1990). However, such programs may never reach the parent–child dyads who need it the most and in whom communication is the worst (see also Donohue, 1987; Weed, Olsen, & Tanas, 1988). Little is known about whether such approaches are effective in increasing knowledge, family comfort, or contraceptive use. Finally, parents may be involved in community programs, such as the one by Vincent and his colleagues (1987).

SCHOOL FACTORS. Teenagers who are not doing well in school and have lower educational aspirations are more likely to have sex during adolescence than those faring better in school (Hofferth & Hayes, 1987). School functioning itself is mediated by education, job, and welfare status of the mother (Furstenberg et al., 1987; Spenner & Featherman, 1978), such that children in poverty are clearly at risk for both school failure and early sexuality. If students do not expect to complete or do well in school, the motivation to avoid pregnancy may be lower.

Providing the means to reach otherwise unattainable goals (i.e., going to college when the family is unable to pay or when others in the neighborhood or school are unlikely to attend) is a means to enhance the desirability of delaying pregnancy (and perhaps sexual activity) by focusing on schooling (see the Youth Incentive Entitlement Pilot Program and the Summer Training and Education Program in Table 9.1).

Around 80% of American high school students have taken a sex education course and have received AIDS education in school (Dawson, 1990). Such programs often increase knowledge regarding reproduction and pregnancy risk, but do not necessarily influence behavior (Kirby, 1984, 1988; U. S. Congress, 1991).

A growing number of schools provide reproductive health-related services such as counseling and, in some cases, access to contraceptives and gynecological examinations. Use of these clinics is high, especially among adolescents without other sources of health care. The use of clinics for counseling regarding sexual and contraceptive decision making only appears to take place in clinics that offer contraceptive services (Kirby, Waszak, & Ziegler, 1990). However, the effects of clinics on contraceptive behavior have yielded mixed findings.

Interventions to Promote Sexual Well-Being

We have chosen to list interventions in the context of risk factors for several reasons. First, the health promotion literature distinguishes between intervention strategies that are person focused and environmentally or contextually focused. By pairing interventions with one or several risk factors, the explicit links to both individual and environmental factors are made. Indeed, many interventions have been faulted for being so individually oriented that they seem to espouse a "blame the victim" approach. Interventions need to pay more attention to the situations in which sex occurs; the role of families, peers, and schools; and the mixed messages of the cultural milieu. We wish to strengthen such trends, which informed our decision to discuss interventions in the sections on antecedent risk factors.

Second, intervention programs vary as to their outcomes, with some focusing on specific outcomes, such as delay of the onset of intercourse or use of contraception, while others focus on more inclusive outcomes, such as school academic and behavioral success, as well as delay of intercourse. In the sexual health promotion literature, both specific and general paradigms are represented. Often the specific approaches are based on public health models, with heavy doses of information dissemination or specific change agents specified, such as peer modeling. Such paradigms tend to overemphasize single risk factors, or a limited set of them, as being responsible for a particular behavior (Feiner & Felner, 1989). They also focus on prevention more than health promotion. The more general paradigms are likely to conceptualize healthy behavior as multidetermined and different domains of healthy behavior as interrelated (i.e., students who are doing well in school and motivated to stay in school are less likely to engage in behaviors that lead to unsafe sex). A focus on multiple antecedent risk conditions might help overcome the narrow etiological models used previously, while a consideration of the similarities and differences in factors that lead to various domains of health might broaden the scope of intervention programs to include health promotion.

Third, interventions have been notoriously deficient in helping youth to manage risky behavior and to anticipate risky situations in advance. Since risk factors cannot always be eliminated or altered, individuals need to learn to manage risk. Given that being an early maturer is a risk factor for early onset of intercourse (and timing of maturation is not particularly amenable to change, except via extreme changes in diet and exercise; Brooks-Gunn, 1988), the sexually oriented situations that an early maturer might encounter need to be identified, and then the individual needs to be given information or skill training on how to either avoid the situation (delay dating older boys) or manage it (avoid drinking, being alone, or discussing the ground rules for sex early on). As another example, risk factors for sexual abuse in girls include parents who are heavy drinkers, who use illegal substances, and who smoked as teenagers (Moore et al., 1989). While youth cannot alter their parents' past behavior, they can learn to avoid parents in certain situations. Programs might also consider helping adolescents anticipate the situation in which their judgment and control might be compromised.

Fourth, thus far in this chapter, we have not distinguished between health promotion and disease prevention. We have taken the 1979 report *Healthy People: The Surgeon General's Report on Health Promotion and Disease Prevention* as an exemplar of the need to consider both simultaneously in order to define sexual health or wellbeing (see also Bond & Compas, 1989; Mechanic, 1990). The developmental challenges to sexual well-being with which we began the chapter are based on current notions of health promotion. The fourth aspect of sexual well-being—safe sex— also is considered vis-à-vis disease prevention. Most of the interventions reviewed here (Hofferth & Hayes, 1987; Paikoff & Brooks-Gunn, in press) have as their express goal preventing pregnancy. The educational campaigns against the HIV infection also are preventative in nature (Turner et al., 1989; U. S. Congress, 1991). However, a few of the recent initiatives stress healthy sexuality, as well as pregnancy prevention. For example, some programs stress feeling good about one's body and about sexual maturation changes. Others focus on helping individuals negotiate sexual encounters with peers, including respect for a potential partner's request for safe sex. Such a broadening of the intervention agenda to include promotion as well as prevention is critical. However, it is unlikely to be accomplished if all aspects of healthy sexuality are not taken into account (i.e., feeling positive about one's body) and if disease prevention is the only goal.

Fifth, given these caveats, the program evaluation literature suggests the following. (1) Most programs increase reproductive knowledge but do not alter the likelihood of early onset of intercourse. Information alone is probably not enough to alter sexual behavior in most teenagers, especially if it is not explicit. (2) School-based clinics, a great hope of the 1970s, have proved to be somewhat disappointing. Clinics that are open only during school hours, that provide multiple services and do not highlight their contraceptive services, that do not have staff specially trained to provide contraceptive services, that do not have outreach (either school or community components), and that do not have wide community support probably will not substantially alter contraceptive use. Perhaps a joint school–community effort, like that in Baltimore (Zabin, Hirsch, Smith, Streett, & Hardy, 1986), will prove to be a better model. (3) Little attention has been paid to approaches that have been used to change other health behaviors, or to the principles underlying behavioral change more generally (exceptions being the Health Belief Model and the Howard and Gilchrist studies cited in Table 9.1), or to experiences in altering adult sex and behavior (see the discussion of changes in homosexual men since the AIDS epidemic in Turner et al., 1989). (4) Pregnancy prevention programs must start by junior high school (see Hamburg, 1986). (5) Mechanisms by which sexual behavior change is initiated or maintained must be examined. Several smoking prevention studies have examined self-efficacy, problem solving, role playing, decision making, and the like in order to see if such factors are altered by and if they are associated with behavior change (Gilchrist & Schinke, 1983). More targeted approaches are needed, particularly to identify groups of students most likely to begin sexual encounters early (the group also most likely to have unprotected intercourse). In many of the studies reviewed, it is unclear whether sexual activity, contraceptive behavior, or pregnancy resolution decisions (e.g., to abort rather than continue) were changed, or how other mediators were associated with sexual behavior.

Conclusions

We recommend that interventions include both individualistic and environmental contextual approaches to altering behavior. Most interventions focus on the individual, either through information dissemination, fear arousal, skill training, or building up motivations regarding school and work. Another set spends more time on the context in which sexuality is expressed, either through peer training efforts, media campaigns, communitywide interventions, or, in a few instances, family interventions. Policy in the area of teenage sexuality has been fragmented and often polarized (witness the recent decision of AT&T to stop funding Planned Parenthood because of its focus on abortion and on teenage pregnancy and the current furor over New York City's Chancellor of Education's desire to provide condoms through the city high schools as a response to the HIV epidemic). This is as true at the national level as it is at the local level.

Multiple pathways to sexual well-being probably exist. Acknowledgment of various routes to healthy sexuality might defuse the political nature of policy debates. We present several such pathways—practicing sexual abstinence but having positive feelings about one's body; not engaging in sexual intercourse with another but engaging in self-exploration; engagement in sexual behavior with another in the context of a committed relationship in middle or late adolescence and using safe sex practices; and engagement in preintercourse behaviors with another during the early and middle adolescent period, which may or may not result in intercourse in later years. More negative pathways might include involuntary sexual behavior/ abuse during childhood or the early adolescent years; intercourse in the beginning of adolescence without contraceptives; multiple partners and unsafe practices; and sexual intercourse as a way of obtaining drugs. Other enhancing and limiting pathways could be specified. The point is that research is needed to identify such pathways, to specify their antecedents, and to track their developmental trajectories (see Jessor & Jessor, 1977, and Powers, Hauser, & Kilner, 1989, for examples in other domains of adolescent behaviors). From a policy perspective, programs could be initiated that discourage the more limiting pathways and encourage those positive pathways acceptable to a specific community.

Acknowledgments

This chapter was written with funding from the National Institutes of Health and the W. T. Grant Foundation, whose support is appreciated. We would like to thank F. F. Furstenberg, Jr., P. L. Chase-Lansdale, S. G. Millstein, and three anonymous reviewers for their comments. Denise Dougherty of the Office of Technology Assessment is also to be thanked.

Notes

1. However, many youth, especially girls, may be pressured to engage in sexual behaviors—incest, rape, and prostitution. Only one current national survey has asked about involuntary and voluntary sexual experience (Moore, Nord, & Peterson, 1989). Using data on 18- to 22-year-olds from the 1987 National Survey of Children, the percentages reporting nonvoluntary sexual intercourse by age 20 were very high (and were probably an underestimate)—12.7% for white females, 8% for black females, 1.9% for white males, and 6.1% for black males. About half of all nonvoluntary sexual experiences occurred before the age of 14 for the girls; such experiences were almost nonexistent for the boys prior to age 14.

2. Most discussions of adolescent sexuality fail to consider homosexual youth. The number of male youth who engage in homosexual acts and in both homosexual and heterosexual acts is limited, although knowledge of such variations is critical to understanding HIV transmission in teenagers and bridges between homosexual and heterosexual partners (Remafedi, 1987; Savin-Williams, 1988). Little is known about adolescent females' practice of lesbian sexual activity as well (Jaffe, Seehaus, Wagner, & Leadbeater, 1988).

3. We have very little information on the prevalence of sexual behavior for Asian American, Native American, or different Hispanic groups. Information from large-scale national surveys on variations in onset of intercourse in adolescents of different social classes and mental or physical health statuses also is rare.

4. Most youth have not stopped having sexual intercourse because of the possibility of being infected with HIV (Brooks-Gunn & Furstenberg, 1990). About 10% of teenagers report this behavior change. Delay of onset of sexual intercourse does not seem to be a response either. The percentage of sexually active boys aged 17 to 19 years in metropolitan areas increased from 66% to 76% from 1979 to 1988 (Sonenstein et al., 1989). The proportion of girls engaging in

intercourse leveled off between 1979 and 1982 but seems to have increased from 1982 to 1988. The most common response of youth is to say that they are more selective in choosing partners. However, we know almost nothing about what it means to teenagers to be more selective.

5. Youth are quite realistic in their perceptions of risk for contracting the virus in that most youth do not believe that they are at high risk. In the 1988 National Survey of Adolescent Males, only 5% reported that they had a high chance of getting AIDS in the next 5 years, with twice as many blacks and Hispanics as whites saying so (Sonenstein et al., 1989). This is a little more than one-half of the boys who would be classified as high risk using their self-reports of behavior rather than of the risk of AIDS (3% had engaged in homosexual activity, 3% reported an STD, 1% had had sex with a prostitute, and 2% had used drugs intravenously or had a sexual partner who had). However, even low-risk teenagers seem to recognize that there is the possibility of infection. In the Philadelphia sample, only one-tenth of the boys and girls indicated that "teens like me don't get AIDS" (Brooks-Gunn & Furstenberg, 1990). Over 80% of the boys in the national survey disagreed with the statement that "AIDS is so uncommon that it is not a big worry" (Sonenstein et al., 1989).

References

American School Health Association (1988). *National adolescent student health survey*. Washington, DC: American Alliance for Health, Physical Education, Recreation and Dance, American School Health Association, Association for the Advancement of Health Education, and Society for Public Health Education.

Attie, I., & Brooks-Gunn, J. (1989). The development of eating problems in adolescent girls: A longitudinal study. *Developmental Psychology, 25,* 70–79.

Attie, I., Brooks-Gunn, J., & Petersen, A. C. (1990). The emergence of eating problems: A developmental perspective. In M. Lewis & S. Miller (Eds.), *Handbook of developmental psychopathology* (pp. 409–420). New York: Plenum Press.

Bernstein, A. C., & Cowan, P. A. (1975). Children's concepts of how people get babies. *Child Development, 46,* 77–91.

Blyth, D. A., Simmons, R. G., & Zakin, D. F. (1985). Satisfaction with body image for early adolescent females: The impact of pubertal timing within different school environments. *Journal of Youth and Adolescence, 14,* 207–225.

Bond, L. A., & Compas, B. E. (Eds.). (1989). *Primary prevention and promotion in the schools*. Newbury Park, CA: Sage.

Brooks-Gunn, J. (1987). Pubertal processes and girls' psychological adaptation. In R. Lerner & T. T. Foch (Eds.), *Biological–psychosocial interactions in early adolescence: A life-span perspective* (pp. 123–153). Hillsdale, NJ: Erlbaum.

Brooks-Gunn, J. (1988). Antecedents and consequences of variations in girls' maturational timing. *Journal of Adolescent Health Care, 9,* 365–373.

Brooks-Gunn, J. (in press). Why do young adolescents have difficulty adhering to health regimes? In N. Krasnegor (Ed.), *Developmental aspects of health compliance behavior*. Hillsdale, NJ: Erlbaum.

Brooks-Gunn, J., Boyer, C. B., & Hein, K. (1988). Preventing HIV infection and AIDS in children and adolescents: Behavioral research and intervention strategies. *American Psychologist, 43,* 958–964.

Brooks-Gunn, J., Duke-Duncan, P., Ehrhardt, A., Hein, K., & Shafer, M. (1989). Adolescent HIV infection in Special Article: Nicholas, S. W., Sondheimer, D. L., Willoughby, A. D., Yaffe, S. J., & Katz, S. L., Human Immunodeficiency Virus infection in childhood, adolescence, & pregnancy: A status report and national research agenda. *Pediatrics, 83,* 299–301.

Brooks-Gunn, J., & Furstenberg, F. F., Jr. (1989). Adolescent sexual behavior. *American Psychologist, 44,* 249–257. Reprinted in R. E. Muus (Ed.), *Adolescent behavior and society: A book of readings* (4th edition, pp. 243–254). New York: McGraw-Hill.

Brooks-Gunn, J., & Furstenberg, F. F., Jr. (1990). Coming of age in the era of AIDS: Sexual and contraceptive decisions. *Millbank Quarterly, 68,* 59–84.

Brooks-Gunn, J., Petersen, A. C., & Eichorn, D. (Eds.). (1985). Time of maturation and psychosocial functioning in adolescence. *Journal of Youth and Adolescence, 14*(3/4).

Brooks-Gunn, J., & Reiter, E. O. (1990). The role of pubertal processes in the early adolescent transition. In S. Feldman & G. Elliott (Eds.), *At the threshold: The developing adolescent.* Cambridge, MA: Harvard University Press.

Brooks-Gunn, J., & Ruble, D. N. (1982). Menarche: Fact and fiction. In G. C. Hongtadarum, R. McCorkle, & N. F. Woods (Eds.), *The complete book of women's health* (pp. 52–58). Englewood Cliffs, NJ: Prentice-Hall.

Brooks-Gunn, J., & Warren, M. P. (1988). The psychological significance of secondary sexual characteristics in 9- to 11-year-old girls. *Child Development, 59,* 161–169.

Brooks-Gunn, J., & Zahaykevich, M. (1989). Parent–child relationships in early adolescence: A developmental perspective. In K. Kreppner & R. M. Lerner (Eds.), *Family systems and life-span development* (pp. 223–246). Hillsdale, NJ: Erlbaum.

Brown, J. D., Childers, K. W., & Waszak, C. S. (1990). Television and adolescent sexuality. *Journal of Adolescent Health Care, 11,* 62–71.

Brown, L. K., Fritz, G. K., & Barone, V. J. (1989). The impact of AIDS education on junior and high school students: A pilot study. *Journal of Adolescent Health Care, 10,* 386–392.

Chilman, C. S. (1983). *Adolescent sexuality in a changing American society: Social and psychological perspectives for the human service professions. (2nd ed.).* New York: Wiley.

Chilman, C. S. (1986). Some psychosocial aspects of adolescent sexual and contraceptive behaviors in a changing American society. In J. B. Lancaster & B. A. Hamburg (Eds.), *School-age pregnancy and parenthood: Biosocial dimensions* (pp. 191–217). New York: Aldine de Gruyter.

Clark, S. D., Jr., Zabin, L. S., & Hardy, J. B. (1984). Sex, contraception and parenthood: Experience and attitude among urban Black young men. *Family Planning Perspectives, 16,* 77–82.

Coles, R., & Stokes, G. (1981). *Sex and the American teenager.* New York: Harper & Row.

Damon, W. (1977). *The social world of the child.* San Francisco: Jossey-Bass.

Dawson, D. A. (1986). The effects of sex education on adolescent behavior. *Family Planning Perspectives, 18,* 162–170.

Dawson, D. A. (1990). AIDS knowledge and attitudes for January–March 1990: Provisional data from the National Health Interview Survey. *Advance data, 193.* DPHHS, PHS, CDC, National Center for Health Statistics, Washington, DC.

DiClemente, R. J., Boyer, C. B., & Morales, E. S. (1988). Minorities and AIDS: Knowledge, attitudes and misconceptions among black and Latino adolescents. *American Journal of Public Health, 78,* 55–57.

DiClemente, R. J., Pies, C. A., Stoller, E. J., Straits, C., Olivia, G. E., Haskin, J., & Rutherford, G. W. (1989). Evaluation of school-based AIDS education curricula in San Francisco. *The Journal of Sex Research, 26,* 188–198.

Donahue, M. J. (1987). *Human sexuality: Values and choices.* Minneapolis: Technical report of the National Demonstration Project Field Test, Search Institute.

Eisen, M., Zellman, G. L., & McAlister, A. (1985). A health brief model approach to adolescents' fertility control: Some pilot program findings. *Health Education Quarterly, 12,* 185–210.

Eisen, M., Zellman, G., & McAllister, A. (1990). Evaluating the impact of a theory-based sexuality and contraceptive education program. *Family Planning Perspectives, 22,* 61–171.

Feldman, S. D., & Elliot, G. (Eds.). (1990). *At the threshold: The developing adolescent.* Cambridge, MA: Harvard University Press.

Felner, R. D., & Felner, T. Y. (1989). Primary prevention programs in the educational context: A transactional-ecological framework and analysis. In L. A. Bond & B. E. Compas (Eds.), *Primary prevention and promotion in the schools* (pp. 13–49). Newbury Park, CA: Sage.

Fine, M. (1988). Sexuality, schooling, and adolescent females: The missing discourse of desire. *Harvard Educational Review, 58,* 29–53.

Fischhoff, B. (1989). Making decisions about AIDS. In V. M. Mays, G. W. Albee, & S. F. Schneider (Eds.), *Primary prevention of AIDS* (pp. 168–205). Newbury Park, CA: Sage.

Fisher, W., Byrne, D., & White, L. (1983). Emotional barriers to contraception. In D. Byrne & W. Fisher (Eds.), *Adolescents, sex, and contraception* (pp. 207–239). Hillsdale, NJ: Erlbaum.

Flay, B. R. (1987). Mass media and smoking cessation: A critical review. *American Journal of Public Health, 77,* 153–160.

Furby, L., & Beyth-Marom, R. (1992). Risk taking in adolescence: A decision-making perspective. *Developmental Review,* pps. 1–44.

Furstenberg, F. F., Jr., Brooks-Gunn, J., & Morgan, S. P. (1987). *Adolescent mothers in later life.* New York: Cambridge University Press.

Furstenberg, F. F., Jr., Moore, K. A., & Peterson, J. L. (1986). Sex education and sexual experience among adolescents. *American Journal of Public Health, 75,* 1331–1332.

Gaddis, A., & Brooks-Gunn, J. (1985). The male experience of pubertal change. *Journal of Youth and Adolescence, 14,* 61–69.

Gardner, W. (1990). A life-span theory of risk-taking. Paper presented at the *Eighth Texas Tech Symposium on interfaces in psychology,* Lubbock, Texas.

Gardner, W., Scherer, D., & Tester, M. (1989). Asserting scientific authority: Cognitive development and adolescent legal rights. *American Psychologist, 44,* 895–902.

Gargiulo, J., Attie, I., Brooks-Gunn, J., & Warren, M. P. (1987). Girls' dating behavior as a function of social context and maturation. *Developmental Psychology, 23,* 730–737.

Garmezy, N., & Rutter, M. (1988). *Stress, coping, and development in children.* Baltimore: Johns Hopkins Paperbacks.

Gfellner, B. M. (1986). Concepts of sexual behavior: Construction and validation of a developmental model. *Journal of Adolescent Research, 1,* 327–347.

Gilchrist, L. D., & Schinke, S. P. (1983). Coping with contraception: Cognitive and behavioral methods with adolescents. *Cognitive Therapy and Research, 7,* 379–388.

Goldman, R. J., & Goldman, J. D. (1982). How children perceive the origin of babies and the roles of mothers and fathers in procreation: A cross-national study. *Child Development, 53,* 491–504.

Gross, R. T. (1984). Patterns of maturation: Their effects on behavior and development. In M. D. Levine & P. Satz (Eds.), *Middle childhood: Development and dysfunction* (pp. 47–62). Baltimore: University Park Press.

Hamburg, B. A. (1986). Subsets of adolescent mothers: Developmental, biomedical, and psychosocial issues. In J. B. Lancaster & B. A. Hamburg (Eds.), *School-age pregnancy and parenthood: Biosocial dimensions* (pp. 115–145). New York: Aldine de Gruyter.

Hardy, A. M., & Dawson, D. (1989). AIDS knowledge and attitudes for December, 1988. *Advance Data.* Vital and Health Statistics of the National Center for Health Statistics, Number 175. Washington, DC: U. S. Department of Health and Human Services.

Hayes, C. D. (Ed.). (1987). *Risking the future: Adolescent sexuality, pregnancy, and childbearing, Volume I.* Washington, DC: National Academy of Sciences Press.

Hofferth, S. L., & Hayes, C. D. (Eds.). (1987). *Risking the future: Adolescent sexuality, pregnancy, and childbearing, Volume II.* Washington, DC: National Academy of Sciences Press.

Howard, M., & McCabe, J. B. (1990). Helping teenagers postpone sexual involvement. *Family Planning Perspectives, 22,* 21–26.

Huszti, H. C., Clopton, J. R., & Mason, P. J. (1989). Acquired immunodeficiency syndrome educational program: Effects on adolescents' knowledge and attitudes. *Pediatrics, 84,* 986–994.

Jaffe, L. R., Seehaus, M., Wagner, C., & Leadbeater, B. J. (1988). Anal intercourse and knowledge of acquired immunodeficiency syndrome among minority-group female adolescents. *Journal of Pediatrics, 112,* 1005–1007.

Janz, N. K., & Becker, M. H. (1984, Spring). The health belief model: A decade later. *Health Education Quarterly, 11,* 1–47.

Jessor, R., & Jessor, S. L. (1977). *Problem behavior and psychosocial development.* New York: Academic Press.

Jones, E., Forrest, J., Goldman, N., Henshaw, S., Lincoln, R., Rosoff, J., Westoff, C., & Wulf, D. (1985). Teenage pregnancy in developed countries: Determinants and policy implications. *Family Planning Perspectives, 17,* 53–63.

Katchadourian, H. (1990). Sexuality. In S. A. Feldman & G. Elliott (Eds.), *At the threshold: The developing adolescent* (pp. 330–351). Cambridge, MA: Harvard University Press.

Kegeles, S. M., Adler, N. W., & Irwin, C. E. (1988). Sexually active adolescents and condoms: Changes over one year in knowledge, attitude, and use. *American Journal of Public Health, 78,* 460–461.

Kinsey, A. C., Pomeroy, W. B., & Martin, C. E. (1948). *Sexual behavior in the human male.* Philadelphia: W. B. Saunders.

Kirby, D. (1984). *Sexuality education: An evaluation of programs and their effects.* Santa Cruz, CA: Network Publications.

Kirby, D. (1988). *The effectiveness of educational programs to help prevent school-age youth from contracting HIV: A review of relevant research.* Washington DC: Center for Population Options.

Kirby, D., Harvery, P. D., Claussenius, D., & Novar, M. (1989). A direct mailing to teenage males about condom use: Its impact on knowledge, attitudes and sexual behavior. *Family Planning Perspectives, 21,* 12–18.

Kirby, D., Waszak, C., & Ziegler, J. (1990). *An assessment of six school-based clinics: Their reproductive health services and impact upon sexual behaviors.* Washington, DC: Center for Population Options.

Kirby, P., & Paradise, L. V. (1987). *Fertility appreciation for families: Prevention services demonstration project.* Unpublished manuscript, University of New Orleans, New Orleans, LA.

Luker, K. (1975). *Taking chances: Abortion and the decision not to contracept.* Berkeley: University of California Press.

Magnusson, D., Strattin, H., & Allen, V. L. (1985). Biological maturation and social development: A longitudinal study of some adjustment processes from mid-adolescence to adulthood. *Journal of Youth and Adolescence, 14,* 267–283.

Marsiglio, W., & Mott, F. (1986). The impact of sex education on sexual activity, contraception use and premarital pregnancy among American teenagers. *Family Planning Perspectives, 18,* 151–161.

Mechanic, D. (1990, January–February). Promoting health. *Society,* 16–22.

Melton, G. B. (1990). Knowing what we do know: APA and adolescent abortion. *American Psychologist, 45,* 1171–1173.

Miller, H. G., Turner, C. F., & Moses, L. E. (Eds.) (1990). *AIDS: the second decade.* Washington, DC: National Research Council.

Miller, L., & Downer, A. (1987, June). Knowledge and attitude change in adolescents following one hour of AIDS instruction. Paper presented at the III International Conference on AIDS, Washington, DC.

Moore, K. A., Nord, C. W., & Peterson, J. L. (1989). Nonvoluntary sexual activity among adolescents. *Family Planning Perspectives, 21,* 110–114.

Morrison, D. M. (1985). Adolescent contraceptive behavior: A review. *Psychological Bulletin, 98,* 538–568.

National Adolescent Student Health Survey. (1988). *National survey reveals teen behavior, knowledge and attitudes on health, sex topics.* Washington, DC: Association for the Advancement of Health Education.

Newcomer, S. F., Gilbert, M., & Udry, J. R. (1980, September). *Perceived and actual same sex peer behavior as determined of adolescent sexual behavior.* Paper presented at the annual meeting of the American Psychological Association, Los Angeles.

Newcomer, S. F., & Udry, J. R. (1985). Parent–child communication and adolescent sexual behavior. *Family Planning and Perspective, 17,* 169–174.

Nicholson, H. J., & Postrado, L. T. (1990). Girls Clubs of America, "Preventing adolescent pregnancy": Effectiveness of two components of a comprehensive approach. In J. J. Card (Chair), *Preventing adolescent pregnancy: Evaluating the methods and results of experimental prevention programs.* Symposium conducted at the biennial meeting of the Society for Research on Adolescence, Atlanta, GA.

Olsen, T. J., & Farkas, G. (1987, May). *The effect of economic opportunity and family background on adolescent fertility among low-income Blacks.* Final report to NICHD, Grant # R01-HD-19153. Columbus, Ohio: Ohio State University. Revised.

Paige, K. E., & Paige, J. M. (1985). *Politics and reproductive rituals*. Berkeley: University of California Press.

Paikoff, R. L. (1990). Attitudes toward consequences of pregnancy in young women attending a family planning clinic. *Journal of Adolescent Research, 5,* 467–484.

Paikoff, R. L., & Brooks-Gunn, J. (in press). Taking fewer chances: Teenage pregnancy prevention programs. *American Psychologist.*

Petersen, A. C., Tobin-Richards, M., & Boxer, A. (1983). Puberty: Its measurement and its meaning. *Journal of Early Adolescence, 3,* 47–62.

Philliber, S., & Allen, J. P. (1992). Life options and community service: Teen outreach program. In B. C. Miller, J. J. Card, R. L. Paikoff, J. L. Peterson (Eds.), *Preventing adolescent pregnancy* (pp. 139–155). Newbury Park, CA: Sage.

Powers, S. I., Hauser, S. T., & Kilner, L. A. (1989). Adolescent mental health. *American Psychologist, 44,* 200–208.

Pratt, B. (1989). *National survey of family growth—Cycle IV.* Unpublished tabulations. Washington, DC: National Center for Health Statistics.

Pratt, S. G., & Pollard, C. R. (1988, Jan.). *Youth health service of Elkins, West Virginia: Evaluation of the primary prevention program.* Morgantown, W. VA: West Virginia University, Office of Health Services Research.

Remafedl, G. (1987). Adolescent homosexuality: Psychosocial and medical implications. *Pediatrics, 79,* 331–337.

Richards, M. H., Boxer, A. M., Petersen, A. C., & Albrecht, R. (1990). The relationship of weight to body image in pubertal girls and boys from two communities. *Developmental Psychology, 26,* 313–321.

Savin-Williams, R. C. (1988). Theoretical perspectives accounting for adolescent homosexuality. *Journal of Adolescent Health Care, 9,* 95–104.

Savin-Williams, R. C., & Berndt, T. J. (1990). Friendships and peer relations. In S. Feldman & G. Elliott (Eds.), *At the threshold: The developing adolescent* (pp. 277–307). Cambridge, MA: Harvard University Press.

Selman, R. L. (1980). *The growth of interpersonal understanding: Developmental and clinical analyses.* New York: Academic Press.

Sipe, C., Grossman, J., & Milliner, J. (1988). *Summer training and education program (STEP): A report of the 1987 experience.* Philadelphia, PA: Public Private Ventures.

Smith, E. A, & Udry, J. R. (1985). Coital and non-coital sexual behaviors of white and black adolescents. *American Journal of Public Health, 75,* 1200–1203.

Smith, P. B., Nenney, S. W., Weinman, M. L., & Mumford, D. M. (1982). Factors affecting perception of pregnancy risk in the adolescent. *Journal of Youth and Adolescence, 11,* 207–215.

Sonenstein, F. L., Pleck, J. H., & Klu, L. C. (1989). Sexual activity, condom use and AIDS awareness among adolescent males. *Family Planning Perspectives, 21,* 152–158.

Spenner, K. I., & Featherman, D. L. (1978). Achievement ambitions. *Annual Review of Sociology, 4,* 373–420.

Surgeon General. (1979). *Healthy people.* Washington, DC: U. S. Government Printing Office.

Tan, A. (1979). TV beauty ads and role expectations of adolescent female viewers. *Journalism Quarterly, 56,* 283–288.

Thomas, B. H., Mitchell, A., Devlin, M. G., Goldsmith, C. H., Singer, J., & Watters, D. (1992). Small group sex education at school: The McMaster teen program. In B. C. Miller, J. J. Card, R. L. Paikoff, J. L. Peterson (Eds.), *Preventing adolescent pregnancy* (pp. 28–52). Newbury Park, CA: Sage.

Turner, C. F., Miller, H. G., & Moses, L. E. (Eds.). (1989). *AIDS: Sexual behavior and intravenous drug use.* Washington, DC: National Academy Press.

Udry, J. R. (1988). Biological predispositions and social control in adolescent sexual behavior. *American Sociological Review, 53,* 709–722.

Udry, J. R., & Billy, J.O.G. (1987). Initiation of coitus in early adolescence. *American Sociological Review, 52,* 841–855.

U. S. Congress. (1991). *Adolescent Health, Vols. 1 and 2.* Washington, DC: Office of Technology Assessment.

Vincent, M., Clearie, A. F., & Schluchter, M. D. (1987). Reducing adolescent pregnancy through school and community-based education. *Journal of American Medical Association, 257,* 3382–3386.

Weed, S. E., Olsen, J. A., & Tanas, R. (1988, December). *The teen-aid family life education project.* An evaluation report prepared for the Office of Adolescent Pregnancy Program (OAPP), The Institute for Research and Evaluation, Washington, DC.

Weinstein, N. D. (1987). Unrealistic optimism about susceptibility to health problems: Conclusions from a community-wide sample. *Journal of Behavioral Medicine, 10,* 481–500.

Werner, E. E., & Smith, R. S. (1982). *Vulnerable but invincible: A longitudinal study of resilient children and youth.* New York: McGraw-Hill.

Westney, O. E., Jenkins, R. R., & Benjamin, C. M. (1983). Sociosexual development of pre-adolescents. In J. Brooks-Gunn and A. C. Petersen (Eds.), *Girls at puberty: Biological and psychosocial perspectives* (pp. 273–300). New York: Plenum.

Zabin, L. S., & Clark, S. D., Jr. (1981). Why they delay: A study of teenage family planning clinic patients. *Family Planning Perspectives, 13,* 205–217.

Zabin, L. S., Hirsch, M. B., Smith, E. A., Streett, R., & Hardy, J. B. (1986). Evaluation of a pregnancy prevention program for urban teenagers. *Family Planning Perspectives, 18,* 119–126.

Zelnik, M. (1983). Sexual activity among adolescents: Perspective of a decade. In E. R. McAnarey (Ed.), *Premature adolescent pregnancy and parenthood* (pp. 21–33). New York: Grune and Stratton.

Zelnik, M., & Kantner, J. F. (1977). Sexual and contraceptive experience of young unmarried women in the United States, 1976 and 1971. *Family Planning Perspectives, 9,* 55–71.

Zelnik, M., & Kim, Y. J. (1982). Sex education and its association with teenage sexual activity, pregnancy and contraceptive use. *Family Planning Perspectives, 14,* 117–126.

10

Promoting Healthful Diet
and Physical Activity

James F. Sallis

The year 2000 health objectives developed by the Public Health Service (U. S. Department of Health and Human Services, 1991) recognize the importance of dietary and physical activity behaviors in the maintenance of good health in adolescents (see Table 10-1). In this chapter, dietary and physical activity behaviors are discussed together, a pairing supported by both physiological and behavioral reasons. Physiologically, diet and physical activity in large part determine energy balance in the body and thus influence growth and body composition. Diet and physical activity have been found to be empirically associated in several studies (Blair, Jacobs, & Powell, 1985) and share many behavioral characteristics: they vary widely from one person to the next, they change daily within each individual, they are influenced by multiple variables, they can be performed either alone or in a social milieu and in many different settings, and they are resistant to change.

This chapter begins with a brief summary of the primary potential benefits and risks of promoting healthful diet and physical activity for adolescents and a discussion of prudent goals for this age group. A consideration of the determinants of dietary and physical activity behaviors sets the stage for a section on intervention approaches. Finally, recommendations are made for the development of effective health promotion interventions for the entire adolescent population in the United States.

The Importance of Diet and Physical Activity in Adolescent Health

Potential Benefits

Proper diet and physical activity may be especially important during adolescence, when rapid growth and development create an increased need for many nutrients, and when excessive accumulation of fat may contribute to health problems and psychosocial difficulties for years to come. Dietary and physical activity practices that

209

Table 10.1. Year 2000 National Health Promotion and Disease Prevention Objectives Concerning Adolescent Physical Activity and Diet

Objectives to Increase Physical Activity and Fitness

1.3 Increase to at least 30 percent the proportion of people age 6 and older who engage regularly, preferably daily, in light to moderate physical activity for at least 30 minutes per day. (Baseline: 22 percent of people aged 18 and older were active for at least 30 minutes 5 or more times per week and 12 percent were active 7 or more timer per week in 1985)

1.4 Increase to at least 20 percent the proportion of people aged 18 and older and to at least 75 percent the proportion of children and adolescents aged 6 through 17 who engaged in vigorous physical activity that promotes the development and maintenance of cardiorespiratory fitness 3 or more days per week for 20 or more minutes per occasion. (Baseline: 12 percent for people aged 18 and older in 1985; 66 percent for youth aged 10 through 17 in 1984)

1.5 Reduce to no more than 15 percent the proportion of people aged 6 and older who engaged in no leisure-time physical activity. (Baseline: 24 for people aged 18 and older in 1985)

1.6 Increase to at least 40 percent the proportion of people age 6 and older who regularly perform physical activities that enhance and maintain muscular strength, muscular endurance, and flexibility. (Baseline data available in 1991)

1.7 Increase to at least 50 percent the proportion of overweight people age 12 and older who have adopted sound dietary practices combined with regular physical activity to attain an appropriate body weight. (Baseline: 30 percent of overweight women and 25 percent of overweight men for people age 18 and older in 1985)

1.8 Increase to at least 50 percent the proportion of children and adolescents in 1st through 12th grade who participate in daily school physical education. (Baseline: 36 in 1984–1986)

1.9 Increase to at least 50 percent the proportion of school physical education class time that students spend being physically active, preferably engaged in lifetime physical activities. (Baseline: Students spent an estimated 27 percent of class time being physically active in 1983)

1.11 Increase community availability and accessibility of physical activity and fitness facilities, such as (a) hiking, biking, and fitness trail miles; (b) public swimming pools; (c) acres of park and recreation open space.

Objectives to Improve Nutrition

2.5 Reduce dietary fat intake to an average of 30 percent of calories or less and average saturated fat intake to less than 10 percent of calories among people age 2 and older. (Baseline: 36 percent of calories from total fat and 13 percent from saturated fat for people aged 20 through 74 in 1976–1980; 36 percent and 13 percent for women aged 19 through 50 in 1985)

2.6 Increase complex carbohydrate and fiber-containing foods in the diets of adults to 5 or more daily servings for vegetables (including legumes) and fruits, and to 6 or more daily servings for grain products. (Baseline: 2½ servings of vegetables and fruits and 3 servings of grain products for women aged 19 through 50 in 1985)

2.7 Increase to at least 50 percent the proportion of overweight people aged 12 and older who have adopted sound dietary practices combined with regular physical activity to attain an appropriate body weight. (Baseline: 30 percent of overweight women and 25 percent of overweight men for people aged 18 and older in 1985)

2.8 Increase calcium intake so at least 50 percent of youth aged 12 through 24 and 50 percent of pregnant and lactating women consume 3 or more servings daily of foods rich in calcium, and at least 50 percent of people aged 25 and older consume 2 or more servings daily. (Baseline: 7 percent of women and 14 percent of men aged 19 through 24 and 24 percent of pregnant and lactating women consumed 3 or more servings, and 15 percent of women and 23 percent of men aged 25 through 50 consumed 2 or more servings in 1985–6)

2.9 Decrease salt and sodium intake so at least 65 percent of home meal preparers prepare food without adding salt, at least 80 percent of people avoid using salt at the table, and at least 40 percent of adults regularly purchase foods modified or lower in sodium. (Baseline: 54 percent of women aged 19 through 50 who served as the main meal preparer did not use salt in food preparation, and 68 percent of women aged 19 through 50 did not use salt at the table in 1985; 20 percent of all people aged 18 and older regularly purchased foods with reduced salt and sodium content in 1988)

2.10 Reduce iron deficiency to less than 3 percent among children aged 1 through 4 and among women of childbearing age. (Baseline: 9 percent for children aged 1 through 2, 4 percent for children aged through 4, and 5 percent for women aged 20 through 44 in 1976–80)

2.14 Achieve useful and informative nutrition labeling for virtually all processed foods and at least 40 percent of fresh meats, poultry, fish, fruits, vegetables, baked goods, and ready-to-eat carry-away foods. (Baseline: 60 percent of sales of processed foods regulated by FDA had nutrition labeling in 1988; baseline data on fresh and carry-away foods unavailable)

2.15 Increase to at least 5,000 brand items the availability of processed food products that are reduced in fat and saturated fat. (Baseline: 2,500 items reduced in fat in 1986)

2.16 Increase to at least 90 percent the proportion of restaurants and institutional food service operations that offer identifiable low-fat, low-calorie food choices, consistent with the *Dietary Guidelines for Americans*. (Baseline: About 70 percent of fast food and family restaurant chains with 350 or more units had at least one low-fat, low-calorie item on their menu in 1989)

2.17 Increase to at least 90 percent the proportion of school lunch and breakfast services and child care food services with menus that are consistent with the nutrition principles in the *Dietary Guidelines for Americans*. (Baseline data available in 1993)

2.19 Increase to at least 75 percent the proportion of the Nation's schools that provide nutrition education from preschool through 12th grade, preferably as part of quality school health education. (Baseline data available in 1991)

Source: U.S. Department of Health and Human Services. (1991). Healthy people 2000: National health promotion and disease prevention objectives. DHHS Publication No. (PHS) 91-50212. Washington, DC: U.S. Government Printing Office.

both promote health during adolescence and assist in the prevention of specific diseases in later life can be identified. If teenagers are to be encouraged to say "no" to so many health-damaging behaviors, it is important to emphasize a positive approach to the development of health-promoting dietary and physical activity behaviors.

Recommended dietary and physical activity practices can have immediate health benefits for adolescents in that they help normalize body weight and body composition (Epstein, 1986). Physical activity can promote positive mental health (Brown & Siegel, 1988; Gruber, 1986). Both of these immediate outcomes are highly desirable to adolescents, and focusing on them may be useful in motivating healthful dietary and physical activity practices that also have long-term benefits.

There is considerable interest in the relationship of dietary and physical activity behaviors to chronic diseases later in life. Dietary behaviors affect the risk of cardiovascular diseases, cancers, obesity, and non-insulin-dependent diabetes mellitus (Bray, 1986; National Research Council, 1989; U. S. Department of Health and Human Services, 1989), all of which are major causes of morbidity and mortality. It is widely accepted that regular physical activity reduces risk for cardiovascular diseases (Powell, Thompson, Caspersen, & Kendrick, 1987), obesity, non-insulin-dependent diabetes mellitus, hypertension, and possibly cancers (Bouchard, Shephard, Stephens, Sutton, & McPherson, 1990). Because atherosclerosis begins in childhood or adolescence (Strong, 1983) and eventually causes more than half of all deaths (Kaplan & Stamler, 1983), there is a growing consensus that promoting heart healthy dietary and physical activity patterns in children and adolescents is essential for producing large reductions in the number one cause of death in the United States.

Bone development in adolescence and young adulthood is related to the risk of osteoporosis in later years, especially among women (Broekhoff, 1986). Both adequate calcium intake and regular physical activity during the growth years facilitate the development of calcium-rich bones that are less likely to become osteoporotic (National Research Council, 1989). Adolescence is therefore a critical period for the prevention of osteoporosis.

Matarazzo (1980) convincingly demonstrated that a person cannot be termed truly healthy unless his or her health-related behaviors, including diet and physical activity, are consistent with a low risk of the major causes of morbidity and mortality. Thus, with the choices they make concerning their dietary and physical activity behaviors, adolescents are laying the foundation for their health over a lifetime.

Potential Risks of Dietary and Physical Activity Health Promotion Programs

Adolescents are counseled by the health community to decrease their intake of dietary fats and calories, to increase their physical activity, and to avoid becoming overweight. How are these messages likely to be perceived by adolescents? It is possible that health promotion messages will be misinterpreted and stimulate extreme behavior changes in predisposed individuals.

Already, there are very strong pressures from popular media, commercial interests, and peers to be thin so as to be attractive (Garner, Garfinkel, & Olmsted, 1983). Women, much more than men, desire a thin body (Fallon & Rozin, 1985) and view thinness as the major determinant of physical attractiveness (Miller, Coffman, & Linke, 1980). It is generally presumed that the cultural norm of ever-thinner bodies as the ideal of beauty for women is largely responsible for recent increases in the prevalence of the eating disorders.

Overnutrition is the most common dietary-related problem in the United States, but efforts to manipulate body shape may have serious consequences for adolescents. Anorexia nervosa is characterized by severe weight loss and a relentless obsession to become thinner. This disorder is seen primarily among middle-class adolescent girls, 1% to 4% of whom are affected (Pope, Hudson, Yurgelun-Todd, & Hudson, 1984). Anorexia is not simply an eating disorder, because excessive physical activity is often used to facilitate weight loss and suppress the appetite (Epling & Pierce, 1988).

Bulimia nervosa is characterized by episodes of binge eating and purging through vomiting, laxative use, or diuretic use. Bulimia was not even recognized as a syndrome until the late 1970s, but only 10 years later this disorder had a prevalence of about 8% in women and 1% in men (Connors & Johnson, 1987). Most bulimics are adolescents, and the use of purging behaviors is even more prevalent than bulimia. Thirteen percent of high school students in one study reported occasional use of purging techniques (Killen et al., 1986). The peak period for the onset of both eating disorders is about 15 to 19 years (Lucas, Beard, Kranz, & Kurland, 1983).

The use of anabolic steroids is another disturbing trend among high school students that affects mainly boys. These drugs are used to produce a muscular physique associated with male physical attractiveness, but they have many health-damaging effects. From 5% to 7% of high school boys and less than 2% of high school girls have used anabolic steroids, and athletes have a particularly high rate of use (Buckley et al., 1988; Windsor & Dumitru, 1989). Presumably, the increased prevalence of steroid use among athletes, and of eating disorders among athletes and female ballet dancers, is due to these individuals being under particularly intense pressure to conform to ideal body shapes (Brooks-Gunn, Burrow, & Warren, 1988; Windsor & Dumitru, 1989; Chapter 2).

It is well known that excessive exercise or failure to take safety precautions can increase the risk of injuries and accidents (Siscovick, 1990). This risk is present with individual conditioning activities like jogging, but it is even higher for the contact team sports that are most often played by adolescents (Jones, Rock, & Moore, 1988). Overexercise in women can produce amenorrhea (Prior, 1990).

Apparently benign messages to avoid obesity and be physically fit add the public health community's voice to the din of input about their bodies with which adolescents must contend. Adolescents may be particularly susceptible to undesirable side effects from otherwise reasonable health promotion messages. This does not mean that efforts to prevent obesity and to promote healthful dietary and physical activity behaviors in adolescents are not needed or justified. However, the side effects of health promotion in adolescents must be assessed, and programs should contain components to minimize undesirable outcomes.

Prudent Dietary and Physical Activity Goals for Adolescents

Dietary guidelines to ensure adequate intake of essential nutrients while minimizing risks of chronic diseases have been developed by many national groups, and similar recommendations have recently been published by the National Research Council (1989) and been included in the first *Surgeon General's Report on Nutrition and Health* (U. S. Department of Health and Human Services, 1989) and the year 2000 health objectives (U. S. Department of Health and Human Services, 1991). In most cases, guidelines are virtually identical for adolescents and adults.

Saturated fats and cholesterol, which are related to the risk of cardiovascular diseases, are eaten in excess by most adolescents. Of the nutrients that appear to influence blood pressure, most adolescents eat too much sodium and too little potassium and calcium. Approximately 20% of adolescents are obese (Gortmaker, Dietz, Sobol, & Wehler, 1987), in part because of excessive consumption of calories and fats. Thus, one of the most important recommendations is that adolescents should follow a diet that promotes heart health. There is little evidence that a heart healthy diet will have a detectable negative impact on mental or physical development, provided that calories are adequate and fat is not severely restricted (National Research Council, 1989). The increasing numbers of poor adolescents are likely to have diets lacking in calories and other nutrients, and this group requires concentrated study. However, inadequate caloric consumption and nutritional deficiencies do not affect nearly as many adolescents as do nutritional excesses.

It is estimated that about 30% of all cancers are diet-related (Doll & Peto, 1981). To prevent cancer, the recommendations are to decrease calories and fat and to increase fiber, vitamin A, and cruciferous vegetables such as cauliflower, broccoli, and cabbage.

To promote optimal bone development and prevent osteoporosis, it is important to consume the recommended amount of calcium. Adolescent girls are generally deficient in this nutrient, while adolescent boys are not (U. S. Department of Health and Human Services, 1989). Non-insulin-dependent diabetes can be prevented by maintaining ideal body weight, so caloric intake must be balanced with expenditure. Adolescents girls have a high rate of iron deficiency anemia (National Research Council, 1989), which could be largely avoided through a health promotion approach to nutrition education for all, but the special needs of pregnant teenagers probably require targeted programs.

Physical activity goals for children and adolescents are more controversial, and recommendations are based primarily on the amount of physical activity required for health benefits in adults. The American College of Sports Medicine (1991) and the year 2000 health objectives (U. S. Department of Health and Human Services, 1991) share two recommendations. To improve cardiovascular fitness, it is necessary to engage in repetitive physical activity involving large muscle groups at 60% to 80% of the maximal heart rate at least three times per week for at least 20 minutes per occasion. Recommended activities include running, swimming, cycling, aerobic dance, and racquet sports. Many health benefits can be achieved by regular physical activity that is less vigorous, such as walking, so regular participation in moderate-intensity activities is recommended.

Data on the activity levels of adolescents are inadequate, but several studies using objective monitoring of activity over entire days found that most adolescents may be meeting the current recommendations for vigorous physical activity (Rowland, 1990). However, activity levels decline dramatically over the adolescent period (Rowland, 1990), and the decline continues throughout adulthood. Adolescence is a critical transition period when structured opportunities for physical activity in school are taken away, apparently leading to a rapid decline in the level of physical activity in young adulthood (Stephens, Jacobs, & White, 1985). One of the primary health promotion tasks for adolescents regarding physical activity is to prepare adolescents to maintain regular physical activity in the transition to adult roles.

Determinants of Dietary and Physical Activity Behaviors

Demographic Variables

AGE. In national studies, total fat and saturated fat intakes were generally shown to increase from childhood to adolescence (Kimm, Gergen, Malloy, Dresser, & Carroll, 1990; Salz et al., 1983), indicating that the diets of adolescents are more unhealthy than those of children. There is some evidence that physical activity decreases during adolescence (Rowland, 1990). These trends argue for intervention in early adolescence or childhood.

GENDER. In large national studies, boys tended to consume more calories per kilogram of body weight than girls (Kimm et al., 1990), but fat and sodium intakes did not differ by gender in adolescence (Kimm et al., 1990; Salz et al., 1983). Smaller studies had conflicting findings regarding fat and sodium (Burdine, Chen, Gottlieb, Peterson, & Vacalis, 1984; Perry, Griffin, & Murray, 1985), so there are no consistent gender differences in nutrient intake.

There are important gender differences in weight loss and dieting practices. Adolescent females are more likely than males to restrict eating to control weight. In a recent study almost 70% of young adolescent girls reported that they had attempted to lose weight during the preceding year (Wadden, Foster, Stunkard, & Linowitz, 1989). Male adolescents are more likely to use exercise rather than dieting as a form of weight control (Desmond, Price, Hallinan, & Smith, 1989).

Hsu (1989) believes that a major reason for the gender gap in eating disorders, which is about 10 to 1, is that girls diet much more frequently than boys. The pursuit of thinness may be likely to become exaggerated in girls because they have more depressed moods and a poorer self-image, and because societal pressure to be thin is more intense for females. Thus, there seems to be a greater need among females for diet regulation interventions related to weight control (Hsu, 1989).

Studies have consistently found that adolescent boys are more physically active than girls (Fuchs et al., 1988; Perry et al., 1985; Ross, Dotson, & Gilbert, 1985).

RACE/ETHNICITY AND SOCIOECONOMIC STATUS. It is difficult to disentangle the effects of socioeconomic status and race/ethnicity, because ethnic minorities are more likely to be poor. For this reason, these important variables will be considered together.

With 25% of children and adolescents in the United States living in poverty (Chapter 3), it is important to consider the nutritional adequacy of their diets. National surveys have shown that poor children are likely to be deficient in iron and to have retarded growth and development (Dwyer, 1980). While specific dietary deficiencies are common, malnutrition appears to be rare among U. S. adolescents.

Economic studies have shown that some types of foods are more income elastic, meaning that purchasing of these foods changes a great deal in response to changes in income. The most elastic appear to be snacks and foods eaten away from home (Popkin & Haines, 1981). Because children and teenagers may take 30% or more of their calories from snacks (Frank, Webber, & Berenson, 1982), a decrease in snacks could have more detrimental effects on adolescents than on adults. Fresh fruits, fresh vegetables, and meats were also found to have high income elasticity (Popkin & Haines, 1981). Most U. S. adolescents could benefit from eating less meat, but poor adolescents may be at high risk of being deficient in several micronutrients found in fresh fruits and vegetables.

Black and white adolescents have been found to consume similar amounts of fat and cholesterol (Kimm et al., 1990). However very few studies have examined racial differences in the diets of adolescents, and additional studies are needed to describe ethnic differences in nutrient intake. The most prudent conclusion is that adolescents in all major U. S. ethnic groups eat too much fat and sodium.

Ethnic differences exist in specific types of foods eaten. Each cultural and ethnic group has a tradition of foods that helps define the group's cultural identity. Each cuisine is defined by staple foods, cooking methods, and added flavorings (Rozin, 1984). While some cultural and ethnic eating patterns are generally more health-promoting than others, it is important for nutrition education programs not to discourage cultural dietary patterns. It is usually possible to improve the healthfulness of the cuisine while maintaining its cultural identity.

Insufficient data exist on economic and racial differences in the physical activity patterns of adolescents to make clear statements. However, studies suggest that physical activity in adults is more strongly related to socioeconomic status (SES) than to race/ethnicity (Caspersen, Christenson, & Pollard, 1986; Cauley, Donfield, LaPorte, & Warhaftig, 1991; Folsom et al., 1991; Hazuda, Stern, Gaskill, Haffner, & Gardner, 1983; Roberts & Lee, 1980; White, Powell, Hogelin, Gentry, & Forman, 1987).

Obesity and the eating disorders are associated with SES and race in complex ways. Low-income males tend to be thinner than high-income males from childhood to adulthood (Garn & Clark, 1976), but the situation for women is more complicated. Low-income females are leaner than high-income females in childhood, but by late adolescence low-income females became the fatter of the two (Garn & Clark, 1976; Goldblatt, Moore, & Stunkard, 1965; Stunkard, d'Aquili, Fox, & Filion, 1972). Ethnic effects mirrored the effects of income (Garn & Clark, 1976). At young ages white females are fatter than black females, but by late adolescence, this situation is reversed. For low-income and African-American females, adolescence is a time of special risk for the development of obesity. Mexican-American adults are usually found to be more obese than Anglos (Stern et al., 1981).

The reasons for the increase in obesity for poor and minority adolescent females have not yet been established, but differences in ideal body shape are a suspected factor, and one with implications for the eating disorders. White females are more likely than black ones to perceive themselves as fat and to report being on a diet. These findings were reported in the 1960s (Huenemann, Shapiro, Hampton, & Mitchell, 1966) and the 1980s (Desmond, Price, Hallinan, & Smith, 1989), so this appears to be a stable racial difference. In a study of Latino adolescent females, Pumariega (1986) found that only among those girls who had adopted a mainstream American viewpoint was there a preoccupation with thinness. Among minority girls, obesity rates tend to be high and concern about weight low.

Psychological/Behavioral Variables

Taste is an important factor in food selection, but many adolescents are motivated by health concerns and convenience (Contento, Michela, & Goldberg, 1988). Teenagers readily acknowledge their overconsumption of junk food, and they identify lack of time, poor self-discipline, and a sense of urgency as the most important barriers to dietary change (Story & Resnick, 1986).

Adolescent girls with a negative body image are more likely than others to develop eating problems (Attie & Brooks-Gunn, 1989). The high prevalence of dieting in young girls is of concern because studies of adults have shown that a pattern of restrained eating or stringent dieting often leads to binge eating. Paradoxically, consciously limiting food intake precipitates excessive consumption when the self-imposed restraint is violated (Herman & Polivy, 1975; Polivy & Herman, 1976a, 1976b).

Consistent with adult data on physical activity determinants (Dishman, Sallis, & Orenstein, 1985; Sallis et al., 1989), adolescents' physical activity behavior is more strongly influenced by perceptions of their own confidence and self-identified barriers than by knowledge and other health beliefs. Beliefs of adolescents related to the health threats of inactivity or their own vulnerability to those threats are not strongly associated with their physical activity behaviors (Butcher, 1983; Desmond et al., 1990; O'Connell, Price, Roberts, Jurs, & McKinley, 1985). However, self-identified barriers to exercise, such as time constraints and lack of interest, were associated with activity patterns and fitness (Desmond et al., 1990; Tappe, Duda,

& Ehrnwald, 1989). Cognitive variables directly related to their own behavior, such as the intention to exercise and self-confidence in their ability to exercise predicted the future physical activity of high school students (Reynolds et al., 1990).

Social Variables

PEER INFLUENCES. Social factors such as peer modeling and encouragement are expected to be important to adolescents because of the special value placed on peer relationships in adolescence (Buhrmester & Furman, 1987). What peers eat can influence teenagers to eat either healthy or unhealthy diets (Contento et al., 1988). Peers eat together daily during school and often after school and on weekends, creating ample opportunity for repeated peer influences. Eating serves as an occasion for socialization, but unfortunately, much of adolescents' eating outside of the home and school takes place in fast food restaurants, where it is difficult to eat foods that are low in fat, sodium, and sugar. Adolescents may define some foods as "cool," or acceptable, so there will be pressure to eat those foods. Peer influences to be thin may be intensified in competitive social environments such that the risk of developing eating disorders is heightened (Brooks-Gunn & Warren, 1985).

Social factors have been consistently and strongly associated with physical activity or fitness of adolescents (Desmond et al., 1990; O'Connell et al., 1985; Reynolds et al., 1990). Adolescents perform much of their physical activity in group settings, either at school, in organized community programs, or in informal groups. Team sports are common in adolescence, but the fact that involvement in such sports is relatively rare in adulthood (Stephens et al., 1985) indicates that sports have relatively little carry-over value.

FAMILY INFLUENCES. Although adolescence is generally a time of increasing independence from the family (Buhrmester & Furman, 1987), there are a variety of parental influences on diet (Hertzler, 1983). Rozin (1984) notes that the diets of adolescents and their parents resemble one another because there have been 12 to 17 years of exposure to family influences. Correlations between parental consumption and the intake of calories, fat, and sodium in children and adolescents have been repeatedly reported (Laskarzewski et al., 1980; Patterson, Rupp, Sallis, Atkins, & Nader, 1988). Many of the findings of familial similarities may be due to the fact that families eat a common diet at least part of the time. The foods available in the home are the same for adolescents and parents, and adolescents tend to eat what is convenient and available (Contento et al., 1988).

Parental influences were the strongest correlates of childhood physical activity (Gottlieb & Chen, 1985), and this general result has also been found for adolescent girls (Butcher, 1983). Physical activity habits of parents and young adolescents are correlated (Sallis, Patterson, Buono, Atkins, & Nader, 1988), suggesting that parents can be effective role models. Parental verbal support may be important in adolescence as well (Godin & Shephard, 1984). Parents control access to organized physical activities through transportation, payment of fees, and attendance at athletic events, but this influence has not been directly studied.

Cultural and Environmental Variables

Cultural and environmental influences are pervasive throughout society, and this characteristic makes them both powerful and difficult to study. This discussion focuses on mass media influences and on the availability and proximity of foods and resources related to physical activity.

MASS MEDIA INFLUENCES. It is impossible to understand the world of the adolescent without considering the influence of the mass media, especially television. Wadden and Brownell (1984) summarized a child's typical exposure to television and highlighted possible effects on dietary behavior. Over the course of a year, most children and adolescents spend more time watching television than they spend in a classroom. The average child watches 20,000 commercials per year, and at least 10,000 of them are for food products. Most food commercials are for high-sugar cereals; candy, gum, and cookies are also frequently advertised. Vegetables are essentially never advertised to children. Eighty percent of the foods advertised to children are high in sugar, fat, or sodium, and these findings have been relatively consistent in studies conducted between 1972 and 1987 (Cortugna, 1988).

Food-related messages are delivered during prime-time programs as well as during commercials. While stars of prime-time programs are rarely obese, they make frequent references to nonnutritious foods (Kaufman, 1980), sending the implicit message that there is little relation between the foods eaten and obesity. The modeling literature indicates that the behavior of multiple attractive models is likely to be well learned (Bandura, 1986). This barrage of messages to eat unhealthy foods is designed to be appealing to youth, is produced and broadcast at great expense, and is repeated many times every day.

Television viewing is correlated with snacking between meals, consumption of the types of foods advertised on television, and attempts to influence food purchasing by the mother (Dietz & Gortmaker, 1985). The foods featured in television ads and programs are the same foods that adolescents eat while they are watching television (Gerbner, Morgan, & Signorelli, 1982). It is likely that the true strength of television's influences on the eating habits of children and adolescents is known best to the advertisers.

Time spent watching television is time that cannot be used for physical activity. If an adolescent spends 8 hours sleeping, 6 hours at school, 2 hours on homework, 2 hours on personal care and eating, and 3 hours watching television, there is not much time left for socializing and being physically active. In fact, adolescents complain that they are too busy and have trouble finding time to participate in physical activity (Story & Resnick, 1986).

Dietz and Gortmaker (1985) found that 10% of adolescents who watched less than 1 hour of television per day were obese. Among those who watched more than 5 hours per day, almost 20% were obese.

Television is presenting a strong and consistent message that is jeopardizing the future health of American youth. The content of this programming is determined almost exclusively by commercial interest, with virtually no effective input from health professionals, educators, or consumer advocates. The present situation appears to be a formidable barrier to the effectiveness of the usual health promotion programs.

The influence of other media, such as radio and print, should be considered when planning health promotion programs. Interestingly, though radio has advertisements for foods with low nutritional value, it could play a supportive role in increasing physical activity. Personal radios and tape players are commonly used to provide a sound track during exercise, so physical activity can be promoted to teens as a time to listen to music.

AVAILABILITY AND PROXIMITY. The amount and variety of food available to most of American society are probably unprecedented in the history of humankind. It would be hard enough to regulate food intake in an environment that had unlimited amounts of desirable foods. But the situation is much worse than that. Food is available in almost every conceivable setting. There is food at home, and there are food stores and food vending machines at school. The streets are seemingly lined with food outlets, including fast-food restaurants, convenience stores, and ice cream, candy, and sandwich shops, to mention only a few. Most fast-food outlets not only offer many more high-fat/salt/calorie items than healthful items, but in many establishments it is difficult to select a meal that conforms to dietary recommendations. There is indirect evidence that the different availabilities of healthful foods in fast-food restaurants versus family restaurants affect dietary behavior, because patrons consumed more calories in fast-food restaurants (Klesges, Bartsch, Norwood, Kautzman, & Haugrud, 1984).

Not only is food universally present, but advertising creates unending pressure to enjoy it. The combination of repetitious encouragement to eat unhealthy but appetizing foods that are readily available at prices that many adolescents can afford has obviously been a successful strategy. Health promotion programs will have to be extremely powerful if the successful marketing practices of the food industry are to be countered or altered.

Fast-food restaurants are an integral part of adolescent culture. With over 140,000 U. S. outlets in 1980 (Sheridan & McPherrin, 1983), they are truly ubiquitous. For a small amount of money, adolescents can socialize and eat at the restaurant that seems to be near every school. Fast-food restaurants employ large numbers of young people; an estimated 17% of teenagers in the early 1980s (Lewin-Epstein, 1981). The time spent in restaurants by adolescent employees makes fast food a central focus in the lives of many young people and their friends. These outlets are particularly welcomed into poor and minority communities, because they provide employment and convenience to area residents.

Opportunities for physical activity can be conceptualized as the availability of relevant facilities, supplies, or programs. Many of the activities that adolescents commonly engage in out of school require facilities, such as fields, basketball courts, and dance studios. For adolescents with limited transportation and money, there are sizable barriers to the use of many facilities. Middle-class adolescents may have many types of structured activities available to them, but lower-income ones may have to rely on programs that are organized either by the school or at a convenient public recreation center.

Many healthful physical activities, like walking, running, and frisbee games, can be performed with limited facilities or supplies. These activities require the individual to manage his or her own activity program completely. Because not all adolescents can be expected to maintain a high activity level successfully on their own, structured programs will continue to be needed for many. It is clear that many such programs are already making contributions to the health of teenagers, given that adolescents obtain most of their physical activity out of school in organized community programs (Ross, Dotson, Gilbert, & Katz, 1985b). The challenge for health promotion is to increase the access of all adolescents to these programs and to emphasize the activities that may be carried over into adulthood, that is, those that require only one or two people. This challenge is significant in the current context of shrinking budgets for services targeted to the poor.

There are many attractive sedentary behaviors that compete with physical activity for adolescents' time. With the driver's license comes an overwhelming desire to drive, and alternative modes of transportation become irrelevant. The desire for independent transportation leads many adolescents to get a job so that they can pay for a car and insurance, but employed teenagers have less time for physical activity. Socialization is a preferred recreation for many girls, and this often occurs during sedentary activities such as eating or watching videotapes. This is an opportunity for an intervention to balance sedentary socializing with socializing during periods of physical activity.

Not all environmental factors discourage physical activity. Substantial resources throughout the nation are devoted to promoting physical activity, but there are some indications that current programs and facilities are not successfully meeting the health-related physical activity needs of all adolescents. On a national basis, there is an enormous ongoing commitment to physical education. However, enrollment in physical education declines from over 90% in grade 7 to about 55% in grade 12 (Ross, Dotson, Gilbert, & Katz, 1985a). Despite concerns about the quality of lessons, low participation in high school, and continuing emphasis on team sports as opposed to carryover activities, physical education is a significant stimulus for physical activity in adolescence.

Outside of physical education, the major structured activity for youth is provided by sports teams. There are many benefits to this emphasis on team sports, such as regular activity, enhanced physical skills, and socialization. However, there are a number of risks for adolescent participants. First, reliance on team sports for physical activity may not prepare the adolescent to be active later in life (Paffenbarger, Hyde, Wing, & Steinmetz, 1984). Second, team sports cause many orthopedic injuries to athletes (Jones et al., 1988). Third, in competitive sports one team must lose each game, and some adolescents never learn to cope with the frequent disappointment. Most participants are criticized often for deficiencies in their playing (Rushall & Siedentop, 1972), and this may be one reason why the dropout rate from youth sports is high (Burton & Martens, 1986). Finally, the pressure to excel in sports can motivate health-damaging behaviors such as excessive exercise, dangerous eating patterns (Brooks-Gunn et al., 1988), and use of anabolic steroids (Buckley et al., 1988).

Developmental Issues

The rapid and profound developmental changes occurring during adolescence must be examined for their relevance to the design of diet and physical activity health promotion programs. Biological changes, including growth spurts, changes in body composition, and the onset of puberty, are of concern to adolescents. Regulation of dietary and physical activity behaviors provides adolescents with specific tools for altering these biological outcomes to some degree. The ability to do this may be appealing to many young people, and this motivation could be channeled in health-promoting directions. Caution must be used to define the limits of the effects of healthy dietary and physical activity patterns, and unhealthy behaviors as a means of altering biological development should be explicitly discouraged.

Interventions that teach adolescents both to resist unhealthy peer pressure and to support peers in health behavior change are well suited to adolescents' needs due to the heightened influence of peers during adolescence (Coleman, 1980). Smoking prevention programs based on these principles have been some of the most effective youth health promotion programs (Flay, 1985).

Rapid cognitive development prepares adolescents for the complex daily decision making that is required to maintain healthful dietary and physical activity patterns in a contrary environment. For example, informed food label reading requires knowledge of nutrients and food additives, as well as the ability to integrate information, such as daily requirements and the composition of a normal diet.

Key social cognitive developmental tasks are the formation of a stable personal identity and effective self-regulation skills. Establishing healthy dietary and physical activity behaviors can enhance one's identity, while failure to regulate these behaviors effectively could undermine one's self-concept. This suggests that adolescents may be receptive to training in how to achieve mastery in these tasks of everyday life. The potential negative effects of failed attempts to change behavior indicate that in addition to providing information, interventions must include training in effective methods of changing one's behavior.

Health promotion is anchored in the concept of responsibility for one's own health (Matarazzo, 1980). Adolescents struggle with moral issues such as personal responsibility, so diet and physical activity programs can be concrete examples of how to develop personal values and put them into action.

Possible Biological Adaptations

For heuristic purposes, it is useful to speculate on biological preferences for foods and physical activities that might have adaptive value in the history of the species. In an environment with an unstable food supply, it would be adaptive to have a preference for foods with high nutrient and caloric values. People would be driven to eat many calories efficiently in times of plenty to prepare them for times of famine. The very well documented preference for sweet foods throughout life (Rozin, 1984) and the probable preference for fatty foods are consistent with a hypothesis of biological adaptation. Sweet foods such as fruits typically have high nutrient value. Fatty foods have high caloric content, and because dietary fats are preferentially converted to body fat (Donato & Hegsted, 1985), they help build up fat stores that aid survival in times of limited food.

With modern agriculture, food preservation, and food distribution systems, the food environment has changed, but our food preferences have not. In the current environment of an unlimited supply of a variety of foods on a year-round basis, these apparently biologically based preferences may lead to overconsumption on a mass basis. Sclafani and Springer's (1976) classic rat studies yielded results consistent with this hypothesis. Almost all of the rats on a "supermarket diet" high in fat, sugar, and variety became obese, while control animals on a bland diet maintained normal weight. It is possible that food preferences of adaptive value in the past may be currently presenting health promotion professionals with a potent barrier to dietary alteration.

Does this perspective on biological adaptation have any value in the physical activity domain? In a world characterized by periodic disruptions in the food supply, preferring sedentary behavior is adaptive because it limits the number of calories expended for nonproductive purposes. Hunting, gathering, and growing food required extensive physical activity on a regular basis. Even if people preferred to be sedentary, they were active by necessity.

Industrialization produced drastic changes in requirements for physical activity. Most people do not have to labor to obtain food. An impressive commitment of human ingenuity over the past couple of centuries has been devoted to devising labor-saving and activity-saving devices. The findings that even children are rarely vigorously active when observed on a playground (Hovell, Bursick, & Sharkey, 1978; Sallis, Patterson, McKenzie, & Nader, 1988), that physical activity declines with age (Rowland, 1990; Stephens et al., 1985), and that physically active occupations typically receive the least rewards are consistent with an aversion to physical activity. If physical activity itself is aversive to many people, then programs must make the behavior more pleasant or develop other salient reinforcers.

While these speculations on the adaptiveness of unhealthy dietary and physical activity behaviors point out potentially powerful barriers to health promotion programs in adolescents, it is important for program designers to be fully aware of barriers so that they can be addressed in interventions. This discussion, hopefully, will stimulate research on these issues.

Health Promotion Interventions for Diet and Physical Activity Change

School-Based Educational Interventions

Schools are the obvious site for adolescent health promotion. School programs reach most adolescents, and because there are ongoing health education classes in most secondary schools, dietary and physical activity interventions can be integrated into existing programs. The current generation of interventions emphasizes principles of behavior modification, and specific components are likely to provide knowledge of the foods and activity patterns that promote health, as well as develop cognitive and behavioral skills needed to alter health-related behaviors and maintain those changes over time.

Diet change programs for the general population of adolescents target changes in nutrients related to chronic diseases. Nutrition education programs without specific behavior modification components have failed to produce changes in behavior (Byrd-Bredbenner, O'Connell, Shannon, & Eddy, 1984; Lewis, Brun, Talmage, & Rasher, 1988), but simply setting a specific dietary change goal in the context of nutrition education can be an effective method of change (White & Skinner, 1988). In one study, 14-year-old children taught 10-year-old children how to make diet changes (Holund, 1990). Three diet change programs for high school students have been reported (Coates et al., 1985; King et al., 1988; Podell, Keller, Mulvihill, Berger, & Kent, 1978). All of the successful dietary interventions were structured behavioral programs, but they were extremely brief (five to six sessions). It is encouraging that short-term changes in diet were found in all three studies, but the changes were not maintained, indicating that more than a few educational sessions are needed to overcome the many influences that promote the consumption of high-fat/salt/calorie foods.

Integrated health promotion programs for the prevention of hypertension, heart disease, cancer, and obesity are often recommended, because similar behavior change programs can be effective with these health-related behaviors. Three large-scale multifactorial interventions for adolescents generally produced favorable changes in diet and physical activity, and favorable effects on smoking were also reported in each study (Killen et al., 1988; Perry et al., 1987; Tell & Vellar, 1987). However, the changes were generally modest, not all measures showed improvement, and long-term maintenance has not been demonstrated. These interventions require trained leaders, whether they are regular teachers or peers, and even if they yield measurable health improvements, some schools may resist devoting scarce class time to them. Few school-based studies targeted poor or minority students, so programs that address their needs must be designed and evaluated.

Family-Based Interventions

Recognizing that families exert important influences on adolescents' eating and physical activity patterns (Sallis & Nader, 1988), several of the school-based programs reviewed above included a family component. Other studies have used the family as the central focus of the intervention. Most of these latter studies were conducted with preteenagers, but the results have implications for adolescent health promotion. Family-based behavioral interventions have been effective in producing short-term diet changes (Baranowski, Henske, et al., 1990; Kirks & Hughes, 1986; Nader et al., 1989; Perry et al., 1988; Petchers, Hirsch, & Bloch, 1987), and in some studies, long-term maintenance of changes has been observed

(Kirks and Hughes, 1986; Nader et al., 1989). Family programs have been less effective in changing physical activity (Baranowski, Simons-Morton, et al., 1990; Nader et al., 1989).

Take-home materials, while favored by parents, may not be powerful enough to produce long-term changes (Perry et al., 1988). The small proportion of parents that participated in group sessions, on the other hand, maintained their dietary changes (Nader et al., 1989). Possibly, a staged approach that begins with parent–child homework would stimulate interest in later face-to-face intensive sessions.

Some family-based programs have targeted minority populations. Mexican-American parents made numerous dietary and risk factor improvements, while Mexican-American children made few changes (Nader et al., 1989). Black families made diet changes (Baranowski, Henske, et al., 1990), but they experienced many barriers to attending exercise and educational sessions at a community center (Baranowski, Simons-Morton, et al., 1990). The family intervention concept may be viable for minorities, but program improvements are needed before this can be considered an effective approach.

Environmental Interventions

The effectiveness of educational and skill-enhancing interventions is limited in large part by the formidable environmental cues and pressures to engage in health-compromising behaviors that are confronted as soon as the health promotion lesson is completed. Becker (1986) makes the cogent point that placing all of the responsibility for health behavior change on the individual is a tyrannical aspect of health promotion.

The school environment can be arranged so that it facilitates healthful eating and physical activity. School districts with strong support for health promotion and those without strong support were contrasted (Stevens & Davis, 1988). Attitudes about health education and reported health behaviors of school personnel did not differ between supportive and nonsupportive districts. However, organizational and policy variables were significant discriminators. Cafeterias in supportive districts served healthful foods, staff members received inservice training in health promotion, and district policies encouraged physical activity on site by staff members. The supportive schools made health-promoting behaviors more likely for both students and staff by removing competing cues and barriers.

The North Karelia (Finland) Youth Project (Vartiainen & Puska, 1987) typifies what many health promotion experts would perceive as a state-of-the-science school-based approach. The intensive intervention included risk factor screening, parent participation, and substantial changes in the school lunch. After 2 years of intervention, there were significant differences in some dietary behaviors but little intervention effect on overall nutrient intake. Despite the comprehensiveness of the program, the results, while significant in some cases, were not impressive.

Limitations of the educational approach led a group of investigators in Massachusetts to examine how much dietary and risk factor change could be accomplished in high school students solely by changing the foods served in the cafeteria. The study was carried out in two boarding schools so that the investigators could have maximal control over the total diet of the students (Ellison, Capper, Goldberg, Witschi, & Stare, 1989). Food service personnel were trained to alter their food procurement and preparation practices to lower the sodium and fat content of the meals, but students were given no dietary education. These interventions produced 15–20% decreases in sodium intake and saturated fat, and blood pressures decreased significantly. The dietary changes were well accepted by both food service workers and students.

The Ellison et al. (1989) environmental intervention described above produced more impressive dietary changes than any of the educationally based programs. This study should stimulate other health promotion researchers to develop methods of increasing the availability of health-promoting foods in a variety of environments.

Nutrient information in cafeterias and menu labeling in restaurants produced significant but modest increases in the selection of healthful items (Mayer, Dubbert, & Elder, 1989), but incentive systems whereby patrons received small rebates or coupons when they selected healthful items were more effective than labeling alone (Cinciripini, 1984). These interventions could be targeted to adolescents, but the limited variety of healthful selections available in the restaurants frequented by teenagers would be a major barrier to success.

Labeling programs in supermarkets have generally been unsuccessful in changing patterns of purchasing (Mayer et al., 1989). It is nonetheless encouraging that significant percentages of restaurants and food stores report some nutrition labeling or other health promotion intervention for their patrons (Elder, Sallis Hammond, Peplinski, & Mayer, 1989). Supermarket interventions may be more effectively targeted to parents of teenagers rather than to adolescents themselves.

Regular vigorous exercise programs delivered in physical education classes produce increases in cardiovascular fitness and decreases in body fat in children (Cooper et al., 1975; Maynard, Coonan, Worsley, Dwyer, & Baghurst, 1987), so changes in school policy toward physical education have the potential to promote physical activity effectively for both the poor and the affluent.

Adolescent Obesity Treatment

The literature on obesity treatment in clinical and school settings was recently reviewed by Parcel, Green, and Bettes (1988), who recommended that to achieve lasting results, programs should target long-term changes in diet and increased physical activity. They concluded that obesity treatments were generally more effective in childhood than in adolescence.

Behavioral treatments for obesity are superior to control conditions (Lansky & Vance, 1983), and studies have reported that from 30% (Lansky & Brownell, 1982) to almost 40% (Botvin, Cantlon, Carter, & Williams, 1979) of adolescents in treatment have some weight loss. Weight loss does not appear to have negative effects on adolescent growth. Parental involvement is also important in the treatment of obese adolescents (Coates, Killen, & Slinkard, 1982; Wadden et al., 1990), but it appears that parents and teenagers should be seen separately, rather than together

(Brownell, Kelman, & Stunkard, 1983). Promising programs have been developed for obese black adolescent girls (Wadden et al., 1990). School-based treatments may be preferred for moderately overweight adolescents, while severely obese teenagers may respond better to clinic-based treatments (Foster, Wadden, & Brownell, 1985).

Summary of the Research Findings

The following summary statements seem to be supported by theory and/or the bulk of the existing evidence:

1. Dietary and physical activity habits are not optimal for current and future health promotion in a large proportion of American adolescents, and these behaviors tend to become less healthy throughout the adolescent years.
2. Adolescents are particularly prone to develop eating disorders, exercise excessively, and use steroids to alter body shape.
3. Intakes of key nutrients appear to be similar for boys and girls, but boys are more physically active than girls. Girls are more likely to use dietary restraint to control body shape, and are more prone to obesity and eating disorders. Boys are more likely to use exercise to control body shape and are more likely to use anabolic steroids.
4. Ethnic and socioeconomic differences in nutrient intake and physical activity in adolescents have not been adequately studied. However, poor and minority girls are more likely to be obese, while affluent and white girls are more likely to develop eating disorders.
5. There appear to be stronger and more numerous negative influences on adolescents' unhealthy eating and physical activity habits than positive influences. The most potent influences may be the most pervasive, such as television, the food industry, the automobile, peers, and the family.
6. Relatively few health promotion programs for adolescents have targeted diet and physical activity. The existing studies have generally shown weak but significant effects in middle-class students. There is little evidence that these programs have had long-lasting effects even though the goal of health promotion must be to establish lifelong patterns of behavior.

Recommendations for Effective Programs to Promote Healthful Dietary and Physical Activity Behaviors in Adolescents

Given that there are multiple influences on the dietary and physical activity behaviors of adolescents, the most effective health promotion approach will require multiple components. An effective intervention strategy would likely provide:

1. social and physical environments that make it easy to be physically active;
2. policies and laws that are consistent with and promote healthful behaviors;

3. an adequate variety of mostly tasty, nutritious, low-fat, low-calorie foods;
4. repeated, appealing media messages that encourage healthful dietary and physical activity practices;
5. educational programs that teach decision-making skills, consumer skills, and behavior change skills, as well as facilitate peer and family support.

Adolescent health promotion programs should be conceptualized as part of a total community-based approach to improving the health of the population. The theory and methods of community health promotion are most advanced in the field of cardiovascular disease prevention (Bracht, 1990; Farquhar, Maccoby, & Solomon, 1984), and many of the principles and methods can be applied to promoting healthful diet and physical activity behaviors in adolescents. Every available communication channel should be used to reinforce the health promotion messages. Every setting in which adolescents are found should be considered for involvement in the interventions; for example, the school, the home, religious organizations, medical settings, recreational settings, eating establishments and food stores, the range of community youth organizations, and work sites that employ teenagers. Not only must all settings be involved, but the various points of community intervention must be coordinated and orchestrated (Preston, Baranowski, & Higginbotham, 1988).

Throughout this chapter, important barriers to adolescent health promotion have been identified. This is not to imply that it is futile to attempt to improve adolescent's dietary and physical activity habits; it is suggested that the most successful programs will be those that effectively modify the most powerful determinants of these behaviors. The psychological and behavioral skill variables that are most often targeted in health promotion programs may be among the weakest determinants, so continued reliance on this approach is apt to be disappointing. Some important determinants are not subject to public health intervention, such as biologically based preferences, gender, socioeconomic status, and racial/ethnic group. The strongest modifiable determinants are probably in the environmental domain, so progress in altering such influences as television commericals, limited convenience of healthy foods, and limited availability of exercise programs and facilities must be achieved before important changes in adolescent diet and physical activity patterns can be expected.

Intervention Possibilities

With this big picture in mind, it may be useful to provide specific ideas and suggestions for countering negative influences and strengthening positive influences on adolescents' dietary and physical activity behaviors. These suggestions represent informed opinion and are meant to stimulate research and encourage the development of innovative interventions.

INDIVIDUAL SKILLS. School health education is unlikely to provide a complete solution to the problem of unhealthful diet and physical activity patterns in adolescence, but it is a valuable resource that is probably not being used in an optimal manner. School health education should have as its goal not only to teach students about the recommendations for health-related diet and physical activity, but also to teach them the most effective behavioral skills for adopting those recommendations. This outcome-oriented approach to health education should be followed throughout the school years.

Consumer education may be an important component of school health education for diet and physical activity change. Adolescents need to be more critical media consumers. They should learn how to analyze advertisements, television programs, and movies to identify and evaluate manipulation techniques, such as emotional appeals, half-truths, and concern for consumer health.

Students could also be taught how to cope with eating out. Survival skills in fast-food establishments are relevant to teenagers' lives. Restaurant patrons who are interested in eating a healthful meal must be assertive; thus, as part of nutrition education classes, adolescents could be taught to ask about food preparation methods, request specific modifications, and order sauces and dressings on the side.

Studying adolescents who are already choosing foods based on health considerations may provide hypotheses about diet change interventions that would be particularly effective with adolescents.

SOCIAL ENVIRONMENT. It is well documented that among teenagers, peers exert an exceptionally strong influence on attitudes and behaviors. However, peer support is rarely incorporated into diet and physical activity change programs. Improving peer support could enhance the effectiveness of educational programs, so this area should be a high priority for research.

Family components may be an important part of a comprehensive approach to health promotion for teenagers, but the specific role of the family in such programs needs to be defined.

The role of health professionals and the health care system in promoting healthy dietary and physical activity behaviors is potentially important. The first step in increasing their role is to improve training in nutrition, exercise science, and principles of health behavior change. Primary care physicians should devote some time to assessing and counseling adolescents regarding diet and physical activity behaviors.

Physicians who conduct sports physical examinations should recommend against overexercise and extreme dietary practices. Team physicians should monitor training and dietary habits, as well as steroid use. Health clinics for adolescents, in schools or elsewhere, should adopt health promotion as part of their missions. Clinics can provide some diet and physical activity counseling for all patients, but especially for pregnant teenagers. Public health clinics may be particularly important sources of health promotion intervention for poor and minority youth, because these teenagers have limited access to other sources of information. Health insurance companies and public agencies should provide adequate reimbursement for preventive dietary and physical activity interventions. A change in reimbursement practices would improve access of teenagers and their families to nutritionists and exercise counselors.

PHYSICAL ENVIRONMENT. Environmental alterations are most feasible in the schools, and Ellison et al. (1989) demonstrated that such an approach can significantly impact diet. At present, schools are sources of junk food, possibly because students have demanded vending machines and stores that sell foods that taste better than cafeteria fare. Schools rely on the income from sales of junk food to finance important services, so there is a financial disincentive to remove these items from the environment. The schools are a critical test case for environmental interventions, because if food in schools cannot be made healthy, it is unlikely that other environments will be controlled.

Physical education is a significant national resource devoted to providing students with physical activity, but there are improvements that could be made in both the quantity and quality of physical education. Almost half of twelfth-grade students do not participate, yet physical education may have a particular role to play at this grade by preparing students to continue physical activity while making the transition from high school to either college or work. If physical education professionals were to adopt the goal of promoting lifetime physical activity, then physical education could become a more effective health promotion intervention. This goal could be facilitated by providing physical education teachers with training in health-related physical activity and by emphasizing in the curriculum activities that can be carried over into adulthood.

All organizations involved in youth activity, including sports leagues, should address the health-related physical activity needs of participants. Youth athletic organizations should put a higher value on participation by all than on individual excellence.

Fast food is undoubtedly here to stay, but consumer demand can influence restaurant chains to develop a variety of low-fat/salt/calorie foods that are tasty and attractive to patrons. There is currently a trend toward providing more healthful items in fast-food restaurants, illustrated by salad bars and reduced-fat burgers, but this trend could be accelerated. It is important that healthful items be developed with as much careful market research as the regular fare, and consumer acceptance cannot be expected unless there is serious promotion of new healthful products.

Reducing reliance on automobiles and other labor-saving devices and cutting down on consumption of processed foods are measures with both health and ecological benefits. Many of the behavior changes recommended for health promotion are also recommended by ecologists for environmental protection and energy conservation. With this natural alliance between these two constituencies, cooperative programs in the educational and political arenas may improve the effectiveness of both groups.

MASS MEDIA. The effects of mass media on the dietary habits of adolescents deserve more study (Flora & Wallack, 1990), both to understand the effects of current practices and to explore the effectiveness of mass media approaches to adolescent health promotion. Society must decide whether powerful media influences will continue to be controlled only by food companies that can buy expensive television advertising time or pay to have their products featured in movies. Alternatives to the present situation, such as mandated public service announcements on healthful diets, need to be considered, and it is likely that political action and organized consumer pressure will be required to bring about changes in current practices.

It is difficult to envision effective methods of reducing the negative impact of television on physical activity. Self- or parent-imposed restrictions or the use of television as a reward for physical activity are likely to be of limited effectiveness due to the immense appeal of sitting in front of the set. Devising entertainment shows that stimulate participation in physical activity and are shown during popular viewing times is an approach that has not been attempted with adolescents. The MTV network could encourage viewers to dance along with videos, or it could broadcast exercise programs with special appeal to teens.

POLICIES AND GOVERNMENTAL ACTION. Many environmental changes depend on governmental action at the local, state, or federal level. At the local level, parks and recreation departments could devote resources to physical activity programs for adolescents. One example of a fruitful partnership between a city parks department and a health promotion program was accomplished as part of the Pawtucket Heart Health Program (Elder et al. 1986). Such public programs are available to all adolescent subgroups, and the structure they provide through activity programs could have beneficial effects on social problems of adolescents such as delinquency.

Inaction on food labeling is often cited by health professionals as a prime example of failure of the federal government to inform and protect the public regarding the health effects of foods (Kessler, 1989). This failure may be largely attributable to bureaucratic rigidity in the Food and Drug Administration, but lobbying by the food industry probably affects governmental policies on food labeling, as well as other issues pertaining to the food industry. Food industry lobbies are very well funded, so their influence is predictably great. The meat, dairy, and egg industry lobbies are particularly active, and federal and state policies toward these major sources of saturated fat and cholesterol tend to be highly favorable.

The President's Council for Physical Fitness and Sport was initiated to stimulate improvements in fitness among American youth. Even though the Council is the main federal agency that deals with physical activity, it has had limited interaction with the public health community. It has been essentially uninvolved with research concerning the promotion of physical activity. The orientation of the Council has historically been to emphasize excellence in athletic performance, rather than to develop or advocate health-related physical activity for the masses. This highly visible office, with access to the president, has contributed to the lack of leadership in the federal government regarding promotion of physical activity in childhood, adolescence, and adulthood. However, recent council actions have begun to reverse this trend.

Special Populations

Adolescents appear to have particular difficulty regulating their dietary and physical activity behaviors, so it may be especially hard for them to achieve the prudent patterns recommended in the year 2000 health objectives (U. S. Department of Health and Human Services, 1991). Health promotion programs for adolescents must specifically address excessive *and* deficient patterns for both types of behaviors, while programs for adults can have a more exclusive focus on excessive dietary habits and deficient levels of physical activity. As discussed previously, increased rates of eating disorders (that may also have an exercise component), activity-related injuries, and anabolic steroid use are potential risks of programs that emphasize only chronic disease prevention in adolescents.

Such risks of health promotion programs have never been reported and would likely affect only a small percentage of teenagers. The prevention of cardiovascular diseases, cancer, diabetes, and osteoporosis, on the other hand, may benefit virtually the entire population. The benefits of health promotion are likely to far outweigh the risks.

Health promotion for adolescents should be planned concurrently with health promotion efforts for children and adults. Prudent behavior patterns should be promoted in childhood, and children should be prepared for the unique demands of adolescence. Health promotion programs for adolescents should address age-related needs, but they should also prepare teens for the independence and responsibilities of adulthood. Environmental changes could benefit the entire age spectrum.

There are specific strengths and needs of subpopulations of adolescents that must be considered when developing a strategy for comprehensive health promotion.

POOR YOUTH. Most societal trends reach the poor last, so efforts must be made to ensure that the economically disadvantaged share equally in the benefits of adolescent health promotion. The primary point of contact with teenagers is the schools, and schools in disadvantaged areas should be among the first to be offered both educational and environmental change programs. Because these groups have the highest school dropout rates, more communitywide programs are needed to reach poor and minority populations.

Poor adolescents may have extra environmental barriers to improved diet and physical activity that should be addressed. In poor communities there is often a lack of food stores with a wide variety of low-fat/salt foods, and public parks and recreation centers may not have adequate facilities (Sallis, Nader, Rupp, Atkins, & Wilson, 1986). High crime rates in poor areas serve as barriers to physical activity, because it may be dangerous to go out on the streets. Compounding the problem, health professionals are often reluctant to initiate health promotion programs for the poor because other life needs (e.g., related to unemployment, crime, and dropping out of school) may be more salient. Failure to adapt programs to the poor merely ensures that this group will become further disadvantaged in their access to health promotion services.

DIFFERENT RACIAL/ETHNIC GROUPS. The tremendous racial and ethnic diversity in the United States is a source of much cultural vitality, but this diversity also creates some challenges for health promotion programs. The need to ensure that dietary interventions do not detract from the cultural integrity of the diets they are intended to alter has already been mentioned. Ethnic groups may also vary in their preferences for types of physical activity, leading to a need to be flexible in the types of activities that are encouraged.

Advertisers have long known the effectiveness of targeting specific ethnic and racial groups with both electronic and print media. Health promotion professionals could learn many lessons from successful advertising campaigns that target particular minority groups (Maxwell & Jacobson, 1989). In addition to producing materials in the correct languages, there are specific images, motivations, sources of information, media habits, and social patterns that must be considered in developing educational programs for each community. When community organization is required to achieve environmental changes, organizing ethnic-specific groups of consumers or organizations to change local or ethnic-specific environmental variables may be more effective than assembling heterogeneous groups.

HANDICAPPED YOUTH. Dietary change interventions may not differ much for handicapped and nonhandicapped individuals. For example, most fast-food restaurants have access for the handicapped. The needs of the handicapped are very different in the area of physical activity, but there is reason to believe that this group is being better served than the nonhandicapped. Most school districts have adapted physical education programs for handicapped students, so these youth are receiving more individualized physical activity programs than are children and adolescents in regular physical education. The Special Olympics program provides motivation and support for handicapped people of all ages to engage in physical activity. The Special Olympics' emphasis on participation by all is a feature that should be adopted by physical activity programs for the nonhandicapped.

What Is the Commitment to Adolescent Health Promotion?

Who should sponsor, organize, and pay for programs to promote healthful dietary and physical activity behaviors in adolescents? A reasonable model is that each segment of society with an interest in adolescents should bear part of the responsibility. Those segments include the health care system, the food industry, the sports industry, the sports- and activity-related equipment industry, the insurance industry, the educational system, governments, social service organizations, and the family. Of course, individual adolescents themselves must bear final responsibility for their own actions.

Although few people will disagree with the goals of adolescent health promotion, there are many who will disagree with specific methods because of philosophical beliefs or vested interests. In American society there are clearly limits on the extent to which healthful diet and physical activity will be promoted through environmental changes and governmental policies. Interventions that involve coercion or restrict freedom of choice are not likely to be tolerated. However, interventions that promote freedom of choice through education, increasing the availability of healthful foods, or encouraging the use of physical activity resources will be supported by large segments of the public. There is likely to be disagreement regarding the important issue of moderating the promotion of unhealthful habits by commercial interests, but with sufficient commitment on the part of the public, even this potent barrier can be overcome.

Even among those who agree that promoting healthful dietary and physical activity behaviors in adolescents is a worthwhile endeavor, there will be disagreement about the priority of this task in relation to many other national needs. Before substantial commitments are made to implementing programs, it is necessary not only to develop more effective interventions than are currently available, but also to plan a coherent strategy to coordinate the various components that will be needed for a successful effort (Preston et al., 1988). A commitment will have to be made to the process of developing a strategy that has a reasonable chance of success at an affordable cost. An even larger national commitment will be needed to put a plan into effect. Those interested in promoting healthful diet and physical activity behaviors in youth must not neglect the need to create and maintain a national commitment to adolescent health promotion.

References

American College of Sports Medicine (1991). *Guidelines for exercise testing and prescription* (4th. ed.). Philadelphia: Lea & Febiger.

Attie, I., & Brooks-Gunn, J. (1989). Development of eating problems in adolescent girls: A longitudinal study. *Developmental Psychology, 25,* 70–79.

Bandura, A. (1986). *Social foundations of thought and action.* Englewood Cliffs, NJ: Prentice-Hall.

Baranowski, T., Henske, J., Simons-Morton, B., Palmer, J., Tiernan, K., Hooks, P. C., & Dunn, J. K. (1990). Dietary change for cardiovascular disease prevention among black-American families. *Health Education Research, 5,* 433–443.

Baranowski, T., Simons-Morton, B., Hooks, P., Henske, J., Tiernan, K., Dunn, J. K., Burkhalter, H., Harper, J., & Palmer, J. (1990). A center-based program for exercise change among black-American families. *Health Education Quarterly, 17,* 179–196.

Becker, M. (1986). The tyranny of health promotion. *Public Health Reviews, 14,* 15–25.

Blair, S. N., Jacobs, D. R., & Powell, K. E. (1985). Relationships between exercise or physical activity and other health behaviors. *Public Health Reports, 100,* 172–180.

Botvin, G. J., Cantlon, A., Carter, B. J., & Williams, C. L. (1979). Reducing adolescent obesity through a school health program. *Journal of Pediatrics, 95,* 1060–1062.

Bouchard, C., Shephard, R. J., Stephens, T., Sutton, J. R., & McPherson, B. D. (Eds.) (1990). *Exercise, fitness, and health: A consensus of current knowledge.* Champaign, IL: Human Kinetics.

Bracht, N. (Ed.) (1990). *Health promotion at the community level.* Newbury Park, CA: Sage.

Bray, G. (1986). Effects of obesity on health and happiness. In K. D. Brownell & J. P. Foreyt (Eds.), *Handbook of eating disorders* (pp. 3–44). New York: Basic Books.

Broekhoff, J. (1986). The effect of physical activity on physical growth and development. In G. A. Stull & H. M. Eckert (Eds.), *Effects of physical activity on children.* (pp. 75–87). Champaign, IL: Human Kinetics.

Brooks-Gunn, J., Burrow, C., & Warren, M. P. (1988). Attitudes toward eating and body weight in different groups of female adolescent athletes. *International Journal of Eating Disorders, 7,* 749–757.

Brooks-Gunn, J., & Warren, M. P. (1985). Measuring physical status and timing in early adolescence: A developmental perspective. *Journal of Youth and Adolescence, 14,* 163–189.

Brown, J. D., & Siegel, J. M. (1988). Exercise as a buffer of life stress: A prospective study of adolescent health. *Health Psychology, 7,* 341–353.

Brownell, K. D., Kelman, J. H., & Stunkard, A. J. (1983). Treatment of obese children with and without their mothers: Changes in weight and blood pressure. *Pediatrics, 71,* 515–523.

Buckley, W. E., Yesalis, C. E., Friedl, K. E., Anderson, W. A., Streit, A. L., & Wright, J. E. (1988). Estimated prevalence of anabolic steroid use among male high school seniors. *Journal of the American Medical Association, 260,* 3441–3445.

Buhrmester, D., & Furman, W. (1987). The development of companionship and intimacy. *Child Development, 58,* 1101–1113.

Burdine, J. N., Chen, M. S., Gottlieb, N. H., Peterson, F. L., & Vacalis, D. (1984). The effects of ethnicity, sex, and father's occupation on heart health knowledge and nutrition behavior of school children: The Texas Youth Health Awareness Survey. *Journal of School Health, 54,* 87–90.

Burton, D., & Martens, R. (1986). Pinned by their own goals: An exploratory investigation into why kids drop out of wrestling. *Journal of Sport Psychology, 8,* 183–197.

Butcher, J. (1983). Socialization of adolescent girls into physical activity. *Adolescence, 18,* 753–766.

Byrd-Bredbenner, C., O'Connell, L. H., Shannon, B., & Eddy, J. M. (1984). A nutrition curriculum for health education: Its effect on students' knowledge, attitude, and behavior. *Journal of School Health, 54,* 385–389.

Caspersen, C. J., Christenson, G. M., & Pollard, R. A. (1986). Status of the 1990 physical fitness and exercise objectives—Evidence from NHIS 1985. *Public Health Reports, 101,* 587–592.

Cauley, J. A., Donfield, S. M., LaPorte, R. E., & Warhaftig. (1991). Physical activity by socioeconomic status in two population based cohorts. *Medicine and Science in Sports and Exercise, 23,* 343–352.

Cinciripini, P. M. (1984). Changing food selections in a public cafeteria. *Behavior Modification, 8,* 520–539.

Coates, T. J., Barofsky, I., Saylor, K. E., Simons-Morton, B., Huster, W., Sereghy, E., Straugh, S., Jacobs, H., & Kidd, L. (1985). Modifying the snack food consumption patterns of inner city high school students: The Great Sensations Study. *Preventive Medicine, 14,* 234–247.

Coates, T. J., Killen, J. D., & Slinkard, L. A. (1982). Parent participation in a treatment program for overweight adolescents. *International Journal of Eating Disorders, 1,* 37–47.

Coleman, J. C. (1980). Friendship and the peer group in adolescence. In J. Adelson (Ed.), *Handbook of adolescent psychology.* (pp. 408–431). New York: Wiley.

Connors, M. E., & Johnson, C. L. (1987). Epidemiology of bulimia and bulimic behaviors. *Addictive Behaviors, 12,* 165–179.

Contento, I. R., Michela, J. L., & Goldberg, C. J. (1988). Food choice among adolescents: Population segmentation by motivations. *Journal of Nutrition Education, 20,* 289–298.

Cooper, K. H., Purdy, J. G., Friedman, A., Bohannon, R. L., Harris, R. A., & Arends, J. A. (1975). An aerobic conditioning program for the Fort-Worth, Texas School District. *Research Quarterly, 46,* 345–350.

Cortugna, N. (1988). TV ads on Saturday morning children's programming—What's new? *Journal of Nutrition Education, 20,* 125–127.

Desmond, S. M., Price, J. H., Hallinan, C., & Smith, D. (1989). Black and white adolescents' perceptions of their weight. *Journal of School Health, 59,* 353–358.

Desmond, S. M., Price, J. H., Lock, R. S., Smith, D., & Stewart, P. W. (1990). Urban black and white adolescents' physical fitness status and perceptions of exercise. *Journal of School Health, 60,* 220–226.

Dietz, W. H., & Gortmaker, S. L. (1985). Do we fatten our children at the television set? Obesity and television viewing in children and adolescents. *Pediatrics, 75,* 807–812.

Dishman, R. K., Sallis, J. F., & Orenstein, D. R. (1985). The determinants of physical activity and exercise. *Public Health Reports, 100,* 158–172.

Doll, R., & Peto, R. (1981). The causes of cancer: Quantitative estimates of avoidable risks of cancer in the United States today. *Journal of the National Cancer Institute, 66,* 1191–1208.

Donato, K., & Hegsted, D. M. (1985). Efficiency of utilization of various sources of energy for growth. *Proceedings of the National Academy of Sciences, U.S.A., 82,* 4866–4870.

Dwyer, J. (1980). Diets for children and adolescents that meet the dietary goals. *American Journal of Diseases of Children, 134,* 1073–1080.

Elder, J. P., McGraw, S. A., Abrams, D. B., Ferreira, A., Lasater, T. M., Longpre, H., Peterson, G. S., Schwertfeger, R., & Carleton, R. A. (1986). Organizational and community approaches to community-wide prevention of heart disease: The first two years of the Pawtucket Heart Health Program. *Preventive Medicine, 15,* 107–117.

Elder, J. P., Sallis, J. F., Hammond, N., Peplinski, S., & Mayer, J. A. (1989). Community-based health promotion: A survey of churches, labor unions, supermarkets, and restaurants. *Journal of Community Health, 14,* 159–168.

Ellison, R. C., Capper, A. L., Goldberg, R. J., Witschi, J. C., & Stare, F. J. (1989). The environmental component: Changing school food service to promote cardiovascular health. *Health Education Quarterly, 16,* 285–297.

Epling, W. F., & Pierce, W. D. (1988). Activity-based anorexia: A biobehavioral perspective. *International Journal of Eating Disorders, 7,* 475–485.

Epstein, L. H. (1986). Treatment of childhood obesity. In K. D. Brownell & J. P. Foreyt (Eds.), *Handbook of eating disorders* (pp. 159–179). New York: Basic Books.

Fallon, A. E., & Rozin, P. (1985). Sex differences in perceptions of desirable body shape. *Journal of Abnormal Psychology, 94,* 102–105.

Farquhar, J. W., Maccoby, N., & Solomon, D. S. (1984). Community applications of behavioral medicine. In W. D. Gentry (Ed.), *Handbook of behavioral medicine* (pp. 437–478). New York: Guilford.

Flay, B. R. (1985). Psychosocial approaches to smoking prevention: A review of findings. *Health Psychology, 4,* 449–488.

Flora, J. A., & Wallack, L. (1990). Health promotion and mass media: Translating research into practice. *Health Education Research, 5,* 73–80.

Folsom, A. R., Cook, T. C., Sprafka, J. M., Burke, G. L., Norsted, S. W., & Jacobs, D. R. (1991). Differences in leisure-time physical activity levels between blacks and whites in population-based samples: The Minnesota Heart Survey. *Journal of Behavioral Medicine, 14,* 1–9.

Foster, G. D., Wadden, T. A., & Brownell, K. D. (1985). Peer-led program for the treatment and prevention of obesity in the schools. *Journal of Consulting and Clinical Psychology, 53,* 538–540.

Frank, G. C., Webber, L. S., & Berenson, G. S. (1982). Dietary studies of infants and children: The Bogalusa Heart Study. In T. J. Coates, A. C. Petersen, & C. Perry (Eds.), *Promoting adolescent health: A dialog on research and practice* (pp. 329–354). New York: Academic Press.

Fuchs, R., Powell, K. E., Semmer, N. K., Dwyer, J. H., Lippert, P., & Hoffmeister, H. (1988). Patterns of physical activity among German adolescents: The Berlin-Bremen Study. *Preventive Medicine, 17,* 746–763.

Garn, S. M., & Clark, D. C. (1976). Trends in fatness and the origins of obesity. *Pediatrics, 57,* 443–456.

Garner, D. M., Garfinkel, P. E., & Olmsted, M. P. (1983). An overview of the socio-cultural factors in the development of anorexia nervosa. In P. L. Darby, P. E. Garfinkel, D. M. Garner & D. V. Coscina (Eds.), *Anorexia nervosa: Recent developments in research* (pp. 65–82). New York: Alan R. Liss.

Gerbner, G., Morgan, M., & Signorelli, N. (1982). Programming health portrayals: What viewers see, say, and do. In D. Pearl, L. Bouthilet, & J. Logan (Eds.), *Television and behavior* (pp. 291–307). U. S. DHHS Publication No. (ADM) 82-1196. Rockville, MD: U. S. Department of Health and Human Services.

Godin, G., & Shephard, R. J. (1984). Normative beliefs of school children concerning regular exercise. *Journal of School Health, 54,* 443–445.

Goldblatt, P. B., Moore, M. E., & Stunkard, A. J. (1965). Social factors in obesity. *Journal of the American Medical Association, 192,* 1039–1044.

Gortmaker, S. L., Dietz, W. H., Sobol, A. M., & Wehler, C. A. (1987). Increasing pediatric obesity in the United States. *American Journal of Diseases of Children, 141,* 535–540.

Gottlieb, N. B., & Chen, M. S. (1985). Sociocultural correlates of childhood sporting activities: Their implications for heart health. *Social Science and Medicine, 5,* 533–539.

Gruber, J. J. (1986). Physical activity and self-esteem development in children: A meta-analysis. In G. A. Stull and H. M. Eckert (Eds.), *Effects of physical activity on children* (pp. 30–48). Champaign, IL: Human Kinetics.

Hazuda, H. P., Stern, M. P., Gaskill, S. P., Haffner, S. M., & Gardner, L. I. (1983). Ethnic differences in health knowledge and behaviors related to the prevention and treatment of coronary heart disease: The San Antonio Heart Study. *American Journal of Epidemiology, 117,* 717–728.

Herman, C. P., & Polivy, J. (1975). Anxiety, restraint, and eating behavior. *Journal of Abnormal Psychology, 84,* 666–672.

Hertzler, A. A. (1983). Children's food patterns—a review: II. Family and group behavior. *Journal of the American Dietetic Association, 83,* 555–560.

Holund, U. (1990). Promoting change of adolescents' sugar consumption: The "learning by teaching" study. *Health Education Research, 5,* 451–458.

Hovell, M. F., Bursick, J. H., & Sharkey, R. (1978). An evaluation of elementary students' voluntary physical activity during recess. *Research Quarterly, 49,* 460–474.

Hsu, L.K.G. (1989). The gender gap in eating disorders: Why are the eating disorders more common among women? *Clinical Psychology Review, 9,* 393–407.

Huenemann, R. L., Shapiro, L. R., Hammpton, M. C., & Mitchell, B. W. (1966). A longitudinal study of gross body composition and body conformation and then association with food and activity in a teenage population. *American Journal of Clinical Nutrition, 18,* 325–338.

Jones, B. H., Rock, P. B., & Moore, M. P. (1988). Musculoskeletal injury: Risks, prevention, and first aid. In S. N. Blair, P. Painter, R. R. Pate, L. K. Smith, and C. B. Taylor (Eds.), *Resource manual for guidelines for exercise testing and prescription* (pp. 285–294). Philadelphia: Lea & Febiger.

Kaplan, N. M., & Stamler, J. (Eds.) (1983). *Prevention of coronary heart disease: Practical management of the risk factors.* Philadelphia: Saunders.

Kaufman, L. (1980). Prime-time nutrition. *Journal of Community Health, 30,* 37–46.

Kessler, D. A. (1989). The federal regulation of food labelling: Promoting foods to prevent disease. *New England Journal of Medicine, 321,* 717–725.

Killen, J. D., Taylor, C. B., Telch, M. J., Saylor, K. E., Maron, D. J., & Robinson, T. N. (1986). Self-induced vomiting and laxative and diuretic use among teenagers. *Journal of the American Medical Association, 255,* 1447–1449.

Killen, J. D., Telch, M. J., Robinson, T. N., Maccoby, N., Taylor, C. B., & Farquhar, J. W. (1988). Cardiovascular disease risk reduction for tenth graders: A multiple-factor school-based approach. *Journal of the American Medical Association, 260,* 1728–1733.

Kimm, S.Y.S., Gergen, P. J., Malloy, M., Dresser, C., & Carroll, M. (1990). Dietary patterns of U. S. children: Implications for disease prevention. *Preventive Medicine, 19,* 432–442.

King, A. C., Saylor, K. E., Foster, S., Killen, J. D., Telch, M. J., Farquhar, J. W., & Flora, J. A. (1988). Promoting dietary change in adolescents: A school-based approach for modifying and maintaining healthful behavior. *American Journal of Preventive Medicine, 4,* 68–74.

Kirks, B. A., & Hughes, C. (1986). Long-term behavioral effects of parent involvement in nutrition education. *Journal of Nutrition Education, 18,* 203–206.

Klesges, R. C., Bartsch, D., Norwood, J. D., Kautzman, D., & Haugrud, S. (1984). The effects of selected social and environmental variables on the eating behavior of adults in the natural environment. *International Journal of Eating Disorders, 3,* 35–41.

Lansky, D., & Brownell, K. D. (1982). Comparison of school-based treatments for adolescent obesity. *Journal of School Health, 8,* 384–387.

Lansky, D., & Vance, M. A. (1983). School-based intervention for adolescent obesity: Analysis of treatment, randomly selected control, and self-selected subjects. *Journal of Consulting and Clinical Psychology, 51,* 147–148.

Laskarzewski, P., Morrison, J. A., Khoury, K., Glatfelter, L., Larsen, R., & Glueck, C. J. (1980). Parent–child nutrient intake relationships in school children ages 6 to 19: The Princeton School District Study. *American Journal of Clinical Nutrition, 33,* 3250–3255.

Lewin-Epstein, N. (1981). *Youth employment during high school.* Washington, DC: National Center for Education Statistics.

Lewis, M., Brun, J., Talmage, H., & Rasher, S. (1988). Teenagers and food choices: The impact of nutrition education. *Journal of Nutrition Education, 20,* 336–339.

Lucas, A. R., Beard, C. M., Kranz, J. S., & Kurland, L. T. (1983). Epidemiology of anorexia nervosa and bulimia. *International Journal of Eating Disorders, 2,* 85–90.

Matarazzo, J. D. (1980). Behavioral health and behavioral medicine: Frontiers for a new health psychology. *American Psychologist, 35,* 807–817.

Mayer, J. A., Dubbert, P. M., & Elder, J. P. (1989). Promoting nutrition at the point of choice: A review. *Health Education Quarterly, 16,* 31–43.

Maynard, E. J., Coonan, W. E., Worsley, A., Dwyer, T., & Baghurst, P. A. (1987). The development of the lifestyle education program in Australia. In B. Hetzel & G. S. Berenson (Eds.), *Cardiovascular risk factors in childhood: Epidemiology and prevention* (pp. 123–149). New York: Elsevier.

Maxwell, B., & Jacobson, M. (1989). *Marketing disease to Hispanics.* Washington, DC: Center for Science in the Public Interest.

Miller, T., Coffman, J., & Linke, R. (1980). Survey on body image, weight and diet of college students. *Journal of the American Dietetic Association, 77,* 561–566.

Nader, P. R., Sallis, J. F., Patterson, T. L., Abramson, I. S., Rupp, J. W., Senn, K. L., Atkins, C. J., Roppe, B. E., Morris, J. A., Wallace, J. P., & Vega, W. A. (1989). A family approach to cardiovascular risk reduction: Results from the San Diego Family Health Project. *Health Education Quarterly, 16,* 229–244.

National Research Council. (1989). *Diet and health: Implications for reducing chronic disease risk.* Washington, DC: National Academy Press.

O'Connell, J. K., Price, J. H., Roberts, S. M., Jurs, S. G., & McKinley, R. (1985). Utilizing the health belief model to predict dieting and exercising behavior of obese and nonobese adolescents. *Health Education Quarterly, 12,* 343–351.

Paffenbarger, R. S., Hyde, R. T., Wing, A. L., & Steinmetz, C. H. (1984). A natural history of athleticism and cardiovascular health. *Journal of the American Medical Association, 252,* 491–495.

Parcel, G. S., Green, L. W., & Bettes, B. A. (1988). School-based programs to prevent or reduce obesity. In N. A. Krasnegor, G. D. Grave, and N. Kretchmer (Eds.), *Childhood obesity: A biobehavioral perspective* (pp. 143–157). Caldwell, NJ: Telford.

Patterson, T. L., Rupp, J. W., Sallis, J. F., Atkins, C. J., & Nader, P. R. (1988). Aggregation of dietary calories, fats, and sodium in Mexican-American and Anglo families. *American Journal of Preventive Medicine, 57,* 150–156.

Perry, C. L., Griffin, G., & Murray, D. M. (1985). Assessing needs for youth health promotion. *Preventive Medicine, 14,* 379–393.

Perry, C. L., Klepp, K.-I., Halper, A., Dudovitz, B., Golden, D., Griffin, G., & Smyth, M. (1987). Promoting healthy eating and physical activity patterns among adolescents: A pilot study of "Slice of Life." *Health Education Research, 2,* 93–103.

Perry, C. L., Luepker, R. V., Murray, D. M., Kurth, C., Mullis, R., Crockett, S., & Jacobs, D. R.

(1988). Parent involvement with children's health promotion: The Minnesota Home Team. *American Journal of Public Health, 78,* 1156–1160.

Petchers, M. K., Hirsch, E. Z., & Bloch, B. A. (1987). The impact of parent participation on the effectiveness of a heart health curriculum. *Health Education Quarterly, 14,* 449–460.

Podell, R. N., Keller, K., Mulvihill, M. N., Berger, G., & Kent, D. F. (1978). Evaluation of the effectiveness of a high school course in cardiovascular nutrition. *American Journal of Public Health, 68,* 573–576.

Polivy, J., & Herman, C. P. (1976a). Clinical depression and weight change: A complex relation. *Journal of Abnormal Psychology, 85,* 338–340.

Polivy, J., & Herman, C. P. (1976b). Effects of alcohol on eating behavior: Disinhibition or sedation? *Addictive Behaviors, 1,* 121–125.

Pope, H. G., Hudson, J. I., Yurgelun-Todd, D., & Hudson, M. S. (1984). Prevalence of anorexia nervosa and bulimia in three student populations. *International Journal of Eating Disorders, 3,* 45–51.

Popkin, B. M., & Haines, P. S. (1981). Factors affecting food selection: The role of economics. *Journal of the American Dietetic Association, 79,* 419–425.

Powell, K. E., Thompson, P. D., Caspersen, C. J., & Kendrick, J. S. (1987). Physical activity and the incidence of coronary heart disease. *Annual Review of Public Health, 8,* 253–287.

Preston, M. A., Baranowski, T., & Higginbotham, J. C. (1988). Orchestrating the points of community intervention: Enhancing the diffusion process. *Policy, Theory, and Social Issues, 9,* 11–34.

Prior, J. C. (1990). Reproduction: Exercise-related adaptations and the health of women and men. In C. Bouchard, R. J. Shephard, T. Stephens, J. R. Sutton, & B. D. McPherson. (Eds.). *Exercise, fitness, and health: A consensus of current knowledge* (pp. 661–675). Champaign, IL: Human Kinetics.

Pumariega, A. J. (1986). Acculturation and eating attitudes in adolescent girls: A comparative and correlational study. *Journal of the American Academy of Child Psychiatry, 25,* 276–279.

Reynolds, K. D., Killen, J. D., Bryson, S. W., Maron, D. J., Taylor, C. B., Maccoby, N., & Farquhar, J. W. (1990). *Preventive Medicine, 19,* 541–551.

Roberts, R. E., & Lee, E. S. (1980). Health practices among Mexican Americans: Further evidence from the Human Population Laboratory Studies. *Preventive Medicine, 9,* 675–688.

Ross, J. G., Dotson, C. O., & Gilbert, G. G. (1985). Are kids getting appropriate activity? *Journal of Physical Education, Recreation, and Dance, 56,* 82–85.

Ross, J. G., Dotson, C. O., Gilbert, G. G., & Katz, S. J. (1985a). What are kids doing in school physical education? *Journal of Physical Education, Recreation, and Dance, 56,* 73–76.

Ross, J. G., Dotson, C. O., Gilbert, G. G., & Katz, S. J. (1985b). After physical education: Physical activity outside of school physical education programs. *Journal of Physical Education, Recreation, and Dance, 56,* 77–81.

Rowland, T. (1990). *Exercise and children's health.* Champaign, IL: Human Kinetics.

Rozin, P. (1984). The acquisition of food habits and preferences. In J. D. Matarazzo, S. M. Weiss, J. A. Herd, N. E. Miller, & S. M. Weiss (Eds.), *Behavioral health: A handbook of health enhancement and disease prevention* (pp. 608–631). New York: Wiley.

Rushall, B. S., & Siedentop, D. (1972). *The development and control of behavior in sport and physical education.* Philadelphia: Lea & Febiger.

Sallis, J. F., Hovell, M. F., Hofstetter, C. R., Faucher, P., Elder, J. P., Blanchard, J., Caspersen, C. J., Powell, K. E., & Christenson, G. M. (1989). A multivariate study of exercise determinants in a community sample. *Preventive Medicine, 18,* 20–34.

Sallis, J. F., & Nader, P. R. (1988). Family determinants of health behavior. In D. S. Gochman (Ed.), *Health behavior: Emerging research perspectives* (pp. 107–124). New York: Plenum.

Sallis, J. F., Nader, P. R., Rupp, J. W., Atkins, C. J., & Wilson, W. C. (1986). San Diego surveyed for heart-healthy foods and exercise facilities. *Public Health Reports, 101,* 216–219.

Sallis, J. F., Patterson, T. L., Buono, M. J., Atkins, C. J., & Nader, P. R. (1988). Aggregation of physical activity habits in Mexican-American and Anglo families. *Journal of Behavioral Medicine, 11,* 31–47.

Sallis, J. F., Patterson, T. L., McKenzie, T. L., & Nader, P. R. (1988). Family variables and physical activity in preschool children. *Journal of Developmental and Behavioral Pediatrics, 9,* 57–61.

Salz, K. M., Tamir, I., Ernst, N., Kwiterovich, P., Glueck, C., Christensen, B., Larsen, R., Pirhonen, D., Prewitt, T. E., & Scott, L. W. (1983). Selected nutrient intakes of free-living white children ages 6–19 years. The lipid research clinics program prevalence study. *Pediatric Research, 17,* 124–130.

Sclafani, A., & Springer, D. (1976). Dietary obesity in adult rats: Similarities to hypothalamic and human obesity syndromes. *Physiology and Behavior, 17,* 461–471.

Sheridan, M., & McPherrin, E. (1983). *Fast food and the American diet.* New York: American Council on Science and Health.

Siscovick, D. S. (1990). Risks of exercising: Sudden cardiac death and injuries. In C. Bouchard, R. J. Shephard, T. Stephens, J. R. Sutton, & B. D. McPherson. (Eds.), *Exercise, fitness, and health: A consensus of current knowledge* (pp. 707–713). Champaign, IL: Human Kinetics.

Stephens, T., Jacobs, D. R., & White, C. C. (1985). A descriptive epidemiology of leisure-time physical activity. *Public Health Reports, 100,* 147–158.

Stern, M. P., Gaskill, S. P., Allen, C. R., Garza, V., Gonzales, J. L., & Waldrop, R. H. (1981). Cardiovascular risk factors in Mexican Americans in Laredo, Texas: I. Prevalence of overweight and diabetes and distributions of serum lipids. *American Journal of Epidemiology, 113,* 546–555.

Stevens, N. H., & Davis, L. G. (1988). Exemplary school health education: A new charge from HOT districts. *Health Education Quarterly, 15,* 63–70.

Story, M., & Resnick, M. D. (1986). Adolescents' views on food and nutrition. *Journal of Nutrition Education, 18,* 188–192.

Strong, W. B. (1983). Atherosclerosis: Its pediatric roots. In N. M. Kaplan and J. Stamler (Eds.), *Prevention of coronary heart disease: Practical management of the risk factors* (pp. 20–32). Philadelphia: Saunders.

Stunkard, A., d'Aquilli, E., Fox, S., & Filion, R.D.L. (1972). Influence of social class on obesity and thinness in children. *Journal of the American Medical Association, 22,* 579–584.

Tappe, M. K., Duda, J. L., & Ehrnwald, P. M. (1989). Perceived barriers to exercise among adolescents. *Journal of School Health, 59,* 153–155.

Tell, G. S., & Vellar, O. D. (1987). Noncommunicable disease risk factor intervention in Norwegian adolescents: The Oslo Youth Study. In B. Hetzel & G. S. Berenson (Eds.), *Cardiovascular risk factors in childhood: Epidemiology and prevention* (pp. 203–217). New York: Elsevier.

U. S. Department of Health and Human Services. (1989). *The Surgeon General's report on nutrition and health.* DHHS (PHS) Publication No. 88-50210. Washington, DC: U. S. Government Printing Office.

U. S. Department of Health and Human Services. (1991). *Healthy people 2000.* Washington, DC: U. S. Government Printing Office.

Vartiainen, E., & Puska, P. (1987). The North Karelia Youth Project 1978–1980: Effects of two years of educational intervention on cardiovascular risk factors and health behavior in adolescence. In B. Hetzel & G. S. Berenson (Eds.), *Cardiovascular risk factors in childhood: Epidemiology and prevention* (pp. 183–202). New York: Elsevier.

Wadden, T. A., & Brownell, K. D. (1984). The development and modification of dietary practices in individuals, groups, and large populations. In J. D. Matarazzo, S. M. Weiss, J. A. Herd, N. E. Miller, & S. M. Weiss (Eds.), *Behavioral health: A handbook of health enhancement and disease prevention* (pp. 608–631). New York: Wiley.

Wadden, T. A., Foster, G. D., Stunkard, A. J., & Linowitz, J. R. (1989). Dissatisfaction with weight and figure in obese girls: Discontent but not depression. *International Journal of Obesity, 13,* 89–97.

Wadden, T. A., Stunkard, A. J., Rich, L., Rubin, C. J., Sweidel, G., & McKinney, S. (1990). Obesity in black adolescent girls: A controlled clinical trial of treatment by diet, behavior modification, and parental support. *Pediatrics, 85,* 345–352.

White, A. A., & Skinner, J. D. (1988). Can goal setting as a component of nutrition education effect behavior change among adolescents? *Journal of Nutrition Education, 20,* 327–334.

White, C. C., Powell, K. E., Hogelin, G. C., Gentry, E. M., & Forman, M. R. (1987). The behavioral risk factor surveys: IV. The descriptive epidemiology of exercise. *American Journal of Public Health, 3,* 304–310.

Windsor, R., & Dumitru, D. (1989). Prevalence of anabolic steroid use by male and female adolescents. *Medicine and Science in Sports and Exercise, 21,* 494–497.

11

Promoting Oral Health in Adolescents

Judith E. N. Albino and Sandra D. Lawrence

In considering the potential health risks of adolescents, oral health issues often remain in the background. Oral health problems generally are not life-threatening, nor are they perceived as having the social impact of high-risk behaviors such as smoking, substance abuse, or unsafe sexual behavior. Yet when 1,400 adolescents were asked about health problems, dental health ranked second in importance, after nervousness (Sternlieb & Munan, 1972). Many oral health behaviors significantly affect physical and psychological health during adolescence, while others have potentially serious effects on future health status. Oral diseases can result in pain, discomfort, and functional problems. Moreover, the teeth and mouth are particularly salient aspects of physical appearance. As the instruments of speech, they play a major role in interpersonal communication, and any defects in appearance are highly visible.

Facial appearance provides information about an individual's identity and influences judgments about intelligence, personality, and other aspects of how individuals perceive, think, and feel about others (Alley, 1988a). Because facial attractiveness almost always has a positive influence, researchers now commonly refer to a *beauty-is-good* stereotype (Dion, Berscheid, & Walster, 1972). Individuals with impaired dental-facial features may be the recipients of social judgments and interactions that potentially have a negative effect on self-image and social adjustment. Consequently, dental problems may negatively influence an individual's developing self-image, which is particularly vulnerable during adolescence.

There is considerable evidence that the most prevalent oral diseases are largely preventable through a combination of community-based programs, accessible professional care, and proper practice of oral self-care behaviors. At the same time, only 55% of Americans have access to fluoridated water and only 57% visit a dentist during any 12-month period (U. S. Department of Health & Human Services, 1990). It is, therefore, readily apparent that better self-care behaviors are necessary to further improve oral health. In addition, oral health promotion activities, because of their potential for demonstrating significant improvement, may offer relatively easily attained success and provide the opportunity for the increases in self-efficacy that commonly accompany self-mastery.

242

Epidemiology of Adolescent Oral Health Problems

Adolescence usually is characterized as a time of heightened vulnerability to the most commonly occurring oral diseases. Yet, over the past three decades, substantial decreases in the general rates of dental caries in young people have been seen, suggesting that their oral health has improved. At the same time, there is no question that oral diseases and conditions continue to represent a major source of risk to the health of this age group. We still see alarmingly high rates of dental caries in children from poor families, including a disproportionate number of American Indian, African-American, and Hispanic children. The rate of untreated caries among minority and otherwise disadvantaged adolescents is almost double the national average; more than 80% of caries in American Indian adolescents are left untreated—almost four times the national average (U. S. Department of Health and Human Services, 1990).

The impact of oral conditions often is underestimated, probably because most oral diseases are not life-threatening. Yet when we consider that these oral diseases account for 20.9 million days of work, study, or other productive activities lost each year, more than 6.4 million days spent in bed, and more than $27 billion spent annually for dental care in the United States, the potential impact of poor oral health becomes obvious (U. S. Department of Health and Human Services, 1990). Although data on days lost as a result of oral health problems are not available for the adolescent population per se, we know that each year white children of all ages lose about 1.0 school days per 100 individuals, and African-American children lose about 3.9 days per 100 persons due to oral health problems (U. S. Department of Health and Human Services, 1988).

The most commonly occurring adolescent oral health problems are caries and malocclusion, although periodontal disease—particularly in its milder manifestations—is also a source of concern in this age group. Oral cancer, while rare, occurs in adolescents as well. Each of these major adolescent oral health problems will be discussed individually.

Caries

Caries has become an almost universal condition. As a result, the phenomenon known as the *cavity-prone years* of adolescence now is part of the public understanding of oral health issues. The incidence of dental caries in many children, however, has been reduced dramatically in recent years, largely as a result of the fluoridation of community water supplies and the increased use of topical fluorides. Since both a suitable fermentable substrate and a vulnerable tooth surface are required for bacteria to produce the acid that leads to decalcification of the tooth structure, or caries, incorporation of fluoride in the enamel can substantially inhibit this process.

Studies have shown that the number of caries-free adolescents increased from 9.7% during the 1960s to more than 17% in the early 1980s. Even so, the mean number of decayed, missing, and filled teeth (DMFT) continues to increase by nearly six surfaces (DMFS) between the ages of 12 and 17, suggesting that dental caries during adolescence is far from being eradicated (U. S. Department of Health and Human Services, 1990). Moreover, a 1979–80 study of the prevalence of dental caries (U. S. Department of Health and Human Services, 1981) showed that the proportion of the DMFS and DMFT measures representing decay was three to four times higher in African-American and ethnic minority children than in white children. The proportion of these measures representing missing teeth was about four times higher in minority groups. These differences, of course, reflect a much greater need for treatment among adolescents of color (a conclusion that is supported by data related to the specific need for crowns or replacement of permanent teeth), especially among those who use public health programs as their primary source of dental care.

Although virtually no epidemiological data are available, dental caries also has been associated with bulimia, an eating disorder that disproportionately tends to affect adolescent and young adult women. Preventive therapies are especially important for this group to avoid enamel destruction, and dental treatment needs to be coordinated with the treatment being provided by other health professionals.

The presence of decayed and missing teeth suggests not only the potential for pain, but also the probability of tooth loss in the future as untreated conditions are allowed to worsen. Improvements in dental caries rates in recent years demonstrate that it is possible to reduce significantly the effects of this oral health problem on adolescents. The regular removal of dental plaque, a predecessor to caries, through conscientious adherence to a basic oral hygiene regimen, good dietary habits including restriction of sweets, and adequate fluoride intake is virtually all that is required to prevent caries in most cases. Yet, improvements in dental self-care behaviors may be difficult to achieve in adolescence. Sustained efforts over a long period of time are required, and the typically insidious progress of caries obscures the relationship between preventive behaviors and oral health.

Periodontal Disease

Although periodontal, or gum, disease is typically associated with adults, nearly two-thirds of adolescents experience gingivitis, or bleeding gums. The prevalence among white children is 55%, and among nonwhite children it is 72%. In addition, about 20% of adolescents have lost at least 2 mm of periodontal attachment on at least one tooth (National Institute of Dental Research, 1989).

Unfortunately, while periodontal disease does seem to be perceived as serious, many people think it is much rarer than is actually the case. Furthermore, neglecting this problem during adolescence may lead to more serious conditions in adulthood, including tooth loss as a function of the bone destruction that accompanies severe periodontal disease.

In addition to the more commonly occurring forms of periodontal disease, a chronic condition called *localized juvenile periodontitis (LJP)* is found in .1–2.3% of adolescents and more frequently in African-American than in whites. This condition can cause considerable periodontal destruction, as well as bone and tooth loss (Zambon, Christersson, & Genco, 1986).

Finally, periodontal symptoms, including gingival recession, have been associated in some studies with the use of smokeless tobacco (Offenbacher & Weathers, 1985). Periodontal consequences should, therefore, be considered when addressing the problems associated with this risk behavior.

Although periodontal disease is not responsive to passive prevention techniques such as fluoridation and sealants (described in a later section), prevention can be substantially effected with proper self-care behaviors. Clearly associated with the presence of microbial colonies in dental plaque, periodontal disease is responsive to scrupulous oral hygiene regimens, particularly in its early stages (Woodall, 1990). Yet adolescents may find it especially difficult to relate to this problem, because they understand the result of untreated periodontal disease, namely tooth loss, to be an adult problem. Consequently, rather than engaging in preventive behaviors, adolescents tend to place this disease in the category of things to be worried about much later.

Oral Cancer

Epidemiologically, oral cancer is a disease of older adults. Yet we have seen a rise in adolescent soft tissue malignant and premalignant conditions, which appears to be associated with the use of smokeless tobacco. Smokeless tobacco use has increased among teenage and young adult males to levels as high as 25% to 35% in some areas. Use on a national basis is estimated at about 16% (U. S. Department of Health and Human Services, 1986).

The problem of health promotion related to smokeless tobacco use is similar to that of smoking. Young people who use tobacco generally do so within a context of social reinforcement that serves to maintain and strengthen this behavior. While adolescents may understand the negative consequences of their actions at an intellectual level, developmental factors, including increased self-consciousness, decreased self-esteem (Simmons, Rosenberg, & Rosenberg, 1973), and increased reliance on peers, may promote substance abuse (Rhodes & Jason, 1988; Chapter 12).

Malocclusion

Malocclusion, or impairment of the normal anatomical relations and associated functioning of the teeth and adjacent craniofacial structures, is most commonly treated during adolescence, after all permanent dentition has erupted but while the potential for growth can still be used to advantage. Although the prevention of rampant caries and periodontal disease can minimize tooth loss and thereby prevent certain malrelations, malocclusion is primarily genetic in origin and in most cases is not considered preventable. For adolescent oral health promotion, two salient questions about malocclusion arise: how to make good decisions about treatment and how to ensure full adherence to treatment recommendations when that course is chosen.

Epidemiological data indicate that as many as 70–75% of the population evidence some deviation from normal occlusion, although most of these cases are not severe. Studies indicate that nearly 30% of adolescents have severe or very severe malocclusion, with the need for treatment described as mandatory (U. S. Department of Health, Education and Welfare, 1977), and that occlusal malrelations tend to worsen during adolescence (McClain & Profitt, 1985). Despite these estimates, only about 25% of white youths and 4% of African-American youths receive treatment for malocclusion, regardless of its severity.

Adolescent Oral Health Promotion

Since adolescent oral health promotion encompasses a wide range of possible interventions, attention should be given to multiple levels of intervention. Not only are public policy and community support important, but development of the adolescent's individual coping and social skills—reinforced by family and health systems—also is required to ensure compliance. Some interventions are more readily available to certain segments of the population than to others. Those adolescents growing up in a disadvantaged environment, whether social or economic, not only have a higher incidence of dental problems, they may not have access to the essential components of good oral health promotion (i.e., treatment and knowledge: Beal, 1989). In addition, utilization of dental services decreases as income decreases (Golden, 1988). Policy and community decisions must, therefore, take into account the differing needs of the many subgroups that comprise our population, including increasing availability of, and motivation for, preventive and curative dental services, particularly for low-income groups (Albino, 1980).

The focus of this section is limited to interventions that are unique in addressing the promotion of oral health during adolescence. The literature related to smoking and the use of smokeless tobacco will not be reviewed in depth, since those problems have been best addressed by strategies designed to deal with substance abuse and the prevention of high-risk behaviors (see Chapter 12 for further discussion).

Community Water Fluoridation

Community water fluoridation may represent the single best means of preventing dental caries. Such programs do not rely on individual compliance, are potentially equally accessible to all, and are highly cost effective. Since community water fluoridation was introduced in the 1940s, dental caries rates in children have decreased by 25–60%, and millions of dollars in dental treatment have been saved (Harris, 1989). It is estimated that water fluoridation in the United States costs less than 50 cents per person annually, and that for every $1 that has been spent on community fluoridation, $50 has been saved in dental treatment costs (Loe, 1983). Even children who have had only limited exposure to fluoridated water show significant declines in caries rates (Burt, Eklund, & Loesche, 1986). Furthermore, fewer root caries are found among adults from fluoridated communities (Stamm, Banting, & Imrey, 1990). Further evidence of the effectiveness of fluoridation has come from data reflecting substantial increases in dental caries for children in two Scottish communities that discontinued water fluoridation, while national rates declined (Attwood & Blinkhorn, 1988; Stephen, McCall, & Tullis, 1987).

While the benefits of community water fluoridation are many, it would be a mistake to think that we can rely completely on this approach. Fluoridated water alone may not be enough to combat caries completely. In fact, most children in fluoridated communities still develop dental caries. Moreover, in 1985 only 55% of Americans had access to fluoridated water, indicating that currently more than 100 million Americans are not being served. At the least, these children should be receiving fluoride supplements; however, only about 1% of adolescents report using fluoride supplements (U. S. Department of Health and Human Services, 1990).

School-based fluoride rinse programs may provide an alternative to fluoridating community water supplies. There is, however, some controversy regarding their effectiveness. Several studies have shown that school fluoridation programs significantly reduce caries rates in children and adolescents even in fluoridated communities (Driscoll, Swango, Horowitz, & Kingman, 1982). Other studies, however, have suggested that the benefits of school fluoride programs are questionable and do not outweigh the costs, especially when compared to the benefits of improved community water fluoridation (Bohannan, Stamm, Graves, Disney, & Bader, 1985).

The above data indicate that not only does fluoride need to be made available to more individuals, but compliance with oral health self-care recommendations also needs to be promoted. Ubiquitous passive use of fluoride cannot yet be assumed, and recent heightened activity by antifluoridationists may decrease the number of people who have access to community fluoridated water. The concern for a link between fluoride ingestion and cancer has many individuals calling for more research on fluoride safety, and some communities are awaiting the results of these studies before implementing water fluoridation practices.

Sealants

Dental sealants, or plastic coatings applied to susceptible tooth surfaces (the pit and fissure surfaces of the molars), provide another effective prevention strategy for caries. The chewing surfaces of children's teeth are highly susceptible to the development of caries. In fact, 84% of the caries experienced by adolescents involve these occlusal pit and fissure tooth surfaces, which are only minimally protected by the use of fluorides (National Institutes of Health, 1984).

Although properly applied dental sealants are recognized as effective in preventing pit and fissure caries in both fluoridated and nonfluoridated communities (National Institutes of Health, 1984), the application of sealants requires professional expertise. Consequently, sealants represent a relatively expensive strategy for enhancing adolescent oral health ($10–15 per child annually: Bohannan et al., 1984). In recent years, the implementation of sealant programs has been severely curtailed by limited public resources, even though treatment of the resulting unprevented caries costs substantially more (Silverstone, 1984). Currently, only

7.6% of school-age children have received dental sealants, and an economic differential clearly exists. Over 12% of children from families earning more than $35,000 a year receive sealants, in contrast to only 2.2% of children from families earning less than $10,000. These numbers break down to 7.5% of white children and 2.1% of African-American children benefitting from dental sealants. With the rising costs of health care and the limited insurance coverage available for preventive procedures, more extensive use of dental sealants does not seem promising.

Self-Care Behaviors

Studies of the initiation and maintenance of oral hygiene self-care behaviors for the prevention of dental caries and periodontal disease comprise the major body of literature related to the enhancement of adolescent oral health through changing individual behaviors. Several trends are observable over the recent history of this work. The most effective approaches have taken into consideration both the cognitive and social developmental aspects of adolescence, utilized peer group approaches, and/or used cognitive-behavioral strategies along with manipulation of environmental cues and supports to enhance performance of oral health behaviors.

BEHAVIORAL STRATEGIES. Oral health behavior patterns, such as brushing, flossing, rinsing, dental appointment keeping, and restriction of sweets, are generally considered resistant to change, and long-term maintenance of desired behaviors has been particularly difficult to achieve (Albino, 1984a; Tedesco & Albino, 1989). Although the task of improving oral hygiene often has been construed as an information problem, educational approaches focused on providing information have been most notable for their lack of success (Kiyak & Mulligan, 1986). Even when supervised skill practice is included, the minimal improvements achieved in oral hygiene status by these interventions have been short-lived. While behavioral approaches employing contingent rewards have been highly effective in producing short-term results with both adults and children (Lund & Kegeles, 1984; Yeung, Howell, & Fahey, 1989), the problem of sustaining these improvements in the absence of reinforcement has not been adequately addressed. The most effective approaches have proved to be those that have used cognitive-behavioral strategies along with manipulation of environmental cues and supports for the performance of oral health behaviors (Albino, 1984b; Tedesco & Albino, 1989).

One of the biggest problems with behavioral interventions in general is the tendency for newly acquired behaviors to disappear over time. The problem of extinction needs to be addressed in terms of the relevance and pattern of the rewards arranged to reinforce desired behaviors. Maintaining acquired oral health behaviors may not require continuation of a particular pattern of reinforcement, since there are indications from the research literature that repeated feedback or other external attention alone may extend learned behaviors.

Obviously, the adaptation of these approaches for adolescents requires special attention to both cognitive and social aspects of development. Developmental issues of adolescence need to be considered in determining effective reinforcers and modes of implementation. The work completed to date has addressed these issues only partially.

COGNITIVE STRATEGIES. Of the approaches generally categorized as cognitive, *fear appeal* was among the first to be tested within the dental context. In summarizing the work on fear arousal and persuasive communication techniques in preventive dentistry, Evans (1978) concluded that increasing the amount of information or the level of emotional arousal cannot be expected to result in positive behavior change related to oral health.

Leventhal (1971), on the other hand, noted that the results of fear arousal studies are not consistent across prevention issues. His *parallel response* hypothesis suggests that there may be two competing responses to messages about health problems intended to evoke fear—one intended to reduce fear and the other to cope with the particular health issue on which the individual is focusing. This model suggests that in order to control irrational responses to these messages, individuals balance not only the amount of fear but also the perceived means for controlling the danger of the health problem presented. Thus, it appears to be of fundamental importance for health practitioners, when attempting to enhance compliance with health recommendations, to understand the value and utility of the information they provide to adolescents. Value and utility, however, are subjective qualities, and we can expect that in adolescence these judgments may be influenced by peer standards and the questioning of parental authority and values that are so typical at this time of life (Rhodes & Jason, 1988).

Both Leventhal's and Evans' approaches appear to return to strategies that focus on information and instruction. However, they indicate that if we depend on instruction, the structure, and perhaps even the context and timing, of preventive messages are as important for successful compliance as the content itself. If this advice is viewed from a developmental perspective, it is not surprising that the adolescents studied thus far generally have not responded to high fear appeals. Such interventions typically have not adequately addressed adolescent developmental issues in either their content or their presentation.

Another approach that incorporates attitudinal responses is the peer group method. Usually involving small group discussions, such programs have attempted, with some success, to mobilize peer influence in preventive dentistry programs (Albino, 1978). Consideration of both cognitive and social developmental aspects of adolescence distinguishes this approach from less successful efforts focused on oral health instruction and skills development.

The *value* placed on oral health, and the beliefs and attitudes related to its maintenance, often are considered the most critical factors in determining the response to prescribed behaviors for preventing dental disease. Kegeles (1975) applied the health belief model to dentistry, suggesting that individuals take preventive oral health action only when they believe (1) that they are susceptible to dental diseases; (2) that dental diseases are serious; (3) that dental diseases can be prevented; and (4) that prevention is no more unpleasant than the disease it is intended to prevent.

The developmental tasks, the cognitive constraints, and the social context of adolescence will substantially limit the responses of this age group to these conditions. For these reasons perhaps, the few interventions that have been developed to deal directly with cognitive and social factors of adolescence have achieved some notable success (Albino, 1978).

Developmental Context for Oral Health Promotion in Adolescence

Self-care behaviors can improve the oral health of most adolescents, even in the presence of water fluoridation and dental sealants, but it is essential to approach the promotion of these behaviors within the context of adolescent developmental issues. The circumstances surrounding behavior change must be understood *from the perspective of the adolescent*. As the preceding section suggests, adolescent oral health issues represent very different problems.

In the cases of caries and periodontal disease, the objective is to initiate and sustain oral health-enhancing and preventive self-care behaviors, while in working to prevent oral cancer, we are seeking abstinence from high-risk behaviors. These differences are extremely important. In both cases, we are asking individuals to make certain behavior changes in order to prevent a problem that the adolescent may not perceive as having a high probability of occurrence. However, in the former instance, we are asking for the adoption of new and time-consuming, but relatively innocuous, behaviors. In the latter, we are asking young people to refrain from behaviors that may be immediately rewarding and may have important social meaning within the adolescent's peer reference group.

With respect to occlusal and other craniofacial conditions, the primary goal is quite different. Here we are attempting to encourage sound decision making related to treatment and, when it is chosen, to achieve cooperation with treatment requirements.

As different as the demands of these various health-enhancing behaviors are, however, all must be carried out within the context of the adolescent's cognitive limits and social realities. Very little research has focused specifically on identifying adolescent developmental factors that influence the acceptance and adoption of oral health or other preventive recommendations. However, a consideration of the literature on other adolescent health topics, combined with our understanding of the difficulties more generally inherent in enhancing oral health behaviors, allows us to develop some sense of the context within which adolescents consider oral health enhancement activities.

As discussed elsewhere in this volume, substantial covariation exists among such adolescent health-related behaviors as cigarette smoking, early and unsafe sexual behavior, and marijuana use (Jessor, 1982). In addition, several recent studies have found an association between engaging in smokeless tobacco use and other risk behaviors, such as cigarette, marijuana, and alcohol use (Ary, Lichtenstein, & Severson, 1987; Dent, Sussman, Johnson, Hansen, & Flay, 1987). Oral health behaviors also are included in such patterns, however. While it is possible that the use of smokeless tobacco, a high-risk behavior for oral cancer, is related to other health risk behaviors, it is not clear that positive and health-enhancing behaviors such as regular tooth brushing and flossing or maintenance of orthodontic appliances are associated with abstinence from alcohol and drugs (Chapter 7).

The potentially negative value of oral health behaviors, then, must be considered along with what we know about the difficulty of instilling oral health behaviors at any age. Kegeles (1963) has attributed this difficulty to the relatively low perceived severity of dental problems such as caries. In adolescents, this problem may be exaggerated by the changes in self-consciousness, self-esteem (Simmons et al., 1973), and importance of peers that accompany adolescent development (Rhodes & Jason, 1988). In addition, adolescents may not identify well with the aging process and, therefore, may not be intimidated by the long-range effects of neglected oral health. In many cases, only the immediate consequences of their actions tend to have a great deal of influence on their behavior.

Chambers (1973) has suggested that the regular and sustained home care required for good oral hygiene simply is incompatible with the lifestyles of many people, and this may be especially so for adolescents. Particularly in early adolescence, young people often are interested in social behaviors and have little time for such mundane things as oral hygiene. This same orientation, however, can make them hypersensitive about personal appearance and overreactive to suggested imperfections of appearance. The physical changes of adolescence interact with social processes and peer standards to further exaggerate this self-focus. For many adolescents, this process can produce situations of great psychological pain. They may, for example, become convinced that their appearance is ruined by some minor deviation from ideal occlusal relations, even though another adolescent may be completely indifferent to an occlusal condition that is actually much more serious. These responses to appearance can be important in influencing adolescents to obtain treatment or engage in oral health self-care behaviors (Albino, 1984a).

Social Meanings of Facial Attractiveness in Adolescence

In addition to causing pain, discomfort, and loss of function, oral health problems may decrease facial attractiveness. A number of dental problems can create mild to severe impairment of facial appearance. Whether this impairment is the result of severe caries, traumatic injury, a birth defect such as cleft lip, or some deviation from ideal tooth alignment, the possibility of psychological distress and social maladjustment must be considered. Evaluating the impact of aesthetic impairment of adolescents' dentofacial features requires an understanding of the social meanings of facial attractiveness during that period of life.

Facial appearance has been described as the most salient stimulus for others' evaluations of both character and ability (Alley & Hildebrandt, 1988; Bull & Rumsey, 1988). The beauty-is-good stereotype strongly influences our thoughts, feelings, and behaviors, and facial attractiveness is probably the most important of our initial perceptions of, and responses to, others (Albino et al., 1990). Individuals within a given culture or society clearly embrace common definitions of facial and physical attractiveness, although these definitions are not necessarily shared across cultures (Alley, 1988b).

In explaining how such cultural standards influence the development of individual assessments of appearance, Adams (1982) has asserted that evaluation and understanding of the self are rooted in daily interactions in which others challenge or confirm the individual's self-knowledge. The transactional processes underlying this explanation are as follows: (1) attractiveness and unattractiveness elicit different social expectations from others; (2) more attractive individuals are the recipients of more favorable social interactions; (3) as a result of these more frequent favorable social experiences, attractive individuals are more likely to develop positive expectations and social images, as well as personality styles and behaviors that reflect this; and (4) as a result of their positive social experiences and greater self-confidence, attractive persons are more likely to initiate and maintain satisfying interpersonal relationships with others. Following similar reasoning, Lerner (1987) suggests that adolescents perceived as less attractive may develop less favorable social and personality styles, as well as a negative self-concept.

The importance of facial appearance may change as a function of age, cognitive development, and social developmental tasks. In adolescence, body and facial characteristics are changing rapidly during a period in which social comparison processes help determine how young people see themselves. This pattern of change renders most young people chronically uncertain about the adequacy of their appearance and particularly sensitive to peer responses. The salience of the mouth in face-to-face interactions with others, therefore, represents enormous potential for anxiety related to personal appearance, and the adolescent with unattractive oral features is particularly vulnerable to negative self-evaluations of his or her appearance (Albino & Tedesco, 1988).

Furthermore, early adolescents rely primarily on facial characteristics in their ratings of physical attractiveness. A number of studies have found that more positive psychosocial characteristics are attributed to those early adolescents who are facially attractive, than to those who are judged unattractive (Adams, 1982; Lerner, 1987). In addition, peer nominations and teachers' ratings of students' social and athletic competence seem to be associated with adolescent self-perceived attractiveness (Lerner et al., 1991).

In summary, there are strong indications that physical attractiveness does affect interpersonal interactions and that adolescents tend to assess their physical attractiveness in terms of facial characteristics. However, there is still much to learn about the ways in which psychosocial development is affected by facial appearance. We need to develop better ways of assessing specific aspects of dental-facial appearance, as well as any effects on psychosocial development. Follow-up assessments that allow enough time for changes in self-perceptions of attractiveness to be internalized and incorporated into the self-image also would make an important contribution to our understanding of these issues.

Dental-Facial Disfigurement and Psychosocial Functioning

In this section, psychosocial problems related to malocclusion and its treatment will be considered as an example of the potential effects of dental-facial disfigurement.

Impact of Malocclusion in Adolescence

Data on the effects of dental-facial disfigurement on adolescent psychosocial functioning is sparse. Macgregor (1970) suggests that children with malocclusion or milder types of facial disfigurement may be at greater risk for developing psychological problems than those with more obvious forms of impairment. The responses of others to individuals with mild impairment may be unpredictable, thereby creating uncertainty and anxiety in the anticipation of social reactions. This situation suggests less consistency in the feedback received from social interactions and the possibility that those affected will develop neither the self-confidence and self-esteem accruing to the physically attractive nor the strong coping skills so often forged by the severely impaired, who must adjust to the inevitable reality of others' responses. Although Macgregor's thesis is intuitively appealing, it has not been tested directly. The work on psychological aspects of malocclusion, however, does provide us with a context within which to explore the impact of dental-facial appearance on adolescents.

Research demonstrates that normal occlusion is perceived as more attractive than various forms of malocclusion (Albino, 1981) and in children is associated with positive evaluations of personality (Shaw, 1981). In addition, one study found that teeth represented the fourth most common target of teasing, after height, weight, and hair, and resulted in strong feelings of upset and sense of harassment (Shaw, Meek, & Jones, 1980).

Although it is clear that normal occlusion is perceived as more attractive than malocclusion, there is little evidence of a direct relationship between dental-facial appearance and psychosocial adjustment. Albino et al. (1981) found no differences in global assessments of self-esteem or self-concept between adolescents seeking orthodontic treatment and those not seeking treatment, even though the former group evaluated their appearance as significantly less attractive. Similarly, no differences in self-esteem or self-concept were found between adolescents who had received treatment and a randomly assigned control group for whom treatment was delayed (Albino, Lawrence, Tedesco, & Cunat, 1990). In addition, Kenealy, Frude, and Shaw (1989) found no negative effects of malocclusion on psychological well-being in a group of 1,018 11- and 12-year-old children. These results are consistent with the research on general physical appearance, however, where little or no direct relationship has been found between actual physical attractiveness and self-esteem. Rather, self-esteem seems to be more strongly associated with self-perception of physical attractiveness, which is a much more subjective judgment (Hatfield & Sprecher, 1986; Patzer, 1985). In summary, then, self-perceptions of occlusal attractiveness, rather than actual malocclusion, may significantly influence an adolescent's well-being. Moreover, this process likely occurs indirectly by influencing the development of self-esteem.

Evaluating Occlusal Appearance

Self-perceptions of occlusal appearance do not necessarily coincide with professional orthodontic assessments. In fact, Albino and Tedesco (1988) reported data demonstrating that while self-assessments of the attractiveness of occlusal features are correlated with both peer ratings and professional ratings of attractiveness, they are more closely related to peer assessments; and professional ratings of appearance are more closely related to objective measures of the severity of mal-occlusion than are self-evaluations or evaluations by peers. It is how the individual evaluates his or her own occlusal attractiveness that is most important in determin-ing psychosocial response, however, and self-perceptions are the most important factor in determining the demand for orthodontic treatment.

Changes in self-perception related to dental-facial appearance do occur as a result of orthodontic treatment (Albino et al., 1989), although these perceptions appear to be rather narrowly focused on dental-facial features. The adolescent who has focused on these problems, however, may begin to perceive them as over-whelming obstacles to social interaction and personal happiness. Others see orth-odontic treatment as a status symbol and press for treatment as an end in itself. In either case, unrealistic expectations can result in disappointment.

Treatment Decisions in Adolescence

It has been suggested that as many as 80% of those who seek orthodontic treatment do so for cosmetic reasons, rather than because of any major impact on health or functioning (Albino, 1984a). Yet precisely because this condition is related to appearance, issues of malocclusion and its treatment may have greater implications for adolescent emotional well-being than for physical and health concerns. Although it is generally assumed that dental-facial disfigurement will reduce self-esteem, and that low self-esteem will lead to poor social adjustment and possibly to affective disorders, the relationships between appearance and psychosocial vari-ables are extremely complex, particularly in adolescence.

The complexity of evaluating the psychological impact of dental-facial disfigure-ment simply underscores the difficulty of treatment decisions. These are not merely clinical decisions, but personal decisions that must be developed within a social framework. Moreover, both the duration of treatment and the ultimate success of treatment can be highly dependent on patient cooperation. In the vast majority of cases where orthodontic correction is not necessary to the physical health and func-tioning of an adolescent, therefore, discussions of treatment decisions should focus on the individual's own perceptions of appearance and desire for treatment.

The decision-making process is likely to be complicated by developmental issues. It is important to know how orthodontic treatment is viewed by the patient's own peer group, since the elective nature of much of this treatment means that it will be more common in some cultural and socioeconomic groups than in others. In addition, the position of the individual's parents on the matter can be an important factor. Recent data on cooperation in orthodontic treatment (Albino, Lawrence, Lopes, Nash, & Tedesco, 1991) indicate that parental influence may be even more important early in treatment. It is possible that some adolescents will refuse treat-ment that they need and want very badly if developmental tasks find them opposing their parents at every turn. On the other hand, another adolescent may inappropriately focus on some minor problem that simply does not warrant the expense of treatment.

The developmental tasks of adolescence have contributed to concern about the aesthetic aspects of occlusion, and no doubt have contributed also to an increasing dilemma regarding the provision of orthodontic treatment in the absence of real functional or health impairment. Some would say that to correct occlusion in such cases creates unrealistic standards for human appearance and that by such over-correction we limit tolerance for, and social responsiveness to, a variety of acceptable forms of facial appearance. For example, the increased use of plastic surgery to "correct" the facial characteristics of children with Down's syndrome has created controversy (May, 1988; Mearig, 1985). Many professionals argue that normalizing the appearance of those with Down's syndrome reduces the social stigma and negative expectations often associated with their physical appearance, thus increasing their chances for better functioning. Others have asserted that surgery is a dangerous and unpleasant procedure, and that instead of subjecting an individual to this experience, we should work to change social values to provide more acceptance of those whose appearance is different.

If these are questions of judgment, the matter becomes one of deciding who is to provide the judgment. Since an individual's desire for treatment is not the same as the need for treatment, professional perceptions and peer perceptions of appearance should be considered along with personal perceptions as part of a social-clinical dynamic within which the adolescent can be helped to develop and maintain his or her self-perception. This sharing of perspectives will be most successful when it includes feedback on peer standards and allows the adolescent to consider and discuss this information, as well as to reflect on his or her parents' roles in the treatment decision (Albino & Tedesco, 1988). In summary, in order to avoid potential problems related to malocclusion in adolescents, sophisticated interdisciplinary approaches to the assessment of need must be developed, as well as the actual provision of orthodontic treatment.

The previous discussion on treatment decisions for malocclusion is further complicated by the problem of availability. Most adolescents in the United States cannot afford elective orthodontic treatment. The cost of a typical course of treatment currently exceeds $2,000. Even when orthodontic treatment is required for functional reasons, it often is delayed and inadequate for disadvantaged segments of society. As acceptable occlusal standards increase, so might the detrimental effects of poor occlusal relations for those for whom treatment is not available.

Summary and Conclusions

Adolescent oral health concerns present some important challenges, both for the young people who are affected and for those who must treat them. In addition to emphasizing the limitations of current community prevention programs, as well as the need for increased personal oral health behaviors and attention to the different demands of our population's subgroups, this chapter underscores how few of the efforts to improve adolescent oral health have taken into serious consideration the relevant developmental and social contexts. Yet studies that have acknowledged the importance of peer influence and rejection of parental values appear to have found an important component for changing health behavior in what previously was believed to be a highly resistant group.

In this chapter, we have looked at several very different problems of oral health that affect adolescents. In every case, however, the key to promoting healthy attitudes and behaviors can be found in understanding the relevant developmental issues. The overarching task of developing one's own identity, separate and apart from that of one's parents, can determine how adolescents will respond to parental wishes. Some adolescents will reject parental demands, including engaging in oral hygiene behaviors. Moreover, because brushing and flossing generally are private activities, young people have no sense of the value placed on these activities by their peers. But since adolescents look to the peer group for standards of behavior, it is most important to find ways to promote these activities in settings that provide peer leadership and support.

The effects of dental problems that impair appearance represent another area in which peer standards and attitudes are critical, and a need exists to assist the adolescent in sorting out these influences. Since there is evidence of some loss of self-esteem associated with early adolescence, any additional stress caused by occlusal disfigurement could be particularly painful. Avoidance of psychological suffering due to malocclusion may be accomplished either through orthodontic treatment or by developing a better understanding of standards for attractiveness and a more accurate assessment of one's own appearance. The manner in which body image and self-perceptions of appearance are developed requires that we interpret others' responses in terms of a standard that must be deduced. This task is not easy, and no systematic approaches have been developed for guiding adolescents through this process. It is just such efforts that are needed, however, if we are to help adolescents, their families, and their dental care professionals make the best decisions about treatment and avoid the danger of creating an artificial demand for treatment, which may result in unrealistic standards for dental-facial appearance. The goal here is to promote the importance of and desire for oral and dental health in adolescents without overemphasizing values of dental-facial attractiveness.

The area of oral health offers an important setting not only for exploring ways of enhancing health, but also for understanding adolescent growth and development. Issues of dental and oral health generally are not as threatening for adolescents to deal with as are high-risk behaviors disapproved of by adults. For this reason, they can provide a relatively safe context within which we can test strategies for helping adolescents to develop self-mastery and decision-making skills that can be useful in many aspects of their lives.

References

Adams, G. R. (1982). Physical attractiveness. In A. Miller (Ed.), *In the eye of the beholder: Contemporary issues in stereotyping* (pp. 253–304). New York: Praeger.

Albino, J. E. (1978). Evaluation of three approaches to changing dental hygiene behaviors. *Journal of Preventive Dentistry, 5,* 4–10.

Albino, J. E. (1980). Motivating underserved groups to use community dental services. In S. L. Silberman & A. F. Tryon (Eds.), *Community dentistry. A problem-oriented approach* (pp. 137–154). Littleton, MA: PSG Publishing.

Albino, J. E. (1981). *Development of methodologies for behavioral measurements related to malocclusion.* Final Report: Contract No. N01-DE-27499. Bethesda, MD: National Institute of Dental Research.

Albino, J. E. (1984a). Psychosocial aspects of malocclusion. In J. D. Matarazzo, N. E. Miller, S. M. Weiss, J. A. Herd, & S. M. Weiss (Eds.), *Behavioral health: A handbook of health enhancement and disease prevention* (pp. 918–929). New York: Wiley.

Albino, J. E. (1984b). Prevention by acquiring health enhancing habits. In M. C. Roberts & L. Peterson (Eds.), *Prevention of problems in childhood: Psychological research and applications* (pp. 200–231). New York: Wiley.

Albino, J. E., Alley, T. R., Tedesco, L. A., Tobiasen, J. A., Kiyak, H. A., & Lawrence, S. D. (1990). Esthetic issues in behavioral dentistry. *Annals of Behavioral Medicine, 12,* 148–155.

Albino, J. E., Cunat, J. J., Fox, R. N., Lewis, E. A., Slakter, M. J., & Tedesco, L. A. (1981). Variables discriminating individuals who seek orthodontic treatment. *Journal of Dental Research, 60,* 1661–1667.

Albino, J. E., Lawrence, S. D., Lopes, C. E., Nash, L. B., & Tedesco, L. A. (1991). Cooperation of adolescents in orthodontic treatment. *Journal of Behavioral Medicine, 14,* 53–70.

Albino, J. E., Lawrence, S. D., Tedesco, L. A., & Cunat, J. J. (1990). *Psychological and social effects of orthodontic treatment.* Paper presented at the annual meeting of the American Association for Dental Research, Cincinnati, OH.

Albino, J. E., Nash, L. B., Lawrence, S. D., Lowrie, G. S., Lewis, E. A., & Tedesco, L. A. (1989). *Changed perceptions of appearance after orthodontic treatment.* Paper presented at the annual meeting of the American Association for Dental Research, San Francisco.

Albino, J. E., & Tedesco, L. A. (1988). The role of perception in treatment of impaired facial appearance. In T. R. Alley (Ed.), *Social and applied aspects of perceiving faces* (pp. 217–237). Hillsdale, NJ: Erlbaum.

Alley, T. R. (1988a). Social and applied aspects of face perception: An introduction. In T. R. Alley (Ed.), *Social and applied aspects of perceiving faces* (pp. 1–8). Hillsdale, NJ: Lawrence Erlbaum.

Alley, T. R. (1988b). Physiognomy and social perception. In T. R. Alley (Ed.), *Social and applied aspects of perceiving faces,* (pp. 167–186). Hillsdale, NJ: Erlbaum.

Alley, T. R., & Hildebrandt, K. A. (1988). Determinants and consequences of facial aesthetics. In T. R. Alley (Ed.), *Social and applied aspects of perceiving faces,* (pp. 101–140). Hillsdale, NJ: Erlbaum.

Ary, D. V., Lichtenstein, E., & Severson, H. H. (1987). Smokeless tobacco use among male adolescents: Patterns, correlates, predictors, and the use of other drugs. *Preventive Medicine, 16,* 385–401.

Attwood, D., & Blinkhorn, A. S. (1988). Trends in dental health of ten-year-old schoolchildren in south-west Scotland after cessation of water fluoridation. *Lancet, 2,* 266–267.

Beal, J. F. (1989). Social factors and preventive dentistry. In J. J. Murray (Ed.), *The prevention of dental disease* (pp. 373–405). New York: Oxford University Press.

Bohannan, H. M., Disney, J. A., Graves, R. C., Bader, J. D., Klein, S. P., & Bell, R. M. (1984). Indications for sealant use in a community-based preventive dentistry program. *Journal of Dental Education, 48*(2), Suppl, 45–55.

Bohannan, H. M., Stamm, J. W., Graves, R. C., Disney, J. A., & Bader, J. D. (1985). Fluoride mouthrinse programs in fluoridated communities. *Journal of the American Dental Association, 111,* 783–789.

Bull, R., & Rumsey, N. (1988). *The social psychology of facial appearance.* New York: Springer-Verlag.

Burt, B. A., Eklund, S. A., & Loesche, W. J. (1986). Dental benefits of limited exposure to fluoridated water in childhood. *Journal of Dental Research, 61,* 1322–1325.

Chambers, D. W. (1973). Susceptibility to preventive dental treatment. *Journal of Public Health Dentistry, 33,* 82–90.

Dent, C. W., Sussman, S., Johnson, C. A., Hansen, W. B., & Flay, B. R. (1987). Adolescent smoke-less tobacco incidence: Relations with other drugs and psychosocial variables. *Preventive Medicine, 16,* 422–431.

Dion, K., Berscheid, E., & Walster, E. (1972). What is beautiful is good. *Journal of Personality and Social Psychology, 24,* 285–290.

Driscoll, W. S., Swango, P. A., Horowitz, A. M., & Kingman, A. (1982). Caries-preventive effects of daily and weekly fluoride mouthrinsing in a fluoridated community: final results after 30 months. *Journal of the American Dental Association, 105,* 1010–1013.

Evans, R. I. (1978). Motivating changes in oral hygiene behavior: Some social psychological per-spectives. *Journal of Preventive Dentistry, 5,* 14–17.

Golden, J. L. (1988). Social aspects of dental care. In A. W. Jong (Ed.), *Community dental health* (pp. 57–69). St. Louis, MO: C. V. Mosby.

Harris, R. R. (1989). Historical perspective—A corner of history: Grand Rapids fluoridation and the prevention of dental caries. *Preventive Medicine, 18,* 541–548.

Hatfield, H., & Sprecher, S. (1986). *Mirror, mirror. . . .* Albany: State University of New York Press.

Jessor, R. (1982). Critical issues in research on adolescent health promotion. In T. J. Coates, A. C. Peterson, & C. Perry (Eds.), *Promoting adolescent health* (pp. 447–465). New York: Academic Press.

Kegeles, S. S. (1963). Why people seek dental care: A test of a conceptual formulation. *Journal of Health and Human Behavior, 4,* 166–173.

Kegeles, S. S. (1975). Public acceptance of dental preventive measures. *Journal of Preventive Den-tistry, 2,* 10–14.

Kenealy, P., Frude, N., & Shaw, W. C. (1989). An evaluation of the psychological and social effects of malocclusion: Some implications for dental policy making. *Social Science Medicine, 6,* 583–591.

Kiyak, H. A., & Mulligan, K. (1986). Behavioral research related to oral hygiene practices. In H. Loe & D. V. Kleinman (Eds.), *Dental plaque control measures and oral hygiene practices* (pp. 225–239). Washington, D. C.: IRL Press.

Lerner, R. M. (1987). A life-span perspective for early adolescence. In R. M. Lerner & T. T. Foch (Eds.), *Biological–psychological interactions in early adolescence* (pp. 9–34). Hillsdale, NJ: Erl-baum.

Lerner, R. M., Lerner, J. V., Hess, L. E., Schwab, J., Jovanovic, J., Talwar, R., & Kucher, J. S. (1991). Physical attractiveness and psychosocial functioning among early adolescents. *Jour-nal of Early Adolescence. 11,* 300–320.

Leventhal, H. (1971). Fear appeals and persuasions: The differentiation of a motivational con-struct. *American Journal of Public Health, 61,* 1208–1224.

Loe, H. (1983). The fluoridation status of U. S. public water supplies. In *Challenges for the eighties: NIDR long-range research plan FY 1985–89.* Publication No. (NIH) 85-860. Bethesda, MD: National Institutes of Health.

Lund, A. K., & Kegeles, S. S. (1984). Rewards and adolescent health behavior. *Health Psychology, 3,* 351–369.

Macgregor, F. C. (1970). Social and psychological implications of dentofacial disfigurement. *Angle Orthodontist, 40,* 231–233.

May, D. C. (1988). Plastic surgery for children with Down syndrome: Normalization or extremism? *Mental Retardation, 26,* 17–19.

McClain, J. B., & Profitt, W. R. (1985). Oral health in the United States: Prevalence of malocclu-sion. *Journal of Dental Education, 49,* 386–396.

Mearig, J. S. (1985). Facial surgery and an active modification approach for children with Down syndrome: Some psychological and ethical issues. *Rehabilitation Literature, 46,* 72–77.

National Institute of Dental Research (1989). *Oral health of United States children. The national survey of dental caries in U. S. school children, 1986–1987.* DHHS Publication No. (NIH) 89-2247. Bethesda, MD: U. S. Department of Health and Human Services.

National Institutes of Health (1984). Consensus development conference statement: Dental seal-ants in the prevention of tooth decay. *Journal of Dental Education, 48*(2), Suppl, 126–131.

Offenbacher, S., & Weathers, D. R. (1985). Effects of smokeless tobacco on the periodontal mucosa and caries status of adolescent molars. *Journal of Oral Pathology, 14,* 162–181.

Patzer, G. L. (1985). *The physical attractiveness phenomena.* New York: Plenum Press.

Rhodes, J. E., & Jason, L. A. (1988). *Preventing substance abuse among children and adolescents.* New York: Pergamon Press.

Shaw, W. C. (1981). Influence of children's dental-facial appearance on their social attractiveness as judged by peers and lay adults. *American Journal of Orthodontics, 79,* 399–415.

Shaw, W. C., Meek, S. C., & Jones, D. S. (1980). Nicknames, teasing, harassment and the salience of dental features among school children. *British Journal of Orthodontics, 7,* 75–80.

Silverstone, L. M. (1984). State of the art on sealant research and priorities for further research. *Journal of Dental Education, 48*(2), Suppl, 107–118.

Simmons, R. G., Rosenberg, R., & Rosenberg, M. (1973). Disturbance in the self-image at adolescence. *American Sociological Review, 38,* 553–568.

Stamm, J. W., Banting, D. W., & Imrey, P. B. (1990). Adult root caries survey of two similar communities with contrasting natural water fluoride levels. *Journal of the American Dental Association, 120,* 143–149.

Stephen, K. W., McCall, D. R., & Tullis, J. I. (1987). Caries prevalence in northern Scotland before, and 5 years after, water defluoridation. *British Dental Journal, 163,* 324–326.

Sternlieb, J. J., & Munan, L. (1972). A survey of health problems, practices, and needs of youth. *Pediatrics, 49,* 177–186.

Tedesco, L. A., & Albino, J. E. (1989). Education en sante buccale: Developpement d'une approche psychologique (Traduction: R. Dupuis). In D. Kandelman (Ed.), *La dentisterie preventive.* Montreal: University of Montreal Press and Mason Press.

U. S. Department of Health, Education, and Welfare, Public Health Service, National Center for Health Statistics (1977). *An assessment of the occlusion of the teeth of youths 12–17 years.* DHEW Publication No. (HRA) 77-1644. Washington, DC: U. S. Government Printing Office.

U. S. Department of Health and Human Services, Public Health Service, National Institutes of Health (1981). *The prevalence of dental caries in United States children, 1979–1980.* NIH Publications No. 82-2245. Washington, DC: U. S. Government Printing Office.

U. S. Department of Health and Human Services, Public Health Service, National Institutes of Health (1986). *The health consequences of using smokeless tobacco: A report of the Advisory Committee to the Surgeon General.* NIH Publication No. 86-2874. Washington, DC: U. S. Government Printing Office.

U. S. Department of Health and Human Services, Public Health Service, National Center for Health Statistics (1988). *Current estimates from the National Health Interview Summary, United States, 1987.* DHHS Publication No. (PHS) 88-1594. Washington, DC: U. S. Government Printing Office.

U. S. Department of Health and Human Services, Public Health Service (1990). *Healthy people 2000: National health promotion and disease prevention objectives: Full report and commentary.* DHHS Publication No. (PHS) 91-50212. Washington, DC: U. S. Government Printing Office.

U. S. Department of Health and Human Services, Public Health Service, National Institutes of Health (1990). Health *United States (and prevention profile), 1989: Fluoridation and dental health.* DHHS Publication No. (PHS) 90-1232. Washington, DC: U. S. Government Printing Office.

Woodall, I. R. (1990). Preventing periodontal disease. In R. J. Genco, H. M. Goldman, & D. W. Cohen (Eds.), *Contemporary periodontics* (pp. 361–370). St. Louis, MO: C. V. Mosby.

Yeung, S.C.H., Howell, S., & Fahey, P. (1989). Oral hygiene program for orthodontic patients. *American Journal of Orthodontics and Dentofacial Orthopedics, 96,* 208–213.

Zambon, J. J., Christersson, L. A., & Genco, R. J. (1986). Diagnosis and treatment of localized juvenile periodontitis. *Journal of the American Dental Association, 113,* 295–299.

12

Promoting Healthy Alternatives
to Substance Abuse

Howard Leventhal and Patricia Keeshan

This chapter attempts to satisfy four objectives: (1) briefly review major approaches to the prevention of substance abuse among adolescents, highlighting key themes and examining outcomes; (2) provide an overview of both the successes and deficiencies of these intervention efforts as a foundation for a transactional analysis of the prevention problem; (3) outline a transactional framework to advance more comprehensive and influential prevention and health promotion efforts; and (4) speculate on potentially effective strategies and policy goals that emerge from the transactional perspective.

Throughout this book, the authors have attempted to *refocus attention on a health promotion perspective.* As this is also our aim, a review of previous intervention strategies, which have focused primarily on creating barriers to substance abuse, may seem unnecessary. However, it is our position that the creation of barriers must remain an integral part of any health promotion strategy. Thus, an overview of current strategies serves as our point of departure. Our analysis will argue that an expansion of current efforts to create barriers, combined with an intensive focus on alternative behaviors, will lead to the development of more effective intervention strategies.

Current Approaches to Prevention of Substance Abuse

Prevention programs targeting adolescents have addressed cigarette smoking (Flay, 1985a; Leventhal, Baker, Brandon, & Fleming, 1989), drug abuse (Sadler & Dillard, 1978), and alcohol dependency (Goodstadt & Sheppard, 1983). Two research traditions have influenced program content: the *informational* and the *behavioral*. Informational strategies were guided first by educational research and later by social psychological theories of communication and attitude change, while behavioral approaches were informed first by behavioral therapy and later by social learning theory. Although we treat informational and behavioral approaches separately, current intervention programs employ techniques that have emerged from each of these traditions in varying proportions and have applied them to diverse target groups. Most recently, there has been greater focus on high-risk groups.

Informational Approaches

At least four types of content are available for use in information programs designed to generate barriers to substance abuse: (1) technical information about the substance, its action, and relevant risks; (2) personalized risk information; (3) action information; and (4) normative information.

Programs are often school based, with the information tailored to the specific substance, the characteristics of the target audience, and the theoretical inclinations of the program designers.

TECHNICAL INFORMATION. The technical information found in programs designed to discourage smoking focuses on facts about the agent, such as the 4,000 or more chemicals generated during cigarette combustion, the negative health outcomes of use (cancer, heart disease, liver disease, etc.), and the rates of disease among smokers compared to nonsmokers (e.g., smokers are 20 times more likely to die of lung cancer and 3 times more likely to die of cardiovascular disease than nonsmokers). Programs designed to deter alcohol or drug abuse also discuss physical effects on the brain and body but focus more often on social consequences. For example, the consequences of specific behaviors, such as the legal and emotional aftermath of a drunk driving accident or arrest, are often stressed (Goodstadt, Sheppard, & Chan, 1982).

There is general agreement among reviewers of programs targeting smoking (Thompson, 1978) and other substances (e.g., Bangert-Drowns, 1988; Rhodes & Jason, 1988; Schaps, DiBartolo, Moskowitz, Palley & Churgin, 1981; Tobler, 1986) that programs presenting only technical information do not produce positive results. Two recent meta-analytic reviews of school-based alcohol and drug programs suggest that strictly informational or educational programs can effect shifts in knowledge of and attitudes toward alcohol and drug use, but these changes rarely produce reductions in the drug-using behaviors of adolescents (Bangert-Drowns, 1988; Tobler, 1986).

PERSONALIZED RISK INFORMATION. The aim of providing information about the hazards associated with substance use is to create a sense of personal vulnerability by attaching use to the occurrence of specific negative outcomes. This sense of vulnerability is expected to translate into avoidance of the particular behavior targeted. Abstract technical information may fail to motivate behavioral change because the target audience does not perceive a clear and present danger. Some investigators have presented more concrete, case-oriented materials accompanied by graphic verbal and visual material to illustrate the consequences of risky behavior and present them as harmful on a personal level (Leventhal & Singer, 1966).

In contrast to programs delivering only technical information about the threat agent and statistical data on its rate of injury, information campaigns using per-

sonalized threat material have been more successful in bringing about both attitude and behavior change (Sutton, 1982). Thus, reductions in the related risk
behavior are seen after a single exposure to certain fear messages, such as movies
depicting cancer surgery (Leventhal, Watts, & Pagano, 1967). Vivid demonstra-
tions of threats to the self appear particularly effective. For example, after observing the redness of their own teeth following the application of a wafer that reveals
areas of plaque buildup, subjects' adherence to regular tooth brushing significantly
increased (Evans, Rozelle, Lasater, Deinbroski, & Allen, 1968). These findings support the more general hypothesis that concrete, case-oriented material is far more
powerful than statistical data in influencing decisions (Borgida & Nisbett, 1977).

While studies such as those cited above are often portrayed as investigations of
the effects of fear-arousing communication, the complex cognitive content of the
messages used is probably as important or more important in initiating change than
the momentary states of fear elicited by them (Leventhal, 1970; Rogers, 1983).
Thus, it is not yet clear precisely what components are effective in producing
change. We suspect, however, that it is information that creates the perception of
an imminent personal threat that changes attitudes and arouses the motivation to
avoid risk (Leventhal, Meyer, & Nerenz, 1980).

ACTION INFORMATION. Although typically viewed as a behavioral rather than an
informational component, action information was explicitly introduced into communication studies over 25 years ago (Leventhal, Singer, & Jones, 1965). A series
of studies demonstrated that the behavioral effects (i.e., actually taking a tetanus
shot or quitting smoking) of both highly and moderately threatening personalized
messages were enhanced when combined with information that provided a plan for
action (Leventhal, 1970; Leventhal, Watts, & Pagano, 1967). The action plan messages contained two critical components. First, they called for an analysis of the
behavioral environment, asking the individual to review his or her daily routine and
identify specific situations in which an action could be easily inserted. For example,
in the antismoking studies, students identified situations where cigarettes were purchased or smoked and generated possible alternative responses. Second, the messages asked the individual to perform a brief mental rehearsal of taking these
actions in the specified situations.

NORMATIVE INFORMATION. The reasoned action model proposes that group
norms play a major role in generating intentions to act and actions (Ajzen & Fishbein, 1973; Fishbein & Ajzen, 1975). Normative beliefs may enhance risky behaviors by leading us to consider a particular behavior as desirable, acceptable, or safe
(Jemmott, Ditto, & Croyle, 1986). Data show that young people misperceive the
prevalence of smoking and drinking among both adults and peers. Indeed, fourth
through twelfth graders overestimate the percentage of adults who smoke by two
to three times the actual rate, and seventh through twelfth graders overestimate
the percentage of peers who smoke by similar rates. Consistent with the hypothesis
that norms may encourage a behavior, youngsters who smoke or intend to smoke

overestimate the percentage of adult and peer smokers to a greater degree than do their nonsmoking peers (Leventhal, Fleming, & Glynn, 1988).

Many alcohol and drug prevention programs have attempted to correct these misperceptions by presenting accurate normative information. They have also tried to shift perceived norms indirectly by using peers as the communicators. Unfortunately, there is little evidence that attempts to alter perceived norms in an experimental situation affect subsequent levels of substance use.

In contrast to experimental studies, longitudinal surveys have found correlations between changes in substance abuse and changes in normative risk perceptions. Both increases in risk perceptions and decreases in the perception of social desirability precede declines in the reported use of marijuana (Johnston, O'Malley, & Bachman, 1987), cocaine (Bachman, Johnston, & O'Malley, 1990) and other substances (Johnston, 1985). Further investigation into these correlations may facilitate health promotion by uncovering factors that mediate the relationships found in longitudinal surveys.

Behavioral (Social Learning) Approaches

Components of current intervention programs with roots in behavioral or social learning ideas are not easily classified. Techniques that are viewed as behavioral in origin are combined with informational approaches to yield complex, multicomponent prevention programs. Programs such as CASPAR (Cambridge and Somerville Program for Alcohol Rehabilitation), the "Here's Looking at You, Two" project, and the STARR (Summer Tobacco and Alcohol Risk Reduction) program include many of the following components: information (e.g., drug effects, alcoholism as treatable); decision making (including an emphasis on problem definition, generation of solutions, evaluation of solutions, taking action, and reevaluation); coping with stress (e.g., identification of stress in one's life and ways of handling); enhancing the self-concept (e.g., identification of strengths and weaknesses, importance of individuality); and refusal skills. The material is presented variously through audiovisuals, group discussion, role play, quiz games, posters, buttons, and catchy phrases (e.g., "Be smart! Don't start!"; U. S. Department of Health and Human Services, 1987a, 1987b; see also National Institute of Drug Abuse, 1983, or Rhodes & Jason, 1988, for detailed presentations of the content of the above programs).

Despite the complexity, certain common themes do emerge. Most programs that can be classified as behaviorally oriented concentrate on the acquisition of skills. Because *social learning ideas* (Bandura, 1977b) are at the core of many programs, most of them emphasize developing skills to control peer pressure for substance use. Project PATH (Programs to Advance Teen Health) encourages adolescents to think of situations in which they may be pressured to smoke and mentally rehearse different ways of saying no, such as changing the topic or telling the person who offers to go ahead and smoke, though the recipient of the offer prefers not to (e.g., Biglan et al., 1987; Biglan, James, LaChance, Zoref, & Joffe, 1988). Rehearsal was also a major component of Stanford's CLASP program, with the adolescents sitting in front of a TV screen and practicing saying no to televised offers of cigarettes (Hops et al., 1986; Perry, Killen, Telch, & Maccoby, 1980).

Not all behavioral programs center primarily on providing skills to avoid use. Others take the *life skills* approach, which is a comprehensive curriculum to train preadolescents in skills that can be applied across many situations (Botvin, Eng, & Williams 1980; Elias et al., 1986). The approach includes practice in problem definition, information search, and response generation, selection, execution, and evaluation. Life skills training is expected to (1) reduce the emotional distress that is thought to be a motivation for substance use; (2) reduce the attractiveness of substance use by increasing the subject's ability to obtain gratification in other areas of life; and (3) enhance skills in refusing inducements to use substances.

EVALUATION OF SOCIAL LEARNING INTERVENTIONS. Results from early social learning programs, particularly those targeting smoking, were sufficiently encouraging to stimulate the funding of several large-scale efforts. Efforts to improve the methodology of these later studies included using the appropriate unit for sampling and analysis, increasing the number of such units, and introducing physiological measures to validate substance use (e.g., Flay, 1985b). In the early 1980s there was a clear expectation that methodological improvements would lead to more robust significant results, supporting the hypothesis that existing programs effectively reduce drug abuse. While the initial results often reinforced this expectation, treatment control differences tended to shrink or vanish in follow-ups conducted 2 or more years after the completion of many programs. This was true of the Waterloo (Flay et al., 1989), Oregon (Ary et al., 1990) and Minnesota studies (Murray, Davis-Hearn, Goldman, Pirie, & Luepker, 1988). Results from longer-term follow-ups of the large-scale life skills program conducted by the Cornell group have been more promising, though it is not clear that positive effects would continue to be seen without the multiple annual booster sessions or if data were included from all participating classrooms (Botvin, Baker, Dusenbury, Tortu, & Botvin, 1990).

Although several recent reviews of programs targeting alcohol or drug use suggest that programs emphasizing social skills produce significant results (Bangert-Drowns, 1988; Schaps et al., 1981), we feel that the outcomes of these programs are less consistent than indicated. There are two reasons for our judgment. First, the programs are often extremely complex, making it difficult to determine precisely what components are the active agents for the reported change.[1] Second, other variables, such as cohort effects, may make it inappropriate to draw conclusions from integrative (or meta-analytic) summaries that fail to consider the changing context in which programs are conducted.

Identifying and Targeting High-Risk Groups

Concerned perhaps with the wisdom of intervening with entire populations of adolescents in school-based programs, where relatively few members are likely to become dangerously involved in substance use, many investigators have urged more precise targeting of prevention efforts.

Efforts to target adolescents at risk are typically aimed at the most visible high-risk group: the inner-city poor, where the economic disadvantages and high rates of school dropping out are thought to place young people at particularly high risk for problems related to substance use. Reported results of endeavors to reach adolescents in this environment are mixed, with some treatment groups even showing increases in substance use compared to controls (Tobler, 1986). Programs designed to provide alternatives to substance abuse show the most promise. In Tobler's (1986) meta-analytic review, programs classified in the "alternatives" modality and applied to economically disadvantaged youngsters exhibited the most robust effects. Interestingly, when applied to higher socioeconomic groups, similar "alternatives" programs showed minimal effects. We believe that these findings point up the need for a reexamination of the various social contexts that can contribute to adolescents' involvement with alcohol and drugs.

Effective targeting of adolescents at risk for substance abuse requires the identification of factors that actually generate risk, rather than simply limiting efforts to those in high-risk environments. Because identifying such factors should advance our understanding of the processes involved, the search has been pursued with some intensity. Factors implicated in the development of substance abuse include disruptive life events, genetic predisposition, family violence, sexual abuse, and poverty. Unfortunately, the lack of specificity of such predictors limits their usefulness.[2] We expect that as our understanding increases, we will be able to design programs that effectively target adolescents at risk.

Lessons from Past Efforts

As our very brief, critical review highlights the deficits in prior programs, it undoubtedly conveys an overly negative picture of what we have learned. Such an impression would be in error, as the lessons of the past serve as a guide and lead us to ask which areas demand increased attention. The following four issues require elaboration.

1. *There is a need to improve conceptualization of the individual in the social context.* To date, the content and format of most programs have been designed to influence individuals. One message emerging from long-term follow-ups of current programs is that they fail to produce lasting changes. Some degree of successful avoidance of substance use can be induced for 1 and sometimes 2 years, but that appears to be the outer limit.

The realization that individuals observe their own performance and can perceive themselves as having the ability to regulate their behavior in a particular domain has led to the incorporation of a higher-order cognitive concept into current intervention programs: the individual's perception of self-efficacy (Bandura, 1977a; Bem, 1967). Presumably, individuals high in feelings of self-efficacy respond to setbacks with continued efforts to change. Consequently, maintenance failure is often attributed to deficiencies in self-efficacy, and enhancing self-efficacy has become a primary focus of skill-based programs.

Another reason for program failures over the long term may be the failure to affect the environment or context in which the adolescent lives. While enhancing perceptions of efficacy may be effective in overcoming certain types of maintenance failure, the flavor of this concept, which is individual in focus, has not influenced investigation of the social factors that encourage the development of sustained efficacy feelings. Moreover, many programs appear to view the individual as passive or reactive rather than active and constructive in response to the social environment.

Current conceptual models must be modified and extended if they are to generate effective operations for directly shaping the social context and the individual's interaction with it. We believe that ecologically focused transactional models, in which environmental conditions are conceptualized as providing situations favorable or unfavorable to both individual growth and subsequent environmental conditions (Felner & Felner, 1990), can make valuable contributions to future efforts.

2. *Providing skills is a partial solution; more emphasis on motivation and goals is required.* Any self-regulative system must have a set point or goal, in addition to having the means to achieve this goal state. As pointed out in our brief review, most current intervention programs tend to focus on the acquisition of skills for avoiding use or resisting peer influence. While these programs effectively provide the means, few give adequate attention to the distinction between what the adolescent can do and what he or she wants to do. Concepts such as self-efficacy tend to incorporate the goal within the skill, that is, to assume that an adolescent will want to avoid substance use simply because he or she can do so. As Cartwright (1949) suggested long ago, communications can succeed in influencing behavior when they combine *motivating* information with information for constructing an action system (Leventhal, 1970). Clearly, without an explicit desire to avoid use, mastering skills becomes irrelevant. Efforts must be directed toward successfully motivating adolescents to make use of the skills provided.

Factors affecting motivation pose complex problems, and certain prerequisities will need to be met before more comprehensive approaches are developed. Undermining the motivations to use substances requires an understanding of what those motivations are. We need a clearer picture of the role that substances play; then we need to identify the kinds of alternatives that are available to the adolescent. What barriers do adolescents perceive as preventing them from trying the alternatives? Perhaps promoting existing alternatives will be insufficient in certain environments, and our focus must shift to creating alternatives. In short, affecting motivation requires an adequate understanding of the adolescents' world: their goals and needs, as well as the various routes perceived as available to attain those goals and satisfy those needs (Dittmann-Kohli, 1986; Chapter 6). This is, of course, a very tall order and has been called for in the past (Globetti, 1974; Kohn, 1974); but we believe that progress can be made, perhaps by exploiting our best source, the adolescents themselves.

3. *Prevention efforts need to be better targeted.* Effective programs designed to meet the needs of specific at-risk subgroups have yet to become a reality. The sources of motivation to use substances among various subgroups clearly differ, as exhibited by the differential impact of alternative programs among high-risk socioeconomic groups versus predominantly white middle-class groups. A more detailed understanding of the variety of motivations within specific subgroups is needed.

Another aspect of targeting involves designing programs whose aims are clearly and narrowly defined. As pointed out by Bacon (1978), multiple intervention targets such as the prevention of alcohol problems (e.g., specific consequences of drunken behavior), the prevention or restriction of alcohol use, and the prevention of alcohol abuse or alcoholism can create ambiguities in the intervention context and lead to a shotgun approach that makes both evaluation and refinement nearly impossible. Because many problems associated with specific substances (e.g., alcohol vs. crack) and specific communities (e.g., the less violent drug trade present in middle-class suburbs than in the inner city) differ, we must be clear about what problems we are aiming to alleviate. Although it is a noble goal, aiming simply to "prevent substance abuse" is too broadly conceived to inform coherent program design.

4. *Methodological improvement alone will not solve the intervention problem.* As mentioned earlier, in spite of widely held expectations, methodological improvements alone have not led to improved outcomes. We see four possible reasons for this situation. First, while one can always find fault, most existent experimental programs have been carefully executed. Second, the data strongly suggest that some methodological worries were unfounded. For example, under the conditions used in these studies, verbal reports of smoking seem sufficiently unbiased to obviate the need for physiological measures. Others, however, have remained worrisome. One of these is the high dropout rate from school and subsequent loss to follow-up in school-based programs. Because users and abusers are more likely to leave school, adolescents in the greatest need of service are lost to evaluation (Pirie, Murray, & Luepker, 1988). Third, in several instances, the absence of a treatment control difference was due to the low rates of smoking in both the treatment and control groups, suggesting perhaps a change in the cultural ethos or a shift in the prevalence of use. Finally, the programs were intensive, using 20 classroom sessions in their first year and 8 to 10 sessions in follow-up years. Indeed, many programs were still in progress at the 2 year postassessment.

The above four general issues lead us to conclude that the severity of substance abuse problems will persist so long as we lack theoretically sound and innovative views of the social psychological processes involved.

A Transactional Analysis of Substance Use

The world of adolescence is complex; understanding the motivations for avoiding or engaging in substance use requires a coherent framework for analysis. This framework should allow for integration of prior work on drug abuse prevention (typically oriented to creating barriers to use), with a focus on promoting healthy alternatives (i.e., attractive involvements and goals that are incompatible with use). Ideally, the framework will embrace the following themes:

1. *Conceptualizing factors affecting adolescent behavior reciprocally in both person and environment.* To treat peer influence as strictly an environmental factor, or sexual drive as solely a person factor, ignores the adolescent's representation of the relationship of peer and self in the first instance, and the representation of the environment–urge (or incentive–drive) relationship in the second. In either case, a nonreciprocal formulation is inadequate.

2. *Viewing the adolescent as active in the construction of his or her own development.* All human beings, adolescents included, actively construct and regulate their environments. Recognition that "young people in action with their context create the basis for their own development" (Silbereisen & Eyferth, 1986, p. 1) is essential. Many programs take the position that substance use is an entirely dangerous and irrational activity and fail to appreciate the degree to which substances may serve important functions in an adolescent's world. These programs may consequently alienate adolescents who actively construct an environment that includes substance use.

An aggressive intervention that takes the position that substance use is without benefit or gain, and focused on teaching refusal skills, may also fail to encourage adolescents to explore the issue of substance use in terms of their own experience (e.g., exploring subjective motives for use, the very real personal risks involved, and the regrets experienced with loss of control). Consequently, adolescents may not be motivated to use the skills offered because they have not developed and internalized vivid and personally relevant reasons to avoid alcohol or drug use.

3. *Incorporating a developmental perspective.* The adolescent's external physical appearance, internal biological condition, and psychological system are in transition, and he or she presents an increasingly adult face to a world whose responses are also dependent upon a changing social or cultural context. This dynamic interchange presents challenges for the adolescent who may find it increasingly difficult to maintain shared expectations with the adult world (Brooks-Gunn & Reiter, 1989; Brooks-Gunn, Rock, & Warren, 1989; Petersen & Taylor, 1980). Research focused on understanding the challenges children and adolescents negotiate in the course of their development must be included in any analysis that aims to encourage the development of more effective interventions.

Additional challenges are posed by the need to keep in touch with and make use of current trends in the social climate. Program evaluation is crucial, as techniques that prove effective at one point in time will not necessarily succeed at another. Program content must undergo creative revision as changing views and specific events provide opportunities to personalize or more vividly portray the frightening aspects of substance use.

The Transactional Framework

Consistent with a reciprocal conceptualization of adolescent behavior, the *structure* of our transactional framework views the adolescent's psychological constructions as a product of reciprocal relationships within a domain of multiple layers extended both internally and externally (Bronfenbrenner, 1986; McAllister, 1983). The *internal extension* concerns the interaction between the adolescent and the drug in creating a personal drug experience. The *external extension* concerns interactions between the adolescent and his or her social and physical contexts. Contexts or "layers" increasingly removed from the adolescent shape interactions at more proximal layers. The adolescent's actions and psychological constructions (e.g., his or her self-concept, aspirations, or temperament), in turn, shape the immediate context. These interactions ultimately influence the adolescent's decisions that lead to avoiding or engaging in substance use.

Within this basic structure, the aim is to incorporate self-regulation models (e.g., Kanfer, 1977; Leventhal & Nerenz, 1983) in a larger "transactional/ecological" context. Thus, the model adds features of symbolic interactionism (e.g., Mead, 1934; Stryker & Statham, 1985) to systems currently evolving in developmental and ecological psychology (Felner & Felner, 1990). We should point out that any truly transactional system cannot be fully detailed, but research that aims to elaborate specific aspects of the framework should provide the basis for the design of more effective intervention programs.

Transactions in the Adolescent World

THE ADOLESCENT ENVIRONMENT: PEERS. The three major end points—introduction to substance use, regular use, and abuse—have been related to active use by peers. Reports of one's best friend smoking and drinking, number of friends smoking and drinking, and members of a self-defined friendship group smoking and drinking (Best et al., 1984; DeVries, 1989; Mosbach & Leventhal, 1988; Sussman et al., 1990) have been used as indices of peer pressure. High correspondence of use patterns between individuals and their cohorts is classically interpreted to reflect peer *pressure*. The assumption that peers generally exert overt pressure to use substances is challenged, however, by data comparing the numbers that have tried or continue to use a variety of substances with those that report experiencing pressure to use (Brown, Clasen, & Eicher, 1986; DeVries, 1989; Sheppard, Wright, & Goodstadt, 1985). While it is possible that adolescents simply do not know what leads them to use drugs (Nisbett & Wilson, 1977), their denial of pressure suggests that peer influence may be based upon a different set of factors than those perceived as pressure (Fischer & Baumann, 1988; Oetting & Beauvais, 1987).

Our transactional analysis suggests that small groups or clusters of adolescents construct shared social environments in which they perceive themselves and other(s) as having mutual cognitive, emotional, and valuative reactions. Psychoactive drugs (e.g., alcohol, marijuana, cocaine) may play an important role in this construction, enhancing the sense of mutuality by creating the perception of sharing a uniquely private emotional experience. We believe the *intersubjectivity* created by sharing generates a sense of "we-ness." This sense of mutuality enhances the attractiveness of the group and may lead to incorporation of the self-image of the others into the image of one's own self (Aron, Aron, Tudor, & Nelson, 1991). The process should result in feelings of self-acceptance and perceived control over the apprais-als of oneself by others. Sharing may be a prime reason why substances are sought out and used in social clusters whose members are best described as intimate (Oet-ting & Beauvais, 1986).

Subgroups try cigarettes, beer, hard liquor, and marijuana at dramatically dif-ferent rates. For example, one predominantly male group prefers to do things with those they themselves have labeled as "druggies" or "dirts." They smoke cigarettes weekly or daily and use hard liquor at least 3 times more often than those that self-identify as associating with the "hot shots" (a predominantly female group of "sophisticated socialites"), and roughly 10 times more often than affiliates of the "jocks" (a group of athletic types) or "regular" kids (a group that does not fit any clear stereotype) (Mosbach & Leventhal, 1988). Given the relatively high level of self-esteem reported by the more frequent users (i.e., the "tough" image of the dirts and the social leader image of the hot shots), it seems that they are more likely to be sources rather than recipients of peer pressure, and hence would not be expected to report using substances in response to pressure. It seems likely that these adolescents have developed, and take pains to project, an image of themselves as tough, independent, adult, and sophisticated. Their substance use helps to pro-ject such an image and serves as a public cue for like-minded others to use in iden-tifying individuals with whom they can establish friendships and share a style of life. That substance abuse creates group cohesion should direct us to acknowledge its influence when we try to design more effective prevention projects.

Conceptualizing peer influence in the above framework suggests that some ado-lescents are likely to interpret substance use—the transitions through initiation and experimentation to regular use—as self-choice and will not experience peer influence as pressure. A key question about future interventions is whether they can help adolescents to create environments for alternative behaviors that are sim-ilar to and have the same motivational power as those for drug use.

THE ADOLESCENT ENVIRONMENT: ADULTS.   Older siblings, parents, members of the extended family, and other adult household residents also play a critical role in socializing attitudes toward drug use. The direct effects of these agents on adoles-cent substance use are seen in certain subgroups. Children who use drugs and alco-hol at the encouragement of adult substance users seem to use substances primarily for self-regulation and the control of emotional distress (Jessor & Jessor, 1977). Another group of children who never experiment with or use drugs because they are raised in tightly regulated family environments appear to have a self-image that is wedded to strongly held religious or moral values and rejects substance users (Shedler & Block, 1990). Their total rejection of use may be integrated into their self-systems well before the age of experimentation. The rigid adherence to family and religious values characteristic of this group illustrates the power, and perhaps the limitations, of combatting substance abuse through the creation of alternatives.

Although the influence of families is often less straightforward, and some ado-lescents react against family models (e.g., pushing the limits of an overprotective environment by using and abusing drugs or adopting a relatively abstemious lifestyle in response to substance use in the family), the lifestyles of family members and other adults in the adolescent's immediate social environment constitute a force that shapes adolescents' psychological constructions. The degree to which the careers and lifestyles portrayed by adults in the immediate social context are attractive or unattractive to adolescents may be partially dependent upon the perceived status and power of the source (Bandura, 1977b; Petty & Cacioppo, 1986). Peers and local gangs will be attractive models if they are viewed as powerful and important by the adult community and the mass media. At the same time, adult models may be rejected if they are seen as having little control over their own lives and low status and importance in the outer world.

Importance may be more closely related to the amount of attention given each group and may be independent of the reasons (negative or positive) for this attention. Once an adolescent's ongoing construction of self is steered toward images projected by a particular reference group, the youth's behavior will reflect the values (including substance use) needed to associate and bond with members of that group. The point we wish to stress is that the larger social system plays an important role in this process by affecting the perceived power and significance of the groups comprising the adolescent's face-to-face relationships. However, given that distal to proximal influences are moderated by a wide range of factors, the linkage from the larger culture to the proximal social group will often be hard to trace and will yield inconsistent findings.

A group of youngsters for whom this issue has received empirical attention are the children of working mothers. These so-called latchkey children are likely to experiment with and use substances if their time alone is spent hanging out with peers at shopping centers (Steinberg, 1986). Latchkey children who return home to report to adult family members, or to be available in case the adult should call, appear more insulated from peer relationships in which substance use is prevalent. These data suggest that family structure and styles of parenting determine cohesion and the bonding of the adolescent to the norms and behaviors of the family unit, and that peer relationships are here less salient to the choices regarding drug use.

THE ADOLESCENT–DRUG INTERACTION. Most adolescents experiment with substances (cigarettes and alcohol more commonly than illicit drugs). What immediate rewards might an adolescent experience with experimentation, and what might counter these positive experiences? A self-regulation model (Leventhal & Cameron, 1989) predicts that adolescents will continue to use substances when the rewards exceed the punishments. The physiological effect of the drug coupled with one's interpretation of the sensations will result in particular moods and emotions. Continued use should be determined in part by the degree to which this initial experience is positive or negative. Beliefs and expectations about future benefits and losses from continued use will also affect the outcome.

In the complex interplay of individual and drug, factors as mundane as the size and age of the individual and the dose of the substance can have powerful effects in creating either a positive or negative experience. Dose effects appear across the board, with small body size and high dose increasing the likelihood of a noxious experience; the unfiltered, high-nicotine cigarette, hard liquor, and more expensive and potent grades of marijuana all produce stronger noxious initial reactions than filtered cigarettes, beer, or cheaper home-grown marijuana. Indeed, low-dose drugs appear to ease the entry into use for initiates (Kandel, Kessler, & Margulies, 1978). The need to develop tolerance to increasingly powerful substances could well be one determinant of the "ladder" of substance abuse, beginning with beer, wine, or cigarettes and moving to hard liquor, marijuana, and more potent drugs (Fleming, Leventhal, Glynn, & Ershler, 1989; Kandel et al., 1978; Kandel & Faust, 1975).

Psychological processes also shape the drug experience. The data show that both previous use of and favorable attitudes toward substances on lower rungs on the ladder can predict later use and misuse of licit and illicit drugs (Smith & Fogg, 1978, 1979). Expectations can direct attention to specific drug effects and lead the individual to interpret them as beneficial and pleasing as opposed to dangerous and distressing. For example, an adolescent who believes that an initial experience will be extremely noxious may delay experimentation with a drug, but if initial use results in a relatively mild experience, the youth may discount other negative expectations (Pearson, 1987).

Transformation from an initially aversive experience to a highly desired and sought-after experience is not limited to the domain of psychoactive drugs. Most people include in their list of favorite foods and drinks a number of items that on first try were aversive. Common examples include highly spiced foods, bitter chocolate, and coffee (Rozin, 1990). However, the mechanisms that allow these transformations are poorly understood. We suspect that all of these transitions are abetted by social contexts that associate positive feelings with use of the substance and create expectations that use will further one's social acceptance and status. Though these may be erroneous beliefs, they encourage experimentation and use, especially when swiftly confirmed by experience without alternatives.

Recommendations for Future Efforts

Our suggestions for intervention are consistent with the transactional framework outlined above. They reflect our view that adolescents actively construct representations of their world and devise adaptive behavioral strategies that make sense within their environments. The framework can be applied whether our target group consists of adolescents residing in the poor inner city or well-to-do suburbs, though the specific content of the intervention will vary with each. It also makes clear that a multilevel program, one that targets each layer, from the remote physical and social environment, through the neighborhood and family, to the individual, is needed for the creation of barriers to substance abuse and essential for promoting alternatives to abuse. Our suggestions also reflect our belief that interventions should be made integral to the adolescent's ordinary life rather than artificially contrived, time-limited events. Finally, we believe the creation of alternatives requires the skillful incorporation of future goals into the adolescent's current life space. When translated into specific initiatives, our formulation leads to several recommendations at the societal, community, and individual levels.

Individually Focused Efforts

As should be obvious by now, we believe that individually focused drug prevention programs will be most effective when nested in societal and community changes. Prevention programs in such a context will have two clearly distinct tasks: the first, to generate the motivations and skills adolescents need to navigate life challenges, including the challenge to not use drugs; the second, to establish stronger linkages between the adolescent and formal and informal social organizations that are opposed to substance abuse.

AFFECTING ADOLESCENT MOTIVES AND SKILLS. Skill training is an important component of individually focused educational efforts. In the first section of this chapter, we reviewed some well-wrought programs that focused upon teaching youngsters how to manage a variety of life situations and say "no" to drugs. In our overview of the lessons learned from these programs, we noted that greater emphasis must be directed to motivating adolescents to use the skills training provided. Communicating realistic and personally relevant risk information is one effective source of motivation. To increase the likelihood that adolescents will internalize risk perceptions, programs will need to address several issues. The proximity of the risks presented must be accessible to the adolescent; long-term consequences such as addiction may not be enough to deter the risk. Outcomes that are viewed as improbable are likely to be disregarded. Further, programs may need to devise ways to undermine adolescents' perceptions of invulnerability and control, challenging beliefs such as "I will be careful, so it won't happen to me." It may be possible to develop messages that stimulate adolescents to identify prior examples of unpleasant experiences involving risky behavior and to use these instances to encourage them to look forward and anticipate the regret they might feel if they take more serious risks in the future (Leventhal, Baker, Brandon, & Fleming, 1989).

As previously pointed out, a comprehensive approach to motivation is predicated on gaining an understanding of the adolescent's world. A key resource is the adolescents themselves. On a similar note, Fine (1988) has advocated opening a discourse of desire in the area of sexuality education. She states that

a discourse of desire, remains a whisper inside the official work of the U. S. public schools. . . . When it is spoken it is tagged with reminders of "consequences"—emotional, physical, moral, reproductive, and/or financial. A genuine discourse of desire would invite adolescents to explore what feels good and bad, desirable and undesirable, grounded in experience, needs, and limits.

Opening such a discourse in the area of drug and alcohol education could serve as an effective component of current interventions, as well as providing background information that is crucial to future efforts to promote alternatives.

ALTERNATIVE COMMITMENTS. Alternative commitments represent another powerful source of motivation for avoiding substance use and abuse. Alternatives create barriers to substance use and other dangerous behaviors when they act as distractors and remove the adolescent from high-risk settings. If an adolescent is busy at work and absent from the sites where drugs are used, he or she is less likely to use them. Conversely, drug use and abuse can be a threat to maintaining those significant social and work relationships that emerge with any commitment to alternatives.

In our judgment, it would be an error, however, to view the generation of commitments as a replacement for induction of risk perceptions. Rather, the benefits of commitments, both the distractions of involvement and the risk of loss of non-drug rewards, should complement the personalized social and health threats used in antidrug programs.

Although there is considerable overlap, creating barriers and promoting alternatives to substance use are substantively different objectives. Questions remain regarding with whom, when, in what sequence, and how each of these components should be used. Involvement in alternative valued goals must be initiated early and sustained throughout the life span. To be successful, the social system must recognize the changing needs and perspectives of the developing individual and communicate this recognition. Communication alone is not enough: the social environment must also provide interpretations or meanings that make desirable particular ways of coping with or adapting to these changing feelings and needs. Thus, socializing agents also must prepare the adolescent for the subjective feelings that will motivate various activities.

Similarly, once substance use is in place and dependence is driving abuse, interventions may have to struggle with the simple fact that in some social contexts, drugs provide stronger positive rewards than do other life experiences. Programs to deal with dependence may have to focus first on motivations that undermine the positive rewards of use (e.g., converting the pleasure of use to a threat) and then move toward increasing the salience of significant alternative involvements. The individual needs to be considered, therefore, in relation to the *stage of substance use,* as well as the social context (Glynn, Leventhal, & Hirschman, 1986; Prochaska & DiClemente, 1983).

LINKING THE ADOLESCENT TO THE SOCIAL CONTEXT. To be more effective in our intervention efforts, we must link the adolescent to his or her social context. Toward this end, a few investigators are planning innovative programs in which they will conduct and assess the traditional, individually focused (school-based) program within a larger communitywide intervention (Pentz et al., 1989). Community involvement includes multiple organizations, such as private and public media (local television, radio, and newspapers); government agencies (police, public health, etc.); private businesses; and church and family groups. The tactics used by these social units include media programs, discussions on abuse at church groups, community planning for teen activities, and family participation in the motivational and skills components of school programs through the assignment of shared parent–adolescent homework. (Johnson et al., 1990). Coordination of efforts across units should enhance success.

What is lacking in these efforts is a conceptual framework that will help investigators to organize and link contextual factors to the behavioral domain of the adolescent. An effective framework will suggest ways of integrating program implementation and ways of assessing this integration. For example, public health and medical institutions could contribute to the creation of barriers by providing occasions on which young adolescents are exposed to evidence on the ravages of drugs. An example might be arranging visits to patients suffering from abuse. The value of such tactics will be minimal, however, if exposure is confined to adolescents who are nonusers or if the experience is not carefully constructed to bring out key lessons. Among these lessons might be demonstrating similarities between the adolescent visitors and these adult patients when they themselves were adolescents. Another lesson would be how the patients' earlier decisions led to drug use that denied them access to alternatives they said they wanted but to which they didn't commit themselves.

In summary, a theory for linking the adolescent to the social context needs to consider a wide range of structural and substantive issues. The structural issues will range from access to the adolescent community (i.e., how we achieve information exposure), to source credibility, to bringing into the adolescents' contemporary life space alternative behaviors that are clearly connected to wanted future goals. Issues of significance will involve ways of matching the content of media and organizational programs to the motivational and skills systems of the individual while dealing with the adolescents' ability to distance the self from the information.

INVITING ADOLESCENTS TO EXPLORE THEIR ASPIRATIONS AND FEARS. As previously stated, connecting attainable and attractive alternatives to the adolescent's current life space requires an understanding of the contents of the life space. A useful tool for examining adolescents' perceptions of the lifestyles available to them is the *possible selves* construct developed by Markus (e.g., Markus & Nirius, 1986). In brief:

Possible selves represent individuals' ideas of what they would like to become, and what they are afraid of becoming. . . . Possible selves are the cognitive components of hope fears goals and threats . . . they function as incentives for future behavior (i.e., they are selves to be approached or avoided) and . . . they provide an evaluative or interpretive context for the current view of self. (p. 956)

Exploring the question "What kind of person would I like to become?" brings the issues home to an adolescent. Some may have a fairly clear picture, while others have only a vague idea. The degree to which an adolescent's behavior is actually guided by his or her possible selves will also vary. More concrete pictures of both the desired and the feared possible selves can be expected to have a greater impact on behavior. But several questions remain, for example, "What aspects of the social context serve to encourage the development of more concrete possible selves?"

Even under the best circumstances, few adolescents have formed elaborate self goals (e.g., career choices). It may be more relevant to help them to define clearly "who I *do not* want to be" while identifying more general themes consistent with "who I would like to be." If we are lucky, the adolescents' self-generated feared selves will include outcomes that are more likely to occur if they become involved with substances. When this is the case, the task will be to make the connections between substance use and the feared outcome undeniable. In any case, encouraging adolescents to connect high-risk behaviors with limited choice in the future, while exploring the environment for alternatives that will further self-generated goals, should provide a powerful means of intervention. Because many adolescents value freedom of choice, framing specific activities incompatible with substance use as increasing freedom of choice can further enhance the attractiveness of pursuing these involvements (Kahneman & Tversky, 1984).

Certain contexts (e.g., the inner city) may provide limited exposure to models engaged in activities valued and rewarded by the society at large. Social structures such as the local gang, with its unique language, music, gender stereotypes, and behavioral roles, often provide the most salient models. The construction of worlds unique to specific groups of adolescents is not limited to the inner city. Although adolescents from economically advantaged backgrounds are more likely to be exposed to a wider variety of future opportunities than those from economically disadvantaged backgrounds, some find behavior considered deviant by mainstream society very attractive. It can be expected that specific attributes of the social context will ease or complicate the task of intervention (Johnson et al., 1990).

A Special Case: Promoting Alternatives in the Inner City

The conditions in America's inner cities pose a variety of complex challenges to intervention. Consequently, a closer look at promoting alternatives within this unique environment clearly illustrates the necessity of a multilevel approach.

According to Wilson and DiIulio (1989), the control of drug abuse in the ghettos of the inner city requires that communities regain the status and power needed to control local space, specifically, to "reassert lawful public control over public space" (p. 24). If a community cannot rid its parks and streets of the drug peddlers and their clients and rid itself of random violence and shootings, individual, attitudinal barriers to involvement in the drug trade will crumble, and the possibility for creating alternatives to drug use will remain little more than an unattainable dream.

EMPOWERMENT AND REORGANIZATION. How can we create the conditions needed to empower communities to reorganize themselves to be free of drugs and violence so that people who do not want to use drugs can avoid doing so? Murray (1990) suggests a series of social and legal changes that allow tenants and landlords, working in concert, to refuse rental to or to evict tenants who are drug users or otherwise disruptive. Murray's position is controversial, but its aim is to allow individuals to create neighborhoods and communities that are isolated from drug dealers and drug users. He claims that "In the rush to rid society of the socially disapproved reasons for discriminating among applicants, starting with race, we threw out as well all the ways in which landlords performed a neighborhood-formation function" (p. 24).

Murray argues that current discrimination laws have operated most effectively against the maintenance of cohesive, community-oriented neighborhoods for those with the fewest financial resources and have little impact on those that can afford to control the makeup of their environment through relocation.

The second component of Murray's thesis, which is also the central thesis of this chapter, is that drug use will persist in an expanded form as long as there are limited alternatives. Creating new opportunities, in addition to identifying and promoting existing ones, is required.

CREATING ALTERNATIVES: OPPORTUNITIES. Mass media images and daily encounters must expose adolescents to individuals from their ethnic and economic backgrounds who have "made it" in one or another socially acceptable pursuit. Retail establishments and professional offices run by managers, doctors, and lawyers from the minority community need to be as frequent and salient in the adolescent's world as drug users and drug dealers. Their presence is important not only for the adolescent, but for the family's interactions. The adolescent's parents, older siblings, and extended family members are unlikely to encourage and reward goals that seem to have no possibility of achievement.

The social system must also specify what rewards can be expected and how much effort is necessary to obtain these rewards. The attractiveness of these rewards will reflect societal values; given that money and material incentives are primary indicators of status and success in our society, it should come as no surprise that youngsters may prefer the entrepreneurial tasks of selling heroin or crack to the tasks of studying mathematics and English as steps toward developing career options. The media focuses little attention on many careers (e.g., in engineering, biology, or academia), and the government provides inadequate support to an educational system that prepares young people for the future by functionally relating curriculum content to relevant and desirable outcomes. For the most part, representatives of the wide variety of lifestyle and career options are absent from the adolescent's life space. This is true whether the adolescent lives in the inner city or in an upper- or middle-class suburb. In contrast to society's poor performance in projecting images of the above careers is its skill in promoting images of sports figures. Stars of our national sports arenas—football, basketball and baseball—are key salespersons for our economy and highly visible to young adolescents. Adolescents understand their work and can imitate and practice it in their neighborhoods. However, while the details of these roles are available for modeling and identification, the probability of becoming a successful professional athlete is small. The scarcity of positions and the intense competition for them do not in themselves minimize the value of practice in this domain, but the instruments of the social system must emphasize those aspects of athletic participation useful in achieving a variety of potential goals (e.g., developing discipline and persistence or skills such as observation and analysis).

The *barriers* to carrying out the changes that can powerfully impact life in our inner cities are many. One significant issue is the readiness of the larger community to attribute problems in the inner-city ghettos to the personal characteristics of the individuals living there, rather than viewing them as expected outcomes of interaction with a disorganized environment. Personal attributions create excuses for denying both financial resources for critical services (e.g., police protection) and the authority for making the decisions that are essential to the safety and empowerment of those residents who wish to form stable, drug-free neighborhoods.

Conclusions

Efforts to improve public health by regulating public behavior are not new. Such efforts surely predate recorded history, waxing and waning with the advent of plagues, population movements, and spiritual practices. Evidence of their antiquity is readily available in religious documents and oral traditions that detail dietary, sexual, family, and community practices. Whorton (1982) provides a lively review of both religious and secular health reform movements in the United States over the past century. He opens by describing the early-nineteenth-century Christian physiologists, with their emphasis on balance and avoidance of excess in diet and sexual behavior, and shows how these same themes informed later health movements such as vegetarianism.

This extended history can and should communicate several significant lessons. First, producing change requires major, culturewide involvement. This means a societal investment at all levels (i.e., from the top down and the bottom up). Drug abuse and other risk behaviors will not be curtailed unless *governmental, religious, and noninstitutional organizations act in concert* for success. Resources, time; and personal effort must be expended to create a cohesive social organization *before* we can comprehensively address adolescent substance abuse.

Second, it is clear that programs will necessarily be complex, working at multiple levels of the social structure and giving adequate attention to understanding and influencing individuals' motives and skills. We need a mix of incentives and skills to accommodate the changing life situations of individuals over time.

Third, the *ways we construe one another* pose obstacles to success. Intervention efforts will surely fail when inhibited by attributions suggesting that abuse is solely a problem of personal or ethnic characteristics, on the one hand, or environmentally induced on the other. The former encourages blaming and attacking individuals and groups, and generates mistrust, which undermines the procedures essential for creating the communities and personal identities needed for effective self management. The latter, an exclusive focus on the environment, creates excuses, dependencies, and failure to self-regulate.

Fourth, to promote alternatives to drugs, these alternatives must be available. They must be embodied by living examples in the adolescents' local communities. Success in this area may require major changes in safety and housing regulations.

Fifth, it is unrealistic to expect that we can eliminate adolescent drug use and abuse. At best, we can reduce the number of users and abusers. The use of harmful substances has never been, nor is it likely ever to be, completely eradicated in any population. Thus, controlling specific problems is a continuing effort, one that began with the human discovery of the grape and will only end with the end of life as we know it.

Finally, and more optimistically, history suggests that epidemics are self-limiting. The virulence of any plague will moderate with changes in the disease agent and the gradual selection of a more resistant host population. The same may be true for drug abuse and its attendant evils. Data obtained over the prior two decades show movement from drug to drug. Substances seen as dangerous are replaced by newer drugs whose risk is unknown. Thus, declines in the use of drugs such as heroin and cocaine do not reflect a general increase in caution or conservatism on the part of adolescents or society; the aversion of risk is specific to each drug, and its damage is limited. This history might encourage a wait-and-see approach given the heavy costs of intervention in money and time. But while activism can produce its own damaging effects, waiting is also risky, as we do not know where the current epidemic will lead and the degree to which it will destabilize and change our social structure. There is no "natural equilibrium" in nature or human affairs: structure, stability, and freedom require continual vigilance.

Acknowledgments

Preparation of this chapter was supported by PHS Grant No. 5 RO1 DA03530 of the National Institute of Drug Abuse.

Notes

1. In fact, classification of prevention programs within reviews exacerbates the problem by emphasizing procedural rather than theoretical differences (Battjes, 1985). Simply extracting the differential impact of particular modalities, for example, knowledge only, peer programs, or alternatives programs, from the intensity with which they are presented (i.e., hours spent) can be problematic (Tobler, 1986).
2. That is, most adolescents identified as possessing particular high-risk traits or experiencing high-risk environments do not subsequently develop substance abuse disorders.

References

Ajzen, I., & Fishbein, M. (1973). Attitudinal and normative variables as predictors of specific behaviors. *Journal of Personality and Social Psychology, 27*, 41–57.

Argyle, M. (1986). Social behavior problems in adolescence. In R. K. Silbereisen, K. Eyferth, & G. Rudinger (Eds)., *Development as action in context: Problem behavior and normal youth development* (pp. 55–86). New York: Springer-Verlag.

Aron, A., Aron, E. N., Tudor, M., & Nelson, G. (1991). Close relationships as including other in the self. *Journal of Personality and Social Psychology, 60*, 241–253.

Ary, D., Biglan, A., Glasgow, R., Zoref, L., Black, C., Ochs, L., Severson, H., Kelly, R., Weissman, W., Lichtenstein, E., Brozovsky, P., Wirt, R., & James, L. (1990). The efficacy of social-influence prevention programs versus "standard care": Are new initiatives needed? *Journal of Behavioral Medicine, 13,* 281–296.

Bachman, J. G., Johnston, L. D., & O'Malley, P. M. (1990). Explaining the recent decline in cocaine use among young adults: Further evidence that perceived risks and disapproval lead to reduced drug use. *Journal of Health and Social Behavior, 31,* 173–184.

Bacon, S. D. (1978). On prevention of alcohol problems and alcoholism. *Journal of Studies on Alcohol,* 39, 1125–1147.

Bandura, A. (1977a). Self-efficacy: Toward a unifying theory of behavioral change. *Psychological Review, 84,* 191–215.

Bandura, A. (1977b). *Social learning theory.* Englewood Cliffs, NJ: Prentice-Hall.

Bangert-Drowns, R. L. (1988). The effects of school based substance abuse education—a meta-analysis. *Journal of Drug Education, 18,* 243–264.

Battjes, R. J. (1985). Prevention of adolescent drug abuse. *International Journal of Drug Addiction, 20,* 1113–1134.

Bem, D. (1967). Self-perception: An alternative interpretation of cognitive dissonance phenomenon. *Psychology Review, 74,* 183–200.

Best, J. A., Flay, B. R., Towson, S.M.J., Ryan, K. B., Perry, C. L., Brown, K. S., Kersell, M. W., & d'Avernas, J. R. (1984). Smoking prevention and the concept of risk. *Journal of Applied Social Psychology, 14,* 257–273.

Biglan, A., Glasgow, R., Ary, D., Thompson, R., Severson, H., Lichtenstein, E., Weissman, W., Faller, C., & Gallison, C. (1987). How generalizable are the effects of smoking prevention programs? Refusal skills training and parent messages in a teacher administered program. *Journal of Behavioral Medicine, 10,* 613–628.

Biglan, A., James, L. E., LaChance, P., Zoref, L., & Joffe, J. (1988). Videotaped materials in a school-based smoking prevention program. *Preventive Medicine, 17,* 559–584.

Borgida, E., & Nisbett, R. E. (1977). The differential impact of abstract vs. concrete information on decisions. *Journal of Applied Social Psychology, 7,* 258–271.

Botvin, G. J., Baker, E., Dusenbury, L., Tortu, S., & Botvin, E. M. (1990). Preventing adolescent drug abuse through a multi-modal cognitive-behavioral program. *Journal of Consulting and Clinical Psychology, 58,* 437–446.

Botvin, G. J., Eng, A., & Williams, C. L. (1980). Preventing the onset of smoking through life skills training. *Preventive Medicine, 9,* 135–143.

Bronfenbrenner, U. (1979). *The ecology of human development: Experiments by nature and by design.* Boston: Cambridge University Press.

Bronfenbrenner, U. (1986). Ecology of the family as a context for human development. *Developmental Psychology, 22,* 723–742.

Brooks-Gunn, J., & Reiter, E. O. (1989). The role of pubertal processes in the early adolescent transition. In S. Feldman & G. Elliott (Eds.), *At the threshold: The developing adolescent* (pp. 16–53). Cambridge, MA: Harvard University Press.

Brooks-Gunn, J., Rock, D., & Warren, M. P. (1989). Comparability of constructs across the adolescent years. *Developmental Psychology, 25,* 51–60.

Brown, B. B., Clasen, D. R., & Eicher, S. A. (1986). Perceptions of peer pressure, peer conformity dispositions and self reported behavior among adolescents. *Developmental Psychology, 22,* 521–530.

Cartwright, D. (1949). Some principles of mass persuasion. Selected findings in the sale of United States war bonds. *Human Relations, 2,* 253–267.

Cox, W. M. (1987). Personality theory and research. In H. T. Blane & K. E. Leonard (Eds.), *Psychological theories of drinking and alcoholism* (pp. 55–89). New York: Gilford Press.

DeVries, H. (1989). *Smoking prevention in Dutch adolescents.* Datawyse, IL: Maastricht.

Dittmann-Kohli, F. (1986). Problem identification and definition as important aspects of adolescents' coping with normative life tasks. In R. K. Silbereisen, K. Eyferth, & G. Rudinger (Eds)., *Development as action in context: Problem behavior and normal youth development* (pp. 19–38) New York: Springer-Verlag.

Elias, M. J., Gara, M., Ubriaco, M., Rothbaum, P. A., Clabby, J. F., & Schuyler, T. (1986). Impact of a preventive social problem solving intervention on children's coping with middle-school stressors. *American Journal of Community Psychology, 14,* 259–275.

Evans, R. I., Rozelle, R. M., Lasater, T. M., Deinbroski, T. M., & Allen, B. T. (1968). New measure of the effects of persuasive communications: A chemical indicator of toothbrushing behavior. *Psychological Reports, 23,* 731–736.

Felner, R. D., & Felner, T. Y. (1990). Primary prevention programs on the educational context: A transactional-ecological framework and analysis. In L. Bond & B. Campas (Eds.), *Primary prevention in the schools* (pp. 116–131). Beverly Hills, CA: Sage.

Fine, M. (1988). Sexuality schooling, and adolescent females: The missing discourse of desire. *Harvard Educational Review, 58,* 29–53.

Fishbein, M., & Ajzen, I. (1975). *Belief, attitude, intention, and behavior.* Reading, MA: Addison-Wesley.

Fisher, J. D., & Baumann, K. E. (1988). Influence and selection in the friend adolescent relationship: Findings from the study of adolescent smoking and drinking. *Journal of Applied Social Psychology, 18,* 289–314.

Flay, B. R. (1985a). Are social-psychological smoking prevention programs effective? The Waterloo study. *Journal of Behavioral Medicine, 8,* 37–59.

Flay, B. R. (1985b). Psychosocial approaches to smoking prevention: A review of findings. *Health Psychology, 4,* 449–488.

Flay, B. R., Koepke, D., Thomson, S. J., Santi, S., Best, A., & Brown, K. S. (1989). Six-year follow-up of the first Waterloo school smoking prevention trial. *American Journal of Public Health, 79,* 1371–1376.

Fleming, R., Leventhal, H., Glynn, K., & Ershler, J. (1989). The role of cigarettes in the initiation and progression of early substance abuse. *Addictive Behaviors, 14,* 261–272.

Globetti, G. (1974). A conceptual analysis of the effectiveness of alcohol education programs. In M. Goodstadt (Ed.), *Research on methods and programs of drug education* (pp. 97–112). Ontario: Addiction Research Foundation of Ontario.

Glynn, K., Leventhal, H., & Hirschman, R. (1986). A cognitive developmental approach to smoking prevention. *NIDA monograph series* (pp. 130–152). Publication No. (ADM) 86-1334. Washington, DC: U. S. Dept. of Health and Human Services.

Goodstadt, M. S., & Sheppard, M. A. (1983). Three approaches to alcohol education. *Journal of Studies on Alcohol, 44,* 362–380.

Goodstadt, M. S., Sheppard, M. A., & Chan, G. C. (1982). An evaluation of two school-based alcohol education programs. *Journal of Studies on Alcohol, 43,* 352–369.

Hirschman, R. S., & Leventhal, H. (1989). Preventing smoking behavior in school children: An initial test of a cognitive-development program. *Journal of Applied Social Psychology, 19,* 559–583.

Hops, H., Weismann, W., Biglan, A., Thompson, R., Faller, C., & Severson, H. (1986). A taped situation test of cigarette refusal skills among adolescents. *Behavioral Assessment, 8,* 45–154.

Jemmott, J. B., Ditto, P. H., & Croyle, R. T. (1986). Judging health status: Effects of perceived prevalence and personal relevance. *Journal of Personality and Social Psychology, 50,* 899–905.

Jessor, R., & Jessor, S. L. (1977). *Problem behavior and psychosocial development: A longitudinal study of youth.* New York: Academic Press.

Johnson, C. A., Pentz, M. A., Weber, M. D., Dwyer, J. H., Baer, N., MacKinnon, D. P., Hansen, W. B., & Flay, B. R. (1990). Relative effectiveness of comprehensive programming for drug abuse prevention with high-risk and low-risk adolescents. *Journal of Consulting and Clinical Psychology, 58,* 447–456.

Johnston, L. D. (1985). Etiology of Drug Abuse: Implications for prevention. DHHS Publication No. (ADM) 85-1335. Rockville, MD: U. S. Dept. of Health and Human Services.

Johnston, L. D., O'Malley, P., & Bachman, J. (1987). *National trends in drug use and related factors among American high school students 1975-1986.* DHHS Publication No. (ADM) 87-1535. Washington, DC: U. S. Government Printing Office.

Kahneman, D., & Tversky, A. (1984). Choices, values, and frames. *American Psychologist, 39,* 341–351.

Kandel, D. B., & Faust, R. (1975). Sequence and stages in patterns of adolescent drug use. *Archives of General Psychiatry, 32,* 923–932.

Kandel, D. B., Kessler, R. C., & Margulies, R. Z. (1978). Antecedents of adolescent initiation into stages of drug use: A developmental analysis. In D. B. Kandel (Ed.), *Longitudinal research and drug use: Empirical findings and methodological issues* (pp. 73–98). Washington, DC: Hemisphere.

Kanfer, F. H. (1977). The many faces of self-control, or behavior modification changes its focus. In R. B. Stuart (Ed.), *Behavioral self-management: Strategies, techniques, and outcomes* (pp. 1–48). New York: Brunner-Mazel.

Kohn, P. (1974). Motivation for drug and alcohol use. In M. Goodstadt (Ed.), *Research on methods and programs of drug education* (pp. 53–84). Ontario: Addiction Research Foundation of Ontario.

Leventhal, H. (1970). Findings and theory in the study of fear communications. *Advances in Experimental Social Psychology, 5,* 119–186.

Leventhal, H., Baker, T., Brandon, T., & Fleming, R. (1989). Intervening and preventing cigarette smoking. In T. Ney & A. Gale (Eds.), *Smoking and human behavior* (pp. 313–336). Oxford: Wiley.

Leventhal, H., & Cameron, L. (in press). Persuasion and health attitudes. In T. Brock & S. Shavitt (Eds.), *Psychology of persuasion.* Needham Heights, MA: Allyn & Bacon.

Leventhal, H., Fleming, R., & Glynn, K. (1988). A cognitive developmental approach to smoking intervention. In S. Macs, C. D. Speilberger, P. B. Defares, & I. G. Sarason (Eds.), *Topics in health psychology: Proceedings of the first annual expert conference in health psychology* (pp. 79–105). New York: Wiley.

Leventhal, H., Meyer, D., & Nerenz, D. (1980). The common sense representation of illness danger. In S. Rachman (Ed.), *Medical psychology. Volume II,* (pp. 7–30). New York: Pergamon Press.

Leventhal, H., & Nerenz, D. R. (1983). A model for stress research with some implications for the control of stress disorders. In T. C. Rosen & L. J. Solomon (Eds.), *Stress reduction and prevention* (pp. 5–38). New York: Plenum Press.

Leventhal, H., & Singer, R. P. (1966). Affect arousal and positioning of recommendations in persuasive communications. *Journal of Personality and Social Psychology, 4,* 137–146.

Leventhal, H., Singer, R., & Jones, S. (1965). Effects of fear and specificity of recommendations upon attitudes and behavior. *Journal of Personality and Social Psychology, 2,* 20–29.

Leventhal, H., Watts, J. C., & Pagano, F. (1967). Effects of fear instructions and how to cope with danger. *Journal of Personality and Social Psychology, 6,* 313–321.

Markus, H., & Nirius, P. (1986). Possible selves. *American Psychologist, 41,* 954–969.

McAllister, A. L. (1983). Social psychological approaches. In T. J. Glynn, C. G. Leukefeld, & J. P. Ludford (Eds.), *Preventing adolescent substance abuse: Intervention strategies* (pp. 36–50). NIDA Research Monograph 47. DHHS Publication No. (ADM) 83-1280. Rockville, MD: U. S. Dept. of Health and Human Services.

Mead, G. H. (1934). *Mind, self, and society.* Chicago: University of Chicago Press.

Mosbach, P., & Leventhal, H. (1988). Peer group identification and smoking: Implications for intervention. *Journal of Abnormal Psychology, 97,* 238–245.

Murray, C. (1990). How to win the war on drugs: The drug free zone solution. *The New Republic, 202,* 19–25.

Murray, D. M., Davis-Hearn, M., Goldman, A. I., Pirie, P., & Luepker, R. V. (1988). Four and five year follow-up results from four seventh grade smoking prevention strategies. *Journal of Behavioral Medicine, 11,* 395–406.

National Institute of Drug Abuse (1983). *Prevention plus: Involving schools, parents, and the community in alcohol and drug education.* DHHS Publication No. (ADM) 83-1256. Rockville, MD: U. S. Dept. of Health and Human Services.

Nisbett, R. E., & Wilson, T. D. (1977). Telling more than we can know: Verbal reports on mental processes. *Psychological Review, 84,* 231–259.

Oetting, E. R., & Beauvais, F. (1986). Peer cluster theory: Drugs and the adolescent. *Journal of Counseling and Development, 65,* 17–30.

Oetting, E. R., & Beauvais, F. (1987). Common elements in youth drug abuse: Peer clusters and other psychological factors. *Journal of Drug Issues, 17,* 137–151.

Pearson, G. (1987). *The new heroin users.* New York: Basil Blackwell.

Pentz, M. A., Dwyer, J. H., MacKinnon, D. P., Flay, B. R., Hansen, W. B., Wang, E.Y.I., & Johnson, C. A. (1989). A multicommunity trial for primary prevention of adolescent drug abuse. *Journal of the American Medical Association, 261,* 3259–3266.

Perry, C., Killen, J., Slinkard, L. A., & McAlister, A. (1980). Peer teaching and smoking prevention among junior high students. *Adolescence, 9,* 277–281.

Perry, C., Killen, J., Telch, M., & Maccoby, N. (1980). Modifying smoking behavior of teenagers: A school based intervention. *American Journal of Public Health, 70,* 722–725.

Petersen, A. C., & Taylor, B. (1980). The biological approach to adolescence: Biological change and psychological adaptation. In J. Adelson (Ed.), *Handbook of adolescent psychology* (pp. 117–155). New York: Wiley.

Petty, R. E., & Cacioppo, J. T. (1986). *Communication and persuasion: Central and peripheral routes to attitude change.* New York: Springer-Verlag.

Pirie, P. L., Murray, D. M., & Luepker, R. V. (1988). Smoking prevalence in a cohort of adolescents, including absentees, dropouts and transfers. *American Journal of Public Health, 78,* 176–178.

Prochaska, J. O., & DiClemente, C. C. (1983). Stages and processes of self-change of smoking: Toward an integrative model of change. *Journal of Consulting and Clinical Psychology, 51,* 390–395.

Rhodes, J. E., & Jason, L. A. (1988). *Preventing substance abuse among children and adolescents.* New York: Pergamon Press.

Rogers, R. W. (1983). Cognitive and physiological processes in fear appeals and attitude change: A revised theory of protection motivation. In J. T. Cacioppo & R. Petty (Eds.), *Social psychology: A sourcebook* (pp.). New York: Guilford Press.

Rozin, P. (1990). Development in the food domain. *Developmental Psychology, 26,* 555–562.

Sadler, O. W., & Dillard, N. R. (1978). A description and evaluation of TRENDS: A substance abuse education program for sixth graders. *Journal of Educational Research, 71,* 171–175.

Scarr, S., & McCartney, K. (1983). How people make their own environment: A theory of genotype—environment effects. *Child Development, 54,* 424–435.

Schaps, E., DiBartolo, R., Moskowitz, J., Palley, C., & Churgin, S. (1981). Primary prevention evaluation research: A review of 127 impact studies. *Journal of Drug Issues, 11,* 17–43.

Shedler, T., & Block, J. (1990). Adolescent drug use and psychological health: A longitudinal inquiry. *American Psychologist, 45,* 612–630.

Sheppard, M. A., Wright, D., & Goodstadt, M. (1985). Peer pressure and drug use: Exploding the myth. *Adolescence, 20,* 949–958.

Silbereisen, R. K., & Eyferth, K. (1986) Development as action in context. In R. K. Silbereisen, K. Eyferth, & G. Rudinger (Eds.), *Development as action in context: Problem behavior and normal youth development* (pp. 3–18). New York: Springer-Verlag.

Smith, G. M., & Fogg, C. P. (1978). Psychological predictors of early use, late use, and nonuse of marijuana among teenage students. In D. B. Kandel (Ed.), *Longitudinal research on drug use: Empirical findings and methodological issues* (pp. 101–113). New York: Hemisphere.

Smith, G. M., & Fogg, C. P. (1979). Psychological antecedents of teenage drug use. In R. G. Simmons (Ed.), *Research in community and mental health, Volume I* (pp. 87–102). Greenwich, CN: JAI Press.

Steinberg, L. (1986). Latchkey children and susceptibility to peer pressure: An ecological analysis. *Developmental Psychology, 22,* 433–439.

Stryker, S., & Statham, A. (1985). Symbolic interaction and role theory. In G. Lindsay & E. Aronson (Eds.), *The handbook of social psychology: Volume I* (3rd ed.) (pp. 311–378). New York: Random House.

Sussman, S., Dent, C. W., Stacy, A. W., Burciaga, C., Raynor, A., Turner, G. E., Charlin, V., Craig, S., Hansen, W. B., Burton, D., & Flay, B. R. (1990). Peer-group association and adolescent tobacco use. *Journal of Abnormal Psychology, 99,* 349–352.

Sutton, S. R. (1982). Fear arousing communications: A critical examination of theory and research. In J. R. Eiser (Ed.), *Social psychology and behavioral medicine* (pp. 303–337). New York: Wiley.

Thompson, E. (1978). Smoking education programs 1960–1976. *American Journal of Public Health, 68,* 250–255.

Tobler, N. S. (1986). Meta-analysis of 143 adolescent drug prevention programs: Quantitative outcome results of program participants compared to a control comparison group. *Journal of Drug Issues, 16,* 537–567.

U. S. Department of Health and Human Services (1987a). *Be smart! Don't start.* DHHS Publication No. (ADM) 87-1502. Rockville, MD: U. S. Dept. of Health and Human Services.

U. S. Department of Health and Human Services (1987b). *Helping your students say no to alcohol.* DHHS Publication No. (ADM) 87-1501. Rockville, MD: U. S. Dept. of Health and Human Services.

Whorton, J. C. (1982). *Crusaders for fitness.* Princeton, NJ: Princeton University Press.

Wilson, J. Q., & DiIulio, J. J. (1989) Crackdown: Treating the symptoms of the drug problem. *The New Republic, 201,* 21–25.

13

The Control of Violence
and the Promotion of Nonviolence
in Adolescents

Felton Earls, Robert B. Cairns, and James A. Mercy

At the outset, we should observe that few specific strategies to achieve the goals of controlling violence or promoting nonviolence have been described in the scientific literature. Yet the dual problems of violence reduction and nonviolence promotion are critical health issues for adolescents. In 1987, homicide was the third leading cause of death in persons 10 to 19 years of age (National Center for Health Statistics, 1988). In that same year, 1 in 16 adolescents was a victim of violent crime. But it is not only victims who are vulnerable. Extreme aggression in adolescence has also been shown to be a reliable predictor of a host of subsequent health problems for the violent individual, from automobile accidents to suicide (Earls, 1991).

An introductory comment is in order on how we employ two key concepts—*violence* and *nonviolence*. In everyday usage, *violence* refers to the exertion of physical force so as to injure or abuse. Consistent with this definition, *interpersonal violence* refers to a class of actions that have qualitatively different consequences from other social behaviors, namely, the intentional infliction of pain and injury through physical force. Nonviolence is ordinarily defined by exclusion: the avoidance of violence, abstention from violence as a matter of principle, or the absence of violence in one's surroundings.

Unfortunately, definition by exclusion is not very useful for precise analysis. Such a definition implies that violent and nonviolent strategies are mutually exclusive; from an alternative perspective, it implies that an increase in violence is associated with a reciprocal decrease in nonviolence and vice versa. There are empirical reasons to question both implications. At the individual level, violent and nonviolent patterns may coexist in the same person, though at different times and in different circumstances. For example, the propensity of a normal individual to deliver painful, life-threatening shocks to an innocent victim, when justified by authority, bears no relation to the subject's level of empathy, intelligence, or gender (Milgram, 1974). In this chapter, the *control of violence* and the *promotion of nonviolence* are seen as being separable though related issues.

An integrating theme for this chapter is our concern with the processes of development and how behaviors are established, maintained, and changed over the life course. Accordingly, we examine age-related trends in populations and ontogenetic trajectories in individuals.

Interpersonal Violence: Perpetrators and Victims

The statistical portrait of violent behavior in adolescence is so dramatic that it deserves at least an introductory presentation here. Violent behavior is far from randomly distributed in the population. It will be useful to review briefly data on the entire age range to underscore how fundamentally important are the adolescent years.

Interpersonal violence, among all behaviors affecting health and longevity, may be the most ubiquitous and sporadic in nature. Demographic factors alone reveal the complexity of its variability. The incidence of violent behavior rises rapidly during adolescence, peaking between the ages of 17 and 19 years. Powerful gender differences in violent crime arrests also appear in late adolescence, with males being 10 times more likely than females to be arrested. Regional variation in homicide rates in the United States is striking, and rates in urban areas exceed those in rural areas. Income and race are also markers of vulnerable subgroups in the population. As if these variables were not sufficient to demonstrate the complexity of associated factors, cross-national data reveal that the United States has rates of violent crime that far exceed those of any other industrialized country (Fingerhut & Kleinman, 1990).

In characterizing interpersonal violence, it is useful to provide evidence on both perpetrators and victims. The FBI's Uniform Crime Reporting Program provides data from police reports on persons arrested for violent crimes. For each of the four categories of violent crime defined by this system (murder, rape, aggravated assault, and robbery), the age-specific rates peak in late adolescence and remain high into early adulthood. By combining all four categories, as shown in Figure 13.1, the distinction is most prominent for males, for whom the rate is severalfold higher than for females.

Given this picture, it is perhaps not surprising that adolescents between the ages of 12 and 19 years have the highest victimization rates of any age group. In 1987, 1,728,120, or 6.2% of adolescents, are estimated to have been the victims of a violent crime (Federal Bureau of Investigation [FBI], 1987). The evidence for victims is derived from two sources: the National Crime Survey conducted by the Department of Justice and mortality reports of the National Center for Health Statistics. Figure 13.2 illustrates victimization rates by age, sex, and race based on findings from the National Crime Survey. Adolescent males, both black and white, have a higher risk for most types of insults. However, the magnitude of the difference

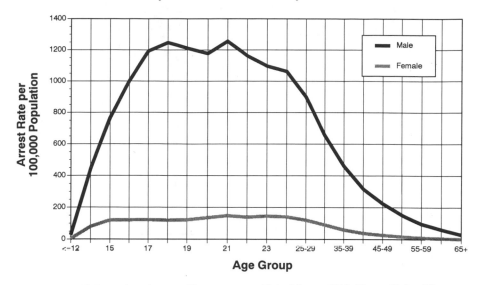

Figure 13.1. Violent crime. Age-specific arrest rates, United States, 1987. (*Source:* Federal Bureau of Investigation, Uniform Crime Reporting Bureau.)

between males and females is much less than the difference in arrest rates as presented in Figure 13.1.

The homicide victimization rates generated by public health agencies for the U. S. population in 1987 parallel the findings from criminal justice agencies. African-American males are at particularly high risk; even the rate for African-American females is distinctly higher than the rate for white females. Homicide constitutes the leading cause of death for African-American males and females between the ages of 15 and 34 years. It is the third leading cause of death among white males and females in the same age range.

While adolescents in America are at considerably higher risk for being both victims and perpetrators than are adolescents in other Western, industrialized societies, the age trajectory of arrest curves for violence are remarkably similar. According to the most recent data from Sweden (*Statistical Abstracts,* 1990), the peak age for arrests for violent crime and the gender ratio in violent crime arrest rate parallel the U. S. findings. Thus, age and gender remain relatively invariant within a picture characterized by dramatic social, cultural, and personal variability.

The Developmental Perspective

The synthetic developmental perspective of the last two decades posits that each individual develops and functions psychologically as a total, integrated organism. Maturational, experiential, and cultural aspects contribute simultaneously and inseparably (Magnusson, 1988; Sameroff, 1983). For our present purposes, the

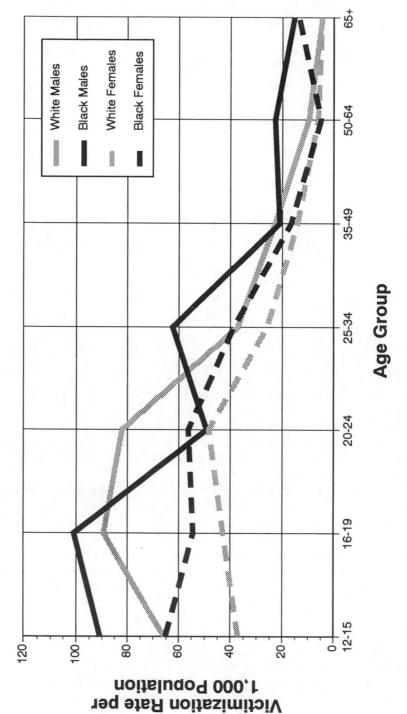

Figure 13.2. Violent crime victimization rates, United States, 1987. (*Source:* U.S. Department of Justice, Bureau of Crime Statistics.)

developmental perspective has special implications for the control of violence and the promotion of nonviolence.

Mechanisms in Development

Until recently, developmental approaches to behavior have had a tendency to "talk past" one another. Different models selectively focused on different mechanisms, and the resultant theories had a patchwork quality. For example, social learning models of adolescent aggression focused on learning processes in the family but explicitly excluded the contributions of biological, maturational, and social-cultural factors (Bandura & Walters, 1963). Similarly, social-cognitive deficit theories of development hold that aggressive individuals have deficiencies in social information processing, which, in turn, lead to aggression and social rejection by peers (Dodge, 1986). Despite such differences in emphasis, there is now a consensus within the modern developmental perspective that violence and nonviolence are multidetermined.

First, investigations of behavioral genetics in animals and humans indicate that such characteristics as impulsivity, thrill seeking, and the propensity to attack are heritable (Cairns, Gariepy, & Hood, 1990; Scarr & McCartney, 1983). Similarly, recent neurobiological investigations have demonstrated the mediational role of neurotransmitters in impulsive violence (Linnoila et al., 1983). While formulations on the neurobiology of violence in humans remain controversial, strong empirical associations have been established in nonhuman mammals, including primates (Lewis et al., in press; McGuire & Raleigh, 1985). The effects are not unidirectional, however, in that social conditions contribute to neurobiological states and vice versa.

Second, while genetic determinants of neurobiological variables certainly exist, the developing brain is also affected by the physical and social environments (Carlson, Earls, & Todd, 1988). These environmental conditions also may contribute importantly to human differences in aggressive behavior. Informative examples are represented by known biomedical hazards. These include head injury, infectious diseases, and prenatal and postnatal exposure to a variety of toxins such as heavy metals, alcohol, and cocaine.

Third, family influences are significant at all ages. Studies of parental influence were originally stimulated by psychodynamic models, and a direct line of influence may be drawn between neoanalytic object relations theory and the contemporary focus on mother–infant attachment (Bowlby, 1969). In turn, the major concerns of social learning theory—frustration-aggression (Dollard, Dobb, Miller, Mowrer, & Sears, 1939); parental rejection and punishment (Patterson, 1982; Sears, Maccoby, & Levin, 1957); identification and modeling of aggression (Bandura & Walters, 1963)—reflect a focus on the family. Empirical studies have strongly confirmed that family influences are pervasive in the origins and support of aggressive behaviors. Virtually all studies of childhood aggression have reported robust associations between punishment and rejection by the parent and heightened aggression in the offspring. Differences in parent–child closeness, parental monitoring, and parental support for aggressive behavior have also been consistently found between violent and nonviolent youth.

Fourth, the influence of social networks and deviant peer groups beyond the family was originally emphasized by sociological accounts of delinquent behavior (Cohen, 1955; Thrasher, 1928). Social control theory (Hirschi, 1969) has emphasized the relationship between individuals and social institutions. In the case of adolescents, the most important institution is the school. Social disorganization theory (Shaw & McKay, 1942) focused attention on structural aspects of communities, such as residential mobility, economic status of families, and ethnic composition. These factors served as markers of disorganization and, in turn, as the predictors of fluctuation in rates of antisocial behavior. As we observe below, the role of microsocial and macrosocial influences have been shown to be powerful in the instigation and control of violent adolescent behavior.

Fifth, cognitive-developmental mechanisms have also been implicated in violent behavior in adolescence. Aggressive, violent adolescents show a variety of cognitive differences, as assessed by neuropsychological tests in comparisons to matched-control, nonaggressive adolescents (Moffitt, 1990). Such shortcomings are consistent with the repeatedly found scholastic failure of aggressive youth, and, potentially, misattribution of the actions of others.

In sum, individual dispositions, familial contributions, and peer social influences on adolescent violence coalesce in development with the values and structure of the society. None of these influences can be ignored in the consideration of health promotion efforts. The larger issue is not whether social behavior is multidetermined; it is how the influences that have been identified can be modified or enhanced to promote adolescent health.

Developmental Views of Violence

Although violence in the United States is concentrated among persons in the second decade of life, developmental considerations hold that it would be folly to divorce the behaviors of adolescence from the events that precede and follow it. Moreover, maturational, experiential, and social forces on adolescence are fused in the course of development (Kuo, 1967; Mason, 1979; Schneirla, 1966). The contributions of separate variables are subsumed by configurations. Understanding these patterns is likely to make the dual tasks of violence control and nonviolence promotion especially challenging.

CHILDHOOD ANTECEDENTS. Borrowing a distinction from developmental psychobiology, we propose that the foundations for violence are organized in childhood and activated in adolescence. The organizational–activational distinction points to the importance of the timing of interventions, and underscores the need to understand both the events that contribute to the consolidation of behavior and the events that trigger its manifestation. But it is important to note that *violence* and *nonviolence* refer to classes of actions, not to single behaviors. For example, the skills required to hit, attack, fight, and injure another person refer to distinct action patterns. Each action pattern and its substrate must be established at some point in development. So must attitudes toward violence as a method for gaining dominance or control. On this score, different aspects of the behaviors classified as violent have a different time course of development. With age, the frequency of aggressive acts tends to diminish, while the intensity and severity of a given aggressive act increase.

The organizational–activational distinction may prove useful in countering the behavioral and emotional events in childhood that are antecedent to adolescent violence. Consider, for example, that interpersonal hostility and the norms for violence are organized in childhood, then activated in adolescence. Hence changes introduced in childhood that diminish the organization of personal hostility or heighten the sanctions for aggressive expression could diminish adolescent violence. Specific prevention programs for the organizational phase include such steps as interventions with dysfunctional or abusive families; establishment of mentoring programs for preadolescents; and rehabilitation of disadvantaged communities through the establishment of schools, jobs, and community services.

Changes may also be introduced at adolescence that directly address activational events. These include working directly with gangs and gang members to achieve a truce or safe areas, establishing more effective handgun control laws, creating a National Service or other alternative job-training and educational programs for at-risk youth, and teaching young men how to communicate peacefully with each other and with women. Initiating change is but the first step. The second step involves maintaining the change. In this regard, the skills required for initiating behavior change are usually different from those required for maintaining it.

DEVELOPMENTAL CONSTRAINTS. Youth violence typically occurs in a pattern of other deviant behaviors, not as a separate characteristic that may be divorced from other problems of adaptation. Consider, for example, the correlated developmental pattern of aggression, school failure, and deviant peer associations. When these factors operate together throughout childhood, violence is more likely to emerge in adolescence. The teenage constellation is likely to include school failure, delinquency, violence, inability to get or hold a job, and rejection even by one's own family.

Benign interventions, whether in the form of special classes or special assistance, may succeed as long as they are active. But if and when they are withdrawn, the multiple factors that combined to bring about this behavior are likely to reinstate the earlier developmental trajectory. Moreover, new constraints emerge in midadolescence when educational, economic, and social options become further closed. Failure in school and difficulties in the community effectively preclude alternative escape routes (rejection for advanced training in school, rejection in employment, rejection by the military). Individuals who need conventional training the most are least likely to qualify for even rudimentary entry positions. And if they are permitted to join, they most likely to fail. The unhappy cycle of failure that begins in childhood accelerates in adolescence (Selman, 1980).

A special issue raised by deviant patterns concerns the interrelations between internal dispositions, on the one hand, and external social, community, and relational factors, on the other. How are internal and external conditions aligned in development? In general, it appears that biological factors tend to bias social affiliations, as well as vice versa. The matching of temperamental biases and aggressive behaviors has been observed in friendship selection in childhood and assortative mating in adolescence (Cairns, Cairns, Neckerman, Gest, & Gariepy, 1988).

Other developmental forces that promote violence involve alignments of social and cultural forces outside the self. In this regard, it has been repeatedly shown that, in childhood and adolescence, highly aggressive males and females tend to affiliate in groups and gangs with other persons who are themselves highly aggressive. Are these behavioral similarities due to selective affiliation of the individuals who join the gang, selection by the gang, or behavioral commonalities that arise during gang involvement? While the data on this issue are not conclusive, they suggest that all three processes typically operate in adolescent groups (Jessor & Jessor, 1977; Kandel, 1978; Magnusson, 1988; Rodgers, Billy, & Udry, 1984).

The correlated nature of developmental forces and external conditions presents a formidable problem for violence prevention. How can the violence be prevented, given the multiple supports for the behavior in some youth? And how can it be changed, once activated in adolescence? In this regard, the finding that *some* persons have "criminal careers" is perhaps not as surprising as the finding that *most* adolescents have their delinquency confined to the teen years (Blumstein, Cohen, Roth, & Visher, 1986). The identification of those adolescents whose antisocial behavior diffuses into adult lifestyles is essential in efforts to reduce violence because they account for a disproportionately large burden of all criminal activity, including violence (Wolfgang, Thornberry, & Figlio, 1987).

What then permits the transitional shift from antisocial behavior? One clue to this process is that considerable social fluidity occurs throughout development in peer affiliations. At every stage, individuals enter new affiliations and become changed by them. Since changes toward nonviolence are promoted by the individual's involvement in conventional institutions, including the military, marriage, and employment (Elder, Caspi, & Burton, 1988; Sampson & Laub, 1990), violence-prone individuals who do not have these options are less likely to desist.

Obstacles to Promoting Nonviolence

American society offers special challenges and obstacles to promoting nonviolence. Our culture has a long history of being fascinated with violence and its marketability. The frequent and dramatic portrayal of violence in newspapers and film, the graphic displays of competition and sport, and the widespread availability and use of alcohol, illicit drugs, and guns cut deeply into our passions. Indeed, an ordinary evening's entertainment in an American home could make one believe that violence is an integral part of the culture and the human condition, regardless of one's class status, rich or poor. A visit to many of the major cities in the United States reveals that neighborhoods that have deteriorated, economically, physically, and socially, are especially vulnerable to interpersonal violence. In this section, such factors that inhibit the promotion of nonviolence in adolescence are briefly reviewed.

Firearm Availability

Most human societies have experimented with the design of weapons with the objective of achieving military superiority. In the modern era, the United States has been a world leader in this respect. But the introduction of the handgun by Samuel Colt in the 1840s suddenly made domestic, interpersonal violence more lethal than it had been before. It is an experience from which American society has still not recovered. This easily concealed weapon provided an instrument that combined the elements of speed, surprise, and finality to the settlement of disputes. The historical account of sharply rising homicide rates in Philadelphia during the middle and latter parts of the nineteenth century was no doubt repeated in other cities as well (Lane, 1979). A century and a half later, the lethality of the handgun is giving way to the more sophisticated technology of automatic assault weapons. Although evidence exists that firearms play a prominent role in producing the comparatively high rates of homicide and nonfatal intentional injuries in the United States, efforts to control their use and limit their production have been modest (Mercy & Houk, 1988).

The information on gun availability and ownership by adolescents in the United States is startling. In one recent investigation, 85% of the adolescent males in a sample representative of a statewide population had immediate access to firearms (Sadowski, Cairns, & Earp, 1989). Moreover, 49% of these teenage males indicated that they owned a gun. The firearms owned by these adolescents ranged from rifles to handguns, including automatic and semiautomatic weapons in some cases. In the majority of instances, the guns were gifts from male relatives, usually the father, grandfather, uncle, or older brother. The median age of first-gun ownership was 12.5 years of age, and there were no reliable differences in this sample in gun ownership between older and young adolescents. Few of the girls in the same sample owned firearms (4%). The failure to find socioeconomic differences in gun ownership is an indication of the pervasiveness of the acceptance of the norm of firearm ownership among adolescent males in this sample.

Access to firearms by adolescents is not always or even typically illegal. Laws that pertain to gun ownership vary markedly across the nation. The primary laws concern the sale and transfer of ownership of guns and ammunition as opposed to their possession and use. In this regard, the Bureau of Alcohol, Tobacco, and Firearms stipulates that retail dealers cannot sell handguns to persons who are less than 21 years of age, and they cannot sell rifles or shotguns to persons who are less than 18 years of age. But there are significant loopholes in the laws concerning the transfer of ownership or making the firearms available to persons who are younger than the age limits stipulated in the law. Gifts of guns, for example, are illegal in North Carolina for children only if they are under 12 years of age.

It must be concluded, then, that our society does not prohibit ready access to weapons of destruction even to persons who, by virtue of their age, may be little qualified for such ownership. To the extent that patterns of availability, interest, and ownership have been studied, the primary constraints appear to be those of social tradition and acceptance, with girls being less likely to become involved with firearms than boys. The patterns of homicide and serious injury that have been observed in the United States appear to parallel the availability and use of firearms. In those regions and settings where firearm ownership is highest, the rates of injury and death by guns are the greatest (Wright, Rossi, & Daly, 1983). What has been less often investigated are the dynamic relationships between gun availability and the escalation of conflicts to serious assault (Cook, 1983). Hence one way to reduce violent entrapment (or, more accurately, the occurrence of serious injury as a consequence of entrapment) would be the adoption of more stringent regulations on weapons availability, accompanied by a shift in societal values about the seriousness of firearm ownership and use, particularly among adolescents.

Alcohol, Drugs, and Violence

That a strong association exists between assaultive behavior and substance abuse cannot be gainsaid. Aggressive teenagers in a national sample were likely to be heavy alcohol and illicit drug users (Elliott, Huizinga, and Ageton, 1985; Elliott, Huizinga, & Menard, 1989), and the same has been observed in samples of urban youths (Earls & Powell, 1989). The longitudinal study of highly aggressive children in adolescence and adulthood reveals a configuration of sequelae, including alcoholism (Anderson, Bergman, & Magnusson, 1989; Magnusson, 1988) and mortality (Cairns & Cairns, in press). It remains to be shown how the involvement in the illicit drug industry by adolescents has contributed to the national rise in teenage homicide rates over the past 5 years. In a recent study of the association between crack cocaine and homicide, it was found that 26% of the homicides that occurred in New York City in 1988 resulted from territorial disputes between rival crack dealers (Goldstein, Brownstein, Ryan, & Belluci, 1988). The recent popularity of crack, an unstable distribution system, and the easy accessibility to firearms combine to produce a lethal climate.

Urban Blight

The significance of achievement in nearly every aspect of American life also produces a social context that is favorable to competition and conflict. Competitiveness sustains a meritocracy that supports a wide socioeconomic gradient within the American population. One consequence of this system is that harsh degrees of poverty are produced and sustained. In the last two decades the entrenchment of very poor, largely African-American and Hispanic groups in central city areas has produced an underclass who appear to be locked into a persistent pattern of disadvantage and despair (Wilson, 1987).

Chronically poor families appear to be part of a spiraling process in which the deterioration of housing leads to a loss of human and economic resources within central urban areas. That the material and social disorganization of such neighborhoods can have pervasive negative effects on health and behavior has been carefully documented for parts of New York City (Wallace, 1990; see also Chapter 3). In New York, it appears that a governmental policy to withdraw municipal services accelerates the deterioration of housing in certain areas. The degree of this decline as measured across many neighborhoods is associated with a plethora of social pathologies and adverse health outcomes, including low birth weight, dropping out of school, substance abuse, interpersonal violence, and, most recently, AIDS. Although it is difficult to disaggregate the multiple effects of such disorganization, good evidence exists to show that a critical feature of such environments explaining the level of crime and violence is the lack of adult supervision and monitoring of youths (Chapter 5; Sampson & Groves, 1989). Thus, it is not simply poverty, but community deterioration and the systematic withdrawal of services and resources, that appear to be specifically linked to violent behavior.

Three questions of special importance for this chapter may be raised with regard to this contemporary state of urban environments: (1) Are the number of families and individuals who are locked into poor, blighted neighborhoods growing, and are these effects being transmitted to the next generation? Current estimates place the size of the underclass at approximately 3 million, with a wide margin of imprecision (Mincy, Sawhill, & Wolf, 1990; Chapter 3). (2) Is this process reversible at either the community or the individual level (i.e., are there routes of escape and, alternatively, what are the attractions)? (3) What are the actual mediational links between community deterioration and the occurrence of violence? That is, do poverty and community blight contribute to the occurrence of violence, or does violence trigger and accelerate urban meltdown? Or, are the individual behaviors inextricably linked to community status? The answers to these questions will be of great importance in evaluating which social policies are likely to be effective in reducing violence and which are likely to fail. There is at least one farsighted research agenda on the horizon to address these issues (Tonry et al., 1990)

American Values

Violence is not particularly disdained in America. In some contexts and circumstances, it is even admired and promoted. Graphic depictions of gunshot wounds, murders, and the killing of animals have become common in motion pictures, even those recommended for children. Beyond drama, violence in professional sports has become increasingly expected, including noncontact games such as basketball. Activities that ordinarily would be deemed assaultive and violent elsewhere become "part of the game" when executed on the playing field or stage. For some children and youth, the boundary between games and real life has become blurred.

The society is at risk of placing a value on competitiveness at any cost. This cultural context is a formidable barrier to the promotion of nonviolence. Indeed, radical efforts may be required to shift American cultural norms toward greater restriction of firearms and less tolerance of violence. Unfortunately, there is still a great deal of misunderstanding on how to achieve these goals. Certain solutions that have been offered may be ineffective or may even have a reverse outcome. Will, for example, less violence in the society lead to less competition or lower achievement aspirations? The preliminary evidence from cross-national comparisons suggests that these characteristics in the society are not closely linked. For a closer look at these issues, we turn now to the development of violence and nonviolence and how they may be controlled (or promoted) in adolescents.

Implications for the Promotion of Nonviolence

The obstacles of easy availability of and access to guns, widespread use of alcohol and drugs, the decay of central city areas, and high cultural tolerance for violence cannot be minimized in any campaign to promote nonviolence among today's youth. In the face of these barriers, efforts in health promotion to decrease violent encounters may be equivalent to trying to control an epidemic of tuberculosis in a densely populated area without adequate sanitation. Antibiotics may be of some value in treating individual cases, and a vaccine would be of even greater value in protecting some groups of individuals, but the environmental conditions that promote the disease would simply overwhelm public resources in combatting it through these means alone. For contemporary America, there are reasons to think in such terms in addressing the problems of controlling interpersonal violence. What we need to promote nonviolence as a health objective is something analogous to what was needed to control infectious diseases toward the end of the last century: vast environmental and policy changes. It is worthwhile to note that improved sanitation was responsible for reducing the prevalence of infectious diseases several decades before antibiotics and vaccines for specific diseases were available (McKeown, 1979). What, we might ask, would the analogous conditions be for controlling violence?

A developmental perspective is useful in pointing to changes that are likely to be most effective. It might be assumed that aggressive and violent behaviors are more readily prevented than they are ameliorated, once established. But the conditions for establishment appear not only in early development but also in middle childhood and adolescence. Moreover, effective prevention demands attention to the several levels of influence—individual, interactional, familial, peer group, and community-cultural. Efforts at control and prevention cannot be limited to a single time frame of development—either in infancy, preschool, middle childhood, or early adolescence. Waiting until the problems of violence emerge full-blown in adolescence may be too late for intervention. From a developmental viewpoint, it is necessary to examine the mechanisms that operate in the different stages of growth from infancy to maturity. Such an examination permits us to draw up a plan for the promotion of nonviolence from infancy to adolescence that extends over the life course and into the next generation.

Prenatal and Early Childhood

In promoting nonviolence, tasks to be accomplished during the early organizational phase of development are straightforward, though accomplishing them requires supportive public policy and political will. These tasks include (1) providing good health care to the mother and child, (2) increasing parental competence in child rearing, (3) minimizing violence within the family and in early social interchanges, and (4) stimulating the development of cooperation and nonconfrontational skills in language and social relations. Obviously, this requires the coordinated activities of parents, health care providers, public health authorities, child care personnel or caregivers, educators, and social workers. To be sure, this broad set of social objectives is related to the promotion of nonviolence only in the most general way. For example, one wants academically skilled children for their own sake. Early school failures and associated problem behaviors can have devastating effects on the subsequent development of children, whether boys or girls. Although females are less likely than males to demonstrate these patterns in early development, when they occur they appear to be as predictive of future difficulties in women as in men (Cairns & Cairns, in press; Robins, 1986).

It has now been well established that intensive educational training and home interventions with infants at high risk for educational failure can result in significant boosts in intelligence (Infant Health and Development Program, 1990). Similarly, evidence from such experiments as the Perry Preschool Program (Berreuta-Clement, Schweinhart, Barnett, & Weikart, 1987) suggests that there may be cumulative benefits to early academic interventions throughout the later phases of child and adolescent development.

Additionally, interventions in the family that diminish coercion tend to alter the likelihood of continued childhood aggression and problems in the home (Patterson, 1986). In this regard, the failure to inhibit or otherwise control blatant attacks of one child on others of the same age or younger is associated with the occurrence of more attacks (Parke & Slaby, 1983). In early childhood, as in adolescence, aggressive acts are reciprocal and escalatory (Holmberg, 1980). Techniques of redirection and nonresponse are effective in reducing the likelihood of further escalation in peer interactions. But when adults fail to intervene in an escalatory sequence, the development of techniques of physical coercion and aggressive control is facilitated. Such early experiences seem to provide important, though not sufficient, conditions for diminishing the likelihood of early failure and the stepping-stone process toward adolescent delinquency and violence (Farrington, 1986) (McGuire and Earls, 1991). More generally, societal investment in the promotion of nonviolence in very young children for later stages in their lives may be expected to have immediate effects on the promotion of nonviolence in their parents, who may themselves be at risk (Earls and Carlson, 1992). Health efforts focused on the infancy period could be a clever way of directly reaching parents and immediately diminishing abuse toward children and others.

Childhood

The links between childhood aggression and adolescent violence have now been studied in some detail. For children, a straight line may be drawn from extreme aggressiveness in late childhood to violence in adolescence (e.g., Stattin & Magnusson, 1989). There are, however, relatively few adolescents for whom problems of violence arise de novo without strong precursors in middle childhood. Direct observations of naturally occurring disputes of childhood indicate that the most common response to provocation is selective nonresponse. This nonaggressive response is observed in virtually all children, including those who have been identified as violent and assaultive (Cairns & Cairns, in press). The problem appears to be that some children also have a low threshold for violent as well as nonviolent reactions.

The childhood constellation of risk factors for violence includes (1) the child's personality predispositions and confrontational behavior patterns, (2) family influences, (3) peer social influences, (4) school adjustment, and (5) neighborhood and community contexts. In addition, social influences (peer, school, and neighborhood-community) act directly upon the child rather than indirectly through the family. As in the preceding stage, such influences are typically not independent. Consider, for example, the role of deviant peer social influences. It has now been established that children tend to affiliate with others who are like themselves with respect to aggressive and acting-out behaviors (Giardano, Cernkovich & Pugh, 1986; Hawkins, Jenson, Catalano, & Lishner, 1988). In schools, ex*.eme acting-out behaviors tend to be associated with poor school performance and low expectations for the child by teachers. Such social clusters of children can become, under some circumstances, dominant gangs in the classroom and school, as well as a problem to teachers, administrators, and parents (Olweus, 1990). In middle childhood, such bully gangs are usually composed of boys, although there is also some tendency for aggressive girls at this age in U. S. schools to form social clusters (Cairns et al., 1988).

There are different perspectives on the nature of relations between family influence, peer rejection, and aggressive behavior. According to one general proposition, disrupted families lead to social-cognitive information processing deficiencies in the child and a lack of social skills that precede peer rejection, and, as a consequence, aggressive actions and further rejection when the child enters school (Dodge, 1986). This *deficit model* thus explains the aggression/violence as being due to the absence of social skills and social information processing ability.

Attention has also been given to events that are present in the aggressive child's environment, rather than to those that are absent. There is often both direct and indirect support for the adoption of aggressive strategies. The family, peer group, social network, and microcommunity may in fact support confrontational, aggressive behaviors as one possible response to a range of settings where aggression by children is justified. This interpretation implies that the task of changing behavior is broader than merely teaching new, nonaggressive strategies. Attempts to intervene with childhood violence have ranged from individually based interventions for conduct disorder to school-based skills development programs. Evaluations of conduct disorders have been equivocal but are most likely to be successful when they use strategies that are focal and behavior based (Kazdin, 1987). School-based intervention in Norway indicates that programs that jointly promote alternative, nonviolent strategies and social sanctions against bullying have had an impact on childhood and adolescent aggression (Olweus, 1990). By pairing new behavior options with community standards, adults effected a change in the youths' activities. Similarly, it should be expected that cooperative learning programs in schools will help foster a sense of cooperation rather than competition.

For a violence prevention program to be effective, a focus on children must be accompanied by a focus on the entire social system in which the children are embedded. Differences in tolerance of aggressive patterns are expressed at several levels, from the family to peer groups and school personnel to the wider society (such as that expressed on national TV). Hence preventive efforts must operate at several levels in childhood in order to be effective.

Adolescence

The study of the development of nonviolence—including cooperation and altruism—is less advanced than the study of violence (Zahn-Waxler, Cummings, & Ianotti, 1986). Nonviolent strategies defy simple classification or developmental description. There are simply more ways to cooperate or be nonviolent than there are ways to be violent.

Nonviolent techniques, including the tactics of ignoring or nonresponse, which are most difficult to sustain in the short term, appear to be highly effective in long-term development. But it should also be noted that the act of nonresponse does not typically occur in isolation. It is usually coupled with behaviors that promote cooperation and diminish frustration and anger. More generally, noncoercive families are characterized not merely by what is missing but also by what is present. Similarly, successful nonviolent youth usually employ strategies that help them detect and avoid violent situations. In this regard, the teaching of nonviolent techniques presupposes the mastering of skills for violence prevention.

In the developmental framework adopted in this chapter, adolescence is considered the activational stage for violence. As in earlier stages, family relationships, peer groups, and community values and organization are woven together in the control of behavior. The difference is that the intensity of the aggressive actions can escalate to assaults, brutality, injury, and death. This is the period, moreover, when peer influences take on strategic importance. By virtue of participation in gang activities, individual members and the gang as a whole become at risk for violence. And when there is access to firearms, gang activities are virtually guaranteed to escalate to violence, including homicide.

Youth gangs may themselves be viewed in a broader framework of social relationships (Thrasher, 1928). Adolescents in general tend to sort themselves into groups that have salient characteristics in common. Acting out and violent behaviors are among the most important. Natural social clusters are also formed around illicit drug usage (Hamburg, Braemer, & Jahnke, 1975; Kandel, 1978; Zank, 1988); and delinquency (Elliott et al., 1989). Females as well as males form groups (Campbell, 1981; Giardano et al., 1986), and gangs are established when groups are formed with only modest external supervision and when violence is permitted to be the primary means of control.

There have been some innovative efforts to intervene with violence at the level of gang activity. The Community Youth Gang Services (CYGS) program in Los Angeles works directly with gang members to settle disputes by nonviolent means.[1] The strategies include agreements on "neutral" territories that are safe to all persons and the establishment of periods of peace. Beyond this implied recognition of gangs as semipolitical units of governance, efforts are made to intervene at the community level to increase school participation and open jobs for at-risk youth. Contacts are made with parents, and attempts are made to increase their involvement in the guidance and supervision of their children. The program is envisioned to work at multiple levels—in the family, at the school, in employment, in the community, and with the gangs themselves.

Evaluations of the CYGS program have been limited but encouraging. In the areas of Los Angeles where the program has been employed (precincts with the highest homicide rates), gang-related homicide rates have sharply diminished. Moreover, the homicide rate was controlled only while the intervention was in place. When the program was shifted to another area of the city, homicides in the targeted areas shot back up beyond the preintervention level.[2] Such an outcome might be expected if the apparent resolution of the gang wars was based upon the immediate peacekeeping activities of the program staff.

While these results are encouraging, not all programs have been successful and intervention remains at an early stage of development. Recent reviews of violence prevention programs (Northrup et al., 1990; Wilson-Brewer, Cohen, O'Donnell, & Goodman, 1990) raise concerns about the paucity of quality evaluation data as well as the lack of attention to issues of maintaining intervention successes over time.

The findings of these reviews should eventually be compared to prevention efforts in the areas of school dropping out, substance abuse, teenage pregnancy, and rape prevention. There has been more progress in these areas, and cross-fertilization of strategies used in such programs with those currently being developed in the area of violence prevention may be beneficial for several reasons. It is important to compare comprehensive, broad-based strategies with more focused efforts. Some evidence exists to show that generic skills training approaches that combine several features are superior to more focused effects that target a single strategy. Such strategies as affect control, peer resistance, stress reduction, or problem solving in reducing the prevalence of substance use in adolescents are better approached as configurations, not as single units (Botvin, Baker, Botvin, Filazzola, & Millman, 1984; Schinke & Gilchrist, 1984). If this is generally the case in preventing undesirable behaviors in adolescents, it would imply that programs designed to promote nonviolence through conflict resolution tactics must be embedded in more comprehensive programs that teach a wider variety of life skills. The comparison of programs can be of benefit in other ways as well. For example, all such programs have similar problems in recruitment and retention of high-risk individuals, in training personnel, and in devising methods to evaluate important outcomes.

Conclusions

Statistics have fueled interest in raising the priority of interpersonal violence on the public health agenda (Mercy & O'Carroll, 1988). Several areas are directly involved in this mission. Efforts to improve community surveillance and the accuracy of reporting fatal and nonfatal injuries due to violent behavior have increased. Government has participated as explicit objectives to reduce the toll of intentional injury due to interpersonal violence over the next decade have been formulated by the Public Health Service (U. S. Public Health Service, 1990). But true health promotion in the area of nonviolence will require coordination of activities at three levels

First, structural obstacles, such as easy availability of firearms and the deteriorating infrastructure of disadvantaged urban communities, must be overcome through policy development. This is a mission that requires the combined endeavors of several agents of society guided by the public health, criminal justice, and social service sectors.

Second, early childhood programs that foster healthy behavioral development and intellectual competence and provide parent training and family support should be expanded. It is in this area that real scientific progress is currently being made.

Finally, school-based and community-based programs to reduce the acceptability of violence and to promote nonviolent lifestyles for adolescents must be refined in content and carefully evaluated. The evidence points to an immediate need to limit access of adolescents to firearms of all sorts and to foster attitudes that would make the use of such weapons cowardly or otherwise unacceptable. These latter two areas are ones in which scientific engagement is promptly needed. For the next decade, this agenda will be one of the most demanding in health promotion (Tonry, Ohlin, & Farrington, 1990).

Notes

1. See Northrup, Jacklin, Cohen, and Wison-Brewer (1990, pp. 8–9) for a description of this program and other community intervention strategies.
2. Steve D. Valdivia, Executive Director of CYGS, also reported these findings to the "Forum on Youth Violence in Minority Communities: Setting the Agenda for Prevention," December 10–12, 1990, Atlanta.

References

Anderson, T., Bergman, L. R., & Magnusson, D. (1989). Patterns of adjustment problems and alcohol abuse in early adulthood: A prospective longitudinal study. *Development and Psychopathology, 1,* 119–131.

Bandura, A., & Walters, R. H. (1963). *Social learning and personality development.* New York: Holt, Rinehart & Winston.

Berreuta-Clement, J. R., Schweinhart, L. P., Barnett, W. S., & Weikart, D. P. (1987). The effects of early educational intervention on crime and delinquency in adolescence and early adulthood. In J. D. Burchard & S. N. Burchard (Eds.), *Prevention of delinquent behavior* (pp. 220–240). Newbury Park, CA: Sage Publishers.

Blumenstein, A., Cohen, J., Roth, A., & Visher, C. A. (1986). *Criminal* careers and career criminals. Washington, DC: National Academy Press.

Botvin, G. J., Baker, E., Botvin, E. M., Filazzola, A., & Millman, R. (1984). Alcohol abuse prevention through the development of personal and social competence: A pilot study. *Journal of Studies on Alcohol, 45,* 550–552.

Bowlby, J. (1969). *Attachment and loss.* New York: Basic Books.

Cairns, R. B., & Cairns, B. D. (in press). *Adolescents in our time: Lifelines and risks.*

Cairns, R. B., Cairns, B. D., Neckerman, H. J., Gest, S., & Gariepy, J.-L. (1988). Social networks and aggressive behavior: Peer support or peer rejection? *Developmental Psychology, 24,* 815–823.

Cairns, R. B., Gariepy, J.-L., & Hood, K. E. (1990). Development, microevolution, and social behavior. *Psychological Review, 97,* 49–65.

Campbell, A. (1981). *Girl delinquents.* New York: St. Martin's Press.

Carlson, M., Earls, F., & Todd, R. (1988). The importance of regressive changes in the development of the nervous system: Towards a neurobiological theory of child development. *Psychiatric Developments, 5,* 1–22.

Cohen, A. K. (1955). *Delinquent boys: The culture of gangs.* Glencoe, IL: Free Press.

Cook, P. J. (1983). The influence of gun availability on violent crime patterns. In M. Tonry & N. Morris (Eds.), *Crime and justice: An annual review of research, Volume 4* (pp. 49–89). Chicago: University of Chicago Press.

Dodge, K. A. (1986). Social information-processing variables in the development of aggression and altruism in children. In C. Zahn-Waxler, E. M. Cummings, and R. Iannotti (Eds.), *Altruism and aggression: Biological and social origins* (pp. 280–302). Cambridge: Cambridge University Press.

Dollard, J., Doob, L. W., Miller, N. E., Mowrer, O. H., & Sears, R. R. (1939). *Frustration and aggression.* New Haven, CT: Yale University Press.

Earls, F. (1991). A developmental approach to understanding and controlling violence. In H. E. Fitzgerald, B. M. Lester, & M. W. Yogman (Eds.), *Theory and research in behavioral pediatrics, Volume 5* (pp. 61–85. New York: Plenum Press.

Earls, F., & Powell, J. (1989). Patterns of substance use and abuse. *Yale Journal of Biology and Medicine, 61,* 233–242.

Earls, F., & Carlson, M. (in press). Towards the sustainability of the American family. *Daedalus.*

Elder, G. H., Jr., Caspi, A., & Burton, L. M. (1988). Adolescent transitions in developmental perspective: Sociological and historical insights. In M. Gunnar (Ed.), *Minnesota symposia on child psychology, Volume 21* (pp. 151–179). Hillsdale, NJ: Erlbaum.

Elliott, D. S., Huizinga, D., & Ageton, S. S. (1985). *Explaining delinquency and drug use.* Beverly Hills, CA: Sage.

Elliott, D. S., Huizinga, D., & Menard, S. (1989). *Multiple problem youth: Delinquency, substance use, and mental health problems.* New York: Springer-Verlag.

Farrington, D. P. (1986). Stepping stones to adult criminal careers. In D. Olweus, J. Block, & M. Radke-Yarrow (Eds.), *Development of antisocial and prosocial behavior: Research, theories, and issues* (pp. 359–384). New York: Academic Press.

Federal Bureau of Investigation (1987). *Uniform crime reports, 1987.* Washington, DC: U. S. Department of Justice.

Fingerhut, L. A., & Kleinman, J. C. (1990). International and interstate comparisons of homicide among young males. *Journal of the American Medical Association, 263,* 3292–3295.

Giardano, P. C., Cernkovich, S. A., & Pugh, M. D. (1986). Friendship and delinquency. *American Journal of Sociology, 91,* 1170–1201.

Goldstein, P. J., Brownstein, H. H., Ryan, P. J., & Belluci, P. A. (1988). Crack and homicide in New York City, 1988: A conceptually based event analysis. *Contemporary Drug Problems, 15,* 65–68.

Hamburg, B. A., Braemer, H. C., & Jahnke, W. A. (1975). Hierarchy of drug use in adolescence: Behavioral and attitudinal correlates of substantial drug use. *American Journal of Psychiatry, 132,* 1155–1167.

Hawkins, J. D., Jenson, J. M., Catalano, R. F., & Lishner, D. M. (1988). Delinquency and drug abuse: Implications for social services. *Social Science Review, 8,* 258–284.

Hirschi, T. (1969). *Causes of delinquency.* Berkeley: University of California Press.

Holmberg, M. C. (1980). The development of social interchange patterns from 12 to 42 months. *Child Development, 51,* 448–456.

Infant Health and Development Program (1990). Enhancing the outcomes of low-birth-weight, premature infants: A multisite, randomized trial. *Journal of the American Medical Association, 263,* 3035–3042.

Jessor, R., & Jessor, S. L. (1977). *Problem behavior and psychosocial development: A longitudinal study of youth.* New York: Academic Press.

Kandel, D. B. (1978). Homophily, selection, and socialization in adolescent friendships. *American Journal of Sociology, 84,* 427–436.

Kazdin, A. E. (1987). Treatment of antisocial behavior in children: Current status and future directions. *Psychological Bulletin, 102,* 187–203.

Kuo, Z.-Y. (1967). *The dynamics of behavioral development: An epigenetic view.* New York: Random House.

Lane, R. (1979). *Violent death in the city: Suicide, accidents and murder in nineteenth Philadelphia.* Cambridge, MA: Harvard University Press.

Lewis, M. H., Devaud, L. L., Gariepy, J. L., Southerland, S. B., Mailman, R. B., & Cairns, R. B. (in press). Dopamine and social behavior in mice bred for high and low levels of aggression. *Brain Research Bulletin.*

Linnoila, M., Virrkunnen, M., Schein, M., Nuntila, A., Rimon, R., & Goodwin, F. K. (1983). Low cerebrospinal fluid 5-hydroxyindoacetic acid concentration differentiates impulsive from non-impulsive violent behavior. *Life Sciences, 33,* 2609–2614.

Magnusson, D. (1988). *Individual development from an interactional perspective: A longitudinal study.* Hillsdale, NJ: Erlbaum.

Mason, W. A. (1979). Ontogeny of social behavior. In P. Marler & J. G. Vandenbergh (Eds.), *Social behavior and communication* (pp. 1–28). New York: Plenum Press.

McGuire, M. T., & Raleigh, M. J. (1985). Serotonin–behavior interactions in vervet monkeys. *Psychopharmacology Bulletin, 21,* 458–463.

McGuire, J., & Earls, F. (1991). Prevention of psychiatric disorder in early childhood. *Journal of Child Psychology and Psychiatry, 32,* 129–153.

McKeown, T. (1979). *The role of medicine.* Princeton, NJ: Princeton University Press.

Mercy, J. A., & Houk, V. N. (1988). Firearm injuries: A call for science. *New England Journal of Medicine, 319,* 1283–1285.

Mercy, J. A., & O'Carroll, P. W. (1988). New directions in violence prediction: The public health arena. *Violence and Victims, 3,* 285–301.

Milgram, S. (1974) *Obedience to authority: An experimental view.* New York: Harper & Row.

Mincy, R. B., Sawhill, I. V., & Wolf, D. A. (1990). The underclass: Definition and measurement. *Science, 248,* 450–453.

Moffitt, T. (1990). The neuropsychology of delinquency: A critical review of theory and research. In N. Morris & M. Tonry (Eds), *Crime and justice: An annual review of research, Volume 12* (pp. 99–169). Chicago: University of Chicago Press.

National Center for Health Statistics (1988). *Health United States, 1987.* DHHS Publication No. (PHS) 88-1232). Hyattsville, MD: U. S. Department of Health, Education and Welfare.

Northrop, D., Jacklin, B., Cohen, S., & Wilson-Brewer, R. (1990). *Violence prevention strategies targeted toward high-risk minority youth.* Background paper prepared for the Forum on Youth Violence in Minority Communities: Setting the Agenda for Prevention, Atlanta, December 10–12.

Olweus, D. (1990). *A national campaign in Norway to reduce the prevalence of bullying behavior.* Paper presented to the Society for Research on Adolescence Biennial Meeting, Atlanta, March 223.

Parke, R. D., & Slaby, R. G. (1983). The development of aggression. In P. H. Mussen (Gen. Ed.) & M. Hetherington (Ed.), *Handbook of child psychology, Volume 4* (4th ed.) (pp. 547–642). New York: Wiley.

Patterson, G. R. (1982). *Coercive family systems.* Eugene, OR: Castalia.

Patterson, G. R. (1986). Performance models for antisocial boys. *American Psychologist, 41,* 432–444.

Robins, L. N. (1986). The consequences of conduct disorder in girls. In D. Olweus, J. Block, & M. Radke-Yarrow (Eds.), *Development of antisocial and prosocial behavior: Research, theories, and issues* (pp. 385–414). New York: Academic Press.

Rodgers, J. L., Billy, J. O. G., & Udry, J. R. (1984). A model of friendship similarity in mildly deviant behaviors. *Journal of Applied Social Psychology, 14,* 413–425.

Sadowski, L. S., Cairns, R. B., & Earp, J. A. (1989) Firearm ownership among nonurban adolescents. *American Journal of Diseases of Children, 143,* 1410–1413.

Sameroff, A. J. (1983). Developmental systems: Contexts and evolution. In P. H. Mussen (Gen. Ed.) and W. Kessen (Vol. Ed.), *Handbook of child psychology, Volume 1: History, theory and methods* (pp. 237–294). New York: Wiley.

Sampson, R. J., & Groves, W. B. (1989). Community structure and crime: Testing social disorganization theory. *American Journal of Sociology, 94,* 774–802.

Sampson, R. J., & Laub, J. H. (1990). Crime and deviance over the life course: The salience of adult social bonds. *American Sociological Review. 55,* 609–627.

Scarr, S., & McCartney, K. (1983). How people make their own environments: A theory of genotype–environment effects. *Child Development, 54,* 426–423.

Schneirla, T. C. (1966). Behavioral development and comparative psychology. *Quarterly Review of Biology, 41,* 283–302.

Schinke, S. P., & Gilchrist, L. D., (1984). Preventing cigarette smoking with youth. *Journal of Primary Prevention, 5,* 48–56.

Sears, R. R., Maccoby, E. E., & Levin, H. (1957). *Patterns of child rearing.* New York: Row Peterson.

Selman, R. L. (1980). *The growth of interpersonal understanding: Developmental and clinical analyses.* New York: Academic Press.

Shaw, C. R., & McKay, H. D. (1942). *Juvenile delinquency and urban areas* (rev. ed.). Chicago: University of Chicago Press.

Stattin, H., & Magnusson, D. (1989). The role of early aggressive behavior in the frequency, seriousness, and types of later crime. *Journal of Consulting and Clinical Psychology, 57,* 710–718.

Statistical Abstracts of Sweden, 1990. Official statistics of Sweden, Volume 76. Stockholm: Statistics Sweden.

Thrasher, F. M. (1928). *The gang.* Chicago: University of Chicago Press.

Tonry, M., Ohlin, L., & Farrington, D. (1990). *Human development and criminal behavior: New ways of advancing knowledge.* New York: Springer-Verlag.

U. S. Public Health Service (1990). *Year 2000 Health Objectives.* Draft copy.

Wallace, R. (1990). Urban decertification, public health and public order: "Planned shrinkage," violent death, substance abuse, and AIDS in the Bronx. *Social Science and Medicine, 31,* 801–813.

Wilson, W. J. (1987). *The truly disadvantaged.* Chicago: University of Chicago Press.

Wilson-Brewer, R., Cohen, S., O'Donnell, L., & Goodman, I. F. (1990). *Violence prevention for early teens: The state of the art and guidelines for future program evaluation.* Newton, MA: Education Development Center.

Wolfgang, M. E., Thornberry, T. P., & Figlio, R. M. (1987). *From boy to man, from delinquency to crime.* Chicago: University of Chicago Press.

Wright, J. D., Rossi, P. H., & Daly, R. (1983). *Under the gun: Weapons, crime, and violence in America.* New York: Aldine de Gruyter.

Zahn-Waxler, C., Cummings, E. M., & Iannotti, R. (Eds.). (1986). *Altruism and aggression: Biological and social origins.* Cambridge: Cambridge University Press.

Zank, S. (1988). *Zur Entwicklung des Losungsmittelschnuffelns bei Jugendlichen und jungen Erwachsenen* [*On the development of solvent-sniffing by adolescents and young adults*]. Berlin: Berlin Verlag Arno Spitz.

14

Promoting Safety in Adolescents

Ralph Hingson and Jonathan Howland

In 1988 more than 96,000 Americans died as a result of unintentional injuries, the fourth leading cause of death in this country (National Safety Council, 1989). Injury disproportionately affects young people and is the greatest killer of persons between the ages of 1 and 37 (National Committee for Injury Prevention and Control, 1989) and the number one cause of loss of productive years prior to age 65. *Injury* refers to damage resulting from acute exposure to physical or chemical agents (Haddon & Baker, 1981). The term *accident* formerly signified "events leading to injuries," but research shows that these events form patterns; they are not random, as the term *accident* implies.

This chapter will focus on persons between the ages of 10 and 19. Injury death rates for adolescents are substantially higher in the United States than in other industrialized nations (U. S. Department of Health and Human Services, 1989; see Table 14.1). Among U. S. adolescents aged 10 to 14 and 15 to 19, injuries are responsible for 57% and 79%, respectively, of all deaths (Runyun & Gerken, 1989). Fatal injuries peak at age 21 and decline gradually in older age groups. For every injury to persons 13 to 19, there are an estimated 41 injury hospitalizations and 1,100 cases treated in emergency departments (Galleghar, Finson, & Guyer, 1984).

This chapter will explore factors associated with injury and interventions to reduce the leading causes of unintentional adolescent injury deaths: motor vehicle crashes, drowning, fires, and burns. Among adolescents between the ages of 10 and 19 in 1987, 8,061 died in motor vehicle crashes, 826 drowned, and 233 died of burns (National Safety Council, 1989). We will also explore major contributors to nonfatal adolescent injury.

Traffic Accidents

Over half of the unintentional injury deaths in the United States are the result of motor vehicle crashes. Every 10 minutes, another American is killed in a traffic crash (National Committee for Injury Prevention and Control, 1989). In 1990, among all age groups there were 44,529 fatalities in 39,779 fatal crashes (U. S. Department of Transportation, 1991). Traffic crashes are not only the greatest sin-

Table 14.1. Death Rates for Teenagers in Selected
Industrialized Nations, 1985

| | Ages 10 to 14 | | Ages 15 to 19 | |
	Male	Female	Male	Female
United States	18.4	7.8	64.1	23.6
Federal Republic of Germany	9.2	4.5	48.4	15.1
France	13.0	5.9	49.9	18.7
Netherlands	7.2	4.8	27.6	9.0
England and Wales	13.9	5.3	35.6	9.9
Sweden	7.0	4.1	35.0	9.9
Canada	16.6	8.3	55.7	21.1
Japan	6.0	2.1	42.5	7.1
Australia	13.1	5.0	67.1	21.3

Note: Death rates per 100,000.

Sources: U.S. Department of Health and Human Services, *Trend and current status in childhood mortalities, United States, 1900–1985* Analytic and Epidemiologic Studies, series *3*, No. *26*, Jan., 1989 Vital and Health Statistics

gle cause of death for every age group between 5 and 34; they further inflict disabling injuries on 1.8 million people each year (National Safety Council, 1989).

Adolescents account for a disproportionate share of the traffic deaths. Though 13- to 19-year-olds comprise only 10% of the U. S. population, 17% of drivers in fatal crashes and 18% of traffic deaths are in that age range. In 1990, more than 40% of the deaths among 13- to 19-year-olds resulted from motor vehicle crashes. Nationally in 1990, half of teenage traffic deaths occurred between 9 P.M. and 6 A.M. and 59% on weekends. Most (81%) were motor vehicle occupants. Eight percent were motorcyclists, 7% pedestrians, 3% bicyclists, and 2% operators of other types of vehicles. Sixty-nine percent of the teenage traffic deaths were males (Insurance Institute for Highway Safety, 1991).

Pedestrian Safety

Pedestrian and bicycle deaths also disproportionately involve adolescents. Nationally in 1990 224 10- to 14-year-olds and 328 15- to 19-year-olds were killed as pedestrians. Based on extrapolation of data from police-reported pedestrian injuries, Rivera (1990) estimates that there are 25,000 pedestrian injuries in the 10- to 19-year-old age group. These injuries result from behaviors of both pedestrians and drivers.

The most common pedestrian error is failure to use crosswalks and sidewalks. According to the U. S. Department of Transportation's Fatal Accident Reporting System (FARS, 1991), over 90% of pedestrian fatalities nationally involve pedestrians crossing streets outside of designated crosswalks. Less than 5% of teenage pedestrian deaths occur on sidewalks or in crosswalks.

Alcohol is also often a factor for both pedestrians and drivers. A police report of alcohol ingestion or a positive blood alcohol level was present among 20% of fatally injured adolescent pedestrians and 17% of drivers nationwide in 1990 (U. S. Department of Transportation, 1991). Because not all pedestrians or drivers are tested, the percentage may be even higher. Among fatally injured pedestrians 10 to 14 years old, 1% had been drinking, while 33% of 15- to 19-year-old pedestrians had been drinking (U. S. Department of Transportation, 1991).

Studies of educational efforts to reduce childhood and adolescent pedestrian deaths have produced inconsistent results, but separating pedestrians from the roadway with sidewalks and crosswalks, conversion of two-way streets to one-way streets to reduce confusion, and motor vehicle design changes all show promise in reducing pedestrian injury (Rivera, 1990).

Bicycle Safety

In 1990 nationwide, 261 bicyclists aged 10 to 19 were fatally injured (U. S. Department of Transportation, 1991). As with pedestrian safety, errors by both bicyclists and drivers contributed to these deaths. While FARS does not record bicyclists' driving errors, among fatally injured bicyclists aged 15–19, 8% had been drinking. Motor vehicle driver violations were issued in 18% of bicycle deaths for teenagers aged 10 to 14 and in 23% of the bicycle deaths for cyclists aged 15 to 19. While only 11% of drivers involved in fatal collisions with bicyclists aged 10 to 14 had been drinking, 19% of drivers in crashes with 16- to 19-year-olds had been drinking.

While considerable attention has recently been devoted to promotion of bicycle helmet use (Bergman, Rivera, Richards, & Roger, 1990; Thompson, Rivera, & Thompson, 1989), instruction in bicycle safety could also help reduce this toll. Bicyclists who disobey traffic laws by not stopping at intersections, weaving through traffic, passing on the right, or failing to signal present motorists with unanticipated driving situations. Research is needed to identify not only the most common bicyclists' behaviors in fatal crashes, but also the most common motor vehicle operators errors, so that all concerned can be educated about these potentially dangerous situations.

Why Are Adolescents Overrepresented in Traffic Fatalities?

ALCOHOL AND DRUGS. Adolescents' driving performance can dip below required levels because of alcohol and drug use. Teenagers are not only the least experienced drivers, they are the least experienced drinkers. Though the adolescent population compared to the adult population has a higher proportion who abstain from alcohol, teenagers more often drink heavily on the occasions when they do drink. Hence, their driving performance can be acutely impaired by alcohol and drugs, particularly if they are fatigued by staying up late (Dement, 1992).

In 1989, an estimated half of all traffic fatalities and 45% of traffic fatalities in the 15 to 19 age group involved someone who was intoxicated, either a driver or a pedestrian (U. S. Department of Transportation, 1990). Epidemiological studies clearly and consistently indicate that impairment is present at a blood alcohol level of 0.05% and increases dramatically at 0.10% and higher (the legal limit of intoxication in most states; National Committee for Injury Prevention and Control, 1989). For younger drivers impairment begins at even lower levels (Agran, 1990; Waller, 1985).

LIFE STRESSES. The adolescent years also include many life stresses, as indicated by higher suicide rates in that age group than in middle age. Recent bereavement, involvement in matrimonial arguments, divorce, and separation, as well as other stressful life events, have been more often reported by adult drivers involved in crashes compared to those not in crashes (Borkenstein, Crowther, Shumoth, Zeil, & Zylman, 1964; Holt, 1981). A World Health Organization Advisory Committee (1980) indicated that individual personality factors such as excessive aggressiveness, overreaction to stimuli, and poor concentration, as well as social factors such as parental/marital discord, separation, substance abuse, serious illness, or parental neglect, may contribute to teenage crash involvement. Though not as well researched as impairment produced by alcohol, it is plausible that life stresses can also impair drivers' performance.

VEHICLE CONDITION. Adolescents often lack the financial resources to buy new automobiles with the latest safety technology. Lack of discretionary income may also make it more difficult for them to keep their vehicles in safe operating condition.

INEXPERIENCE. Because of their inexperience, adolescents may be less likely than older drivers to know how to respond to unexpected driving conditions like icy roads. Studies on driving simulators show that teenage drivers take longer to perceive and respond to dangerous situations (Quimby & Watts, 1981). Teenage drivers may be less likely to know the roads in a given area, particularly when they first start to drive. They may also be less familiar in gauging the distances needed to brake an automobile safely at various driving speeds or road angles, or to gauge the distances needed to pass vehicles.

WILLINGNESS TO TAKE RISKS WHILE DRIVING. Moreover, evidence is clear from a number of studies that adolescent drivers are more likely to engage in risky driving behaviors that greatly increase the difficulty of driving and the likelihood of crashes. A 1988 statewide Massachusetts survey compared 1,762 adolescents aged 16 to 19 (response rate 87%) to 2,385 adults aged 20 and older (response rate 73%; Hingson et al., 1991). Random digit dial sampling was used (Waksberg, 1978), and within each household one respondent in the targeted age group was selected using methods developed by Kish (1965). Adolescent drivers ($N = 1,455$) were significantly more likely than adult drivers ($N = 2,146$) to report that they speed, run red lights, make illegal turns, do not wear safety belts, drive after heavy drinking, drive after marijuana use, and ride with intoxicated drivers (Table 14.2). Not surprisingly, adolescents who reported engaging in these behaviors were more likely to

Table 14.2. The Massachusetts Adolescent (16–19) and Adult (20+) Traffic Survey, 1988.

	Adolescent $N = 1,762$	Adult $N = 2,260$
Past year		
Driver in a crash	25%	12%
Driver in a crash when someone was injured	6	2
Past month		
Drove after 5+ drinks	6	6
Drove after marijuana use	9	3
Rode with a driver who had 5+ drinks	16	8
Previous week		
Sped 20+ miles over the limit	44	29
Made an illegal turn	35	20
Ran a red light	10	3
Did not always wear a safety belt	88	62
Likelihood of being in a crash next year		
High	2	6
Moderate	22	25
Low	76	69

have been involved in crashes in the previous year and crashes that resulted in medical injuries. Compared to adult drivers, adolescent drivers were twice as likely to have been a driver in a crash and three times more likely to have been a driver in a crash resulting in injury.

Jonah and Dawson (1987) conducted a national household survey in Canada (N = 2,207). Sixty-eight percent of those contacted participated. Seventy-seven percent were between the ages of 16 and 20. They also found that adolescent drivers, as well as those in their early twenties, were significantly more likely than older drivers to report engaging in a variety of risky driving behaviors.

Further, many of these risky driving behaviors disproportionately cluster in the same adolescent drivers. For example, among Massachusetts adolescents, those who drove after imbibing five or more drinks in the past month were also much more likely to report speeding, running red lights, making illegal turns, driving after marijuana use, and not wearing safety belts.

Speeding is a particular problem among adolescents especially when they have been drinking. The National Safety Council (1989) estimates that speeding is a factor in 30% of fatal and 25% of nonfatal crashes. Adolescents were disproportionately involved in 20% (2,578/13,199) of fatal crashes involving speeding in 1990, even though they made up only 10% of the driving population (U. S. Department of Transportation, 1991). Increased speed contributes to crashes and fatalities in crashes in several ways. At higher speeds, a driver has less time to respond to unexpected stimuli. Also, at higher speeds, greater distance is needed to brake vehicles. Impact forces are increased exponentially as speed increases, and safety belts are less effective at higher speeds (National Highway Traffic Safety Administration, 1986). States that raised speed limits on rural interstate highways had a significant increase in traffic deaths on those roads relative to other roads in the same states (Baum, Wells, & Lund, 1990). Teenage fatalities have risen more steeply on those rural interstates than have fatalities among adult drivers.

Speeding and drunk driving are a particularly dangerous combination, often exhibited by the same drivers. In 1988, half of the fatalities involving a speeding driver also involved a drunk driver, and half of the fatalities involving a drunk driver also involved a speeder. Because of their poorer sensorimotor coordination and reaction time, drunk drivers are especially dangerous at higher travel speeds. Moreover, speeders are less likely to wear safety belts even when belt use is required by law (Preusser, Lund, & Blomberg, 1988). Like drunk drivers, speeders endanger not only themselves, but others as well, including passengers of the speeding vehicles, occupants of vehicles struck by the speeder, pedestrians, or bicyclists.

Other researchers have reported that risky driving behavior is also associated with other risky health habits, such as smoking, illicit drug use, poor diet, and lack of sleep (Bierness & Simpson, 1988), devoting less time to academic work and sports, staying out late at night, and being dismissed from class (Swisher, 1988). Risky driving and these other risky health behaviors have common underlying psychological, behavioral, and environmental predictors, as outlined in problem behavior theory. These findings have prompted Jessor to question whether prevention/intervention efforts might well be focused at the level of lifestyle (Jessor, 1987) and the psychological, social, and environmental antecedents common to a variety of risky behaviors, rather than being restricted to specific risky driving behaviors (Chapter 7).

Why Do Adolescents Take More Risks?

The health belief model (Becker & Janz, 1984), the theory of reasoned action (Fishbein & Azjen, 1975), social learning theory (Bandura, 1969), and problem behavior theory (Jessor, 1984) offer hypotheses about why adolescents disproportionately engage in risky driving behavior.

According to the health belief model (Becker & Janz, 1984), people who (1) believe they are susceptible to an illness or injury, (2) believe the illness or injury will have severe consequences for them in terms of health, social, or economic functions, (3) believe that preventive actions are effective in reducing the likelihood of injury, or (4) perceive few barriers to engaging in preventive behavior will be more likely to respond to behavioral cues in the environment and to engage in preventive action. In effect, the model suggests that a rational cost/benefit analysis of the risks and benefits may influence driving.

LOWER PERCEIVED RISK OF CRASHING. Although the available data are not entirely consistent, adolescent drivers seem to perceive their risk of crash involvement as lower than that of older drivers. In the Massachusetts survey cited earlier (Hingson, 1991), adolescent drivers were significantly less likely than adults to believe that they would be drivers in crashes in the next year. In the Canadian survey (Jonah, 1987), while adolescents perceived their overall risk of crash involvement during the next year as higher than that of older drivers, they perceived their personal risk of crash involvement as lower when speeding, driving in a snowstorm, driving with one headlight, riding unbelted, driving while intoxicated, driving a small car, or driving with the rear window fogged. Trankle, Gelau, and Metkor (1990) compared 228 18- to 21-year-olds to 70 older drivers in West Germany and found that adolescent drivers reported less risk associated with driving in darkness, on curved roads, or in a rural environment. Yet, younger drivers are disproportionately involved in nighttime fatal crashes on rural roadways, where excessive speed and cutting curves are factors.

LOWER PERCEIVED BENEFITS FROM PREVENTION MEASURES. Jonah and Dawson (1987) found that younger drivers also generally tend to view preventive measures as less effective in reducing crash involvement or injury. Though adolescent drivers viewed air bags and automatic belts as more effective in reducing injuries in crashes, they were less likely than older drivers to believe that increased speeding enforcement, raising the drinking age, lower blood alcohol (BAC) limits for younger drivers, using lights in daytime, or rear seat shoulder belts would reduce injurious traffic crashes. They also considered safety features as less important when purchasing a car than older drivers. Research is also needed regarding adolescent perceptions of the severity of traffic injury consequences and potential barriers to more cautious driving.

DRIVER OVERCONFIDENCE. Social learning theory (Bandura, 1969) suggests that people learn to engage in behaviors that they perceive as rewarding either through personal experience or by watching the experience of others. Atkin and Greenberg (1980) observed that prime-time television commonly portrays illegal and dangerous driving, yet injury and death are rare consequences. Surveys in Sweden (Spolander, 1962) and in New South Wales (Job, 1990) compared the self-reported driving skills of newly licensed drivers, drivers with 1 year of experience, and those with 3 years of experience. While newly licensed drivers rated their skills as poorer than those of the average driver, drivers with 3 or more years of experience judged themselves to be better than average in most respects, and those who rated their skills most highly also reported driving faster and passing other vehicles more often. Job (1990) has hypothesized that adolescents undergo a social learning process that ultimately leads to overconfidence in their perceived driving abilities. The more drivers travel in the absence of a crash involvement, the more they may come to believe that they are better than other drivers.

PEER PRESSURE. Another barrier to safer driving may be teenagers' perceptions of what impresses their peers. Adolescents do not always drive alone. The theory of reasoned action (Fishbein & Azjen, 1975) suggests that not only the individual driver's beliefs but also his or her desire to please others and perceptions of what others value can be important predictors of driving behavior. Social norms among young males do not promote cautious driving. Rather, peer group pressure favors the unrealistic image of a confident, skilled driver who can perform difficult maneuvers at high speeds, sometimes after drinking (Job, 1990).

REWARDS OF RISKY DRIVING. Not only may adolescents be less cognizant of the dangers of risky driving, they may see greater positive rewards in risky driving behavior. Jessor (1984) has pointed out that for adolescents, drinking, drug use, and risky driving can all serve desired psychological functions. They can (1) exhibit control over their lives by acting independently, (2) express opposition to adult authority and conventional norms, (3) be used as a mechanism to cope with anxiety, frustration, or fear of failure at school, and (4) be used to gain and maintain acceptance in peer groups and to demonstrate to others that one has matured and can now engage in adult behaviors (e.g., driving after drinking). Millstein and Irwin (1988) have suggested that adolescent males who reach puberty later may be particularly likely to engage in risky driving behaviors because they lack the physical prowess to assert and gain recognition in other areas such as athletics.

Moreover, in a survey of 1,800 junior and senior high school students, Jessor (1987) found that 60% of males aged 16 to 20 and 33% of females were willing to report that in the past 6 months they had "taken some risks when driving in traffic because it makes driving more fun" (p. 5). Those who reported this were more likely to engage in other risky driving behaviors, such as not wearing a seat belt or driving after drinking.

Injury Prevention

Most of the effort to reduce teenage crash involvement in recent years has focused on reducing drunken driving. For this reason, we focus primarily on interventions to reduce alcohol-related traffic deaths. Three general approaches to injury prevention guide our discussion.

First, systems can be developed to minimize damage from injury (e.g., a swift emergency response and coordinated medical and rehabilitation efforts).

Second, vehicle design or engineering approaches can automatically protect persons from some injury risks (Robertson, 1981): windshield defoggers, performance standards for tires, collapsible steering columns, and fuel system integrity to prevent fires. An analysis by Graham and Garber (1984) suggests that federal safety standards resulted in reductions of 5 to 35% in traffic fatalities.

Roadway design also influences crash rates. On superhighways, fatal crash rates per miles driven are one-third to one-half the rates on other roadways (National Highway Traffic Safety Administration, 1989). One obvious problem on highways other than superhighways is immovable objects near roadways, often utility poles or street lamps. Half of the 23,419 fatal single-vehicle crashes in 1990 involved collision with a fixed object. Other road design improvements include guard rails, cushioned road guards and barriers, embankments, intersection stop signs, and traffic lights. In 1990 35% of the 9,197 total fatal crashes at intersections occurred at sites with no controls (U. S. Department of Transportation, 1991).

Automatic safety belts or air bags are now required in newly manufactured vehicles. It has been estimated that air bags in combination with safety belts can double the protection offered by belts alone (Williams & Lund, 1988). Data from the National Accident Sampling System indicate that belted motor vehicle occupants are one-half as likely to be injured in a crash and one-third as likely to be hospitalized.

Vehicle inspection programs have also been associated with lower traffic fatality rates even after controlling for a variety of confounding variables (Colton & Baxbaum, 1968; McCutchen & Sherman, 1969; Schroer & Peyton, 1979).

Third, efforts to change individuals' behavior may reduce injury. Such efforts may result from individuals being persuaded to change behavior voluntarily or through legal requirements. Each of these behavioral approaches is described below.

Educational Strategies

Numerous educational strategies to inform adolescents about the dangers of drunk driving emerged during the early 1980s. From 1980 to 1985, more than 400 local chapters of citizens groups such as Mothers Against Drunk Driving (MADD) or Remove Intoxicated Drivers (RID) were founded. News stories about the problem increased fifty-fold (McCarthy, Wolfson, & Bolser, 1988). School education programs such as Students Against Drunk Driving (SADD,) were initiated in many locations across the nation. Also, many schools initiated educational programs to discuss the dangers of alcohol and drug use that included the dangers of drunk driving.

Reviews of educational interventions to reduce drunk driving among teenagers have examined both driver education programs and school-based educational programs. Controlled studies of driver education reveal that they do not lower crash rates in adolescent drivers, because any positive effects are offset by the effects of encouraging adolescents to become licensed earlier than they otherwise would (Robertson & Zador, 1978; Shaul, 1975; Williams, 1987).

Controlled studies of school-based programs such as SADD have likewise failed to establish independent effects of particular programs, but the programs studied were introduced at a time when there was unprecedented media and legal attention to the problem of drunk driving in the United States (Klitzner, 1989), and some of the specific programs studied had deficiencies in implementation.

However, school educational programs to reduce adolescent substance abuse, including cigarette smoking (and consumption of alcohol and other drugs, have shown independent effects in reducing or delaying the onset of use of those substances. These programs have introduced several innovations over previous didactic methods. The programs have (1) shown adolescents short-term physiological consequences of substance use (Perry, 1980), (2) used student peer leaders elected by class members and specially trained to lead group discussion, (3) identified social and economic pressures on adolescents to use substances (Botvin et al., 1984; Botvin & Wills, 1985; Klepp, Halper, & Perry, 1986), (4) identified and practiced resistance skills through modeling and role play, and, most recently, (5) developed exercises that involve parents and families with students in an effort to eliminate substance use (Pentz et al., 1989). Whether these programs have also reduced drunk driving was not studied. Systematic investigation is needed that tests the effectiveness of these various strategies in reducing the dangerous habit of driving under the influence of alcohol or drugs.

Legal Strategies

Legislative changes have probably had the most widely recognized impact in reducing drunk driving deaths among teenagers. By 1988, all states had adopted 21 as the minimum purchase age for alcoholic beverages. More than 40 states had adopted criminal per se laws that establish the blood alcohol level that renders the driver under the influence. Over 30 states had also passed administrative per se laws that permit suspension of licenses between the time of arrest and trial (Insurance Institute for Highway Safety, 1991).

These laws attempted to reduce drunk driving in several ways (Nichols & Ross, 1989). First, legal increases in the drinking age sought to reduce adolescent access to alcohol and thereby reduce drunk driving. The criminal and administrative per se laws attempted to deter repeat drunk driving offenses by license suspension or revocation and by increasing penalties—*specific deterrence*. Yet since most adolescents have never been arrested for drunk driving, a potentially more important function of these laws is to deter people from ever driving after drinking in the first place, through *general deterrence* that promotes healthy behaviors rather than punishing crimes. If drivers believe it is very likely that they will be caught, fear of apprehension and punishment may dissuade them from driving after drinking (Nichols & Ross, 1989).

Andeneas (1978) suggested that general deterrence laws can also create moral inhibitions by expressing emerging social norms and making statements to society of new standards of acceptable behavior. The 1988 Massachusetts adolescent survey revealed that peers can monitor each other's behavior and exert *informal social pressure* on each other not to drive while drunk (Hingson & Howland, 1990).

The legislative activity and community-level opposition to drunk driving have had marked and disproportionately beneficial effects on teenage drivers. The legal changes clearly contributed to declines. Although the effects varied considerably from state to state, increases in the legal drinking age were accompanied by a 10–15% reduction in fatal crashes in the age group targeted by those laws (Du Mouchel, Williams, & Zador, 1985; Hingson et al., 1983; Williams, Zador, Harris & Karpf, 1983; U. S. General Accounting Office, 1987). The criminal and administrative per se laws also contributed to declines. When compared to states not passing such laws, administrative per se laws were accompanied by 5% declines in fatal crashes and criminal per se laws by a 2% decline (Zador, Lund, Fields, & Weinburg, 1989). Whether these laws had independent effects in specifically lowering fatal crashes among teenage drunk drivers has not been tested and warrants investigation. Four states have had lowered BAC limits for adolescents long enough for their effects to be monitored. When those states lowered their BAC levels for teenagers, they experienced a significant decline in fatal crashes at night involving teenagers relative to fatal crashes involving adults when compared to other states. There was a 34% decline in night fatalities among teenagers in lower legal BAC states compared to a 26% decline in fatal crashes at night among teenagers in comparison states. In other words, fatal crashes at night among teenagers declined one-third more in states that lowered their BAC limits for teenagers. Fatal crashes at night among adults declined less than 10% in both sets of states (Hingson, Howland, Heeren, & Winter, 1991).

In addition to changes to drinking age and per se laws, other legal and economic strategies also have the potential to reduce teenage involvement in alcohol-related crashes. Increased prices of alcoholic beverages have been associated with reduced drinking, especially among teenagers, and with declines in fatal crashes (Coate & Grossman, 1986; Cook, 1981; Grossman, Coate, & Arluck, 1987; Saffer & Grossman, 1985). These declines were independent of gender, age, demographic characteristics, and driving exposure. Delaying drivers' licensure (Williams, 1987; Williams & Lund, 1987), adopting night curfews (Preusser, Williams, Zador, & Blomberg, 1984), expanding public transportation, and providing other alternatives to driving automobiles are all strategies that apply individually or collectively to reduce alcohol-related adolescent driving and injury. In the United States, mandatory safety belt laws have been typically followed by 5–10% motor vehicle occupant fatality reductions (Campbell & Campbell, 1988).

Sustaining Crash Reductions

It should be noted that most of the declines in teenage single-vehicle night fatal crashes or in the estimated alcohol-involved fatal crashes among drivers occurred during the first half of the 1980s and have risen somewhat since (O'Neill, 1991).

Societal concern about drunk driving may be relaxing slightly, lessening the motivation for adolescents to refrain from concurrent drinking and driving (Hingson, Howland, & Levenson, 1989). For example, media coverage of the drunk driving problem in national periodicals rose sharply in the early 1980s but has slackened since then (McCarthy, Wolfson, & Bolser, 1988). Drunk driving arrests also have declined in recent years (Greenfield, 1988). Although increasing arrests for drunk driving and the extensive use of drunk driving roadblocks can reduce traffic deaths and injuries involving alcohol (Lacey et al., 1986; Voas & House, 1987; Voas, Rhodenizer, & Lynn, 1985), it has been estimated that the likelihood of drunk drivers being stopped by the police in the United States is only one out of five hundred to one out of one thousand drunk driving trips (Voas & Lacey, 1989).

There are gaps in the enforcement of drinking age laws. Raising the legal drinking age in Massachusetts produced a reduction in the proportion of teenagers who themselves purchased alcohol at bars, restaurants, or liquor stores from 63% to 25%. However, the proportion who had others, typically friends or acquaintances just above the legal purchase age, purchase for them increased from 21% to 43% (Hingson et al., 1983). Eighty percent of teenagers interviewed in a 1988 survey in that state reported having consumed alcoholic beverages in the past year—one-third weekly and one-fifth consuming five or more drinks on typical drinking occasions (Hingson et al., 1990). There is a need to restrict liquor sales to minors more actively and to hold adults responsible for encouraging irresponsible drinking and driving behaviors among their adolescent guests.

Further, every year, nearly 5,000 people are killed while riding with a drunk driver and almost one-third are teenagers. In the 1988 Massachusetts survey, twice as many teenagers reported that they rode with a drunk driver than reported personally driving after heavy drinking (Hingson et al., 1990). To better understand the passenger's role, it may be necessary to study the behaviors of adolescents in drinking groups, and not only the drunk driver. How they obtain alcohol, what pressures they place on each other to drink, and how they respond to designated driver campaigns should be explored. Research should also assess the benefit of penalties for drunk drivers who allow others to ride with them.

Can Interventions to Reduce Drunk Driving Inform Other Injury Prevention Efforts?

While motor vehicle accidents secondary to drunk driving have been the focus of our discussion, other sources of injury exist that could probably benefit from intervention. The question, then, is whether we can extend what we know about the prevention of drunk driving to other types of injuries in adolescents, including drownings, burns, and recreational injuries.

There are some clear commonalities across different types of injuries in adolescents. For example, males consistently show higher injury rates across different sources/types of injury than females. Similarly, nonwhites show higher rates than whites (National Committee for Injury Prevention and Control, 1989). Other commonalities include the important role of decision making in safety and the detrimental role that alcohol often plays. For example, decisions about when and where to swim appear to be an important factor in drownings (Baker, O'Neill, & Karpf, 1984). These decisions may be compromised by alcohol, which often accompanies swimming and boating events (Howland & Hingson, 1988; Howland, Mangione, Hingson, Levenson, & Winter, 1990). As many as 40% of adolescent drownings involve alcohol (Wintemute, 1990). It appears that normative prescriptions against the use of alcohol during these recreational events are less developed than those against drinking and driving; drinking in aquatic settings is far more common than drinking and driving (Howland, Mangione, Hingson, Levenson, & Winter, 1990).

Alcohol also plays a role in some burn deaths, both as a result of falling asleep while smoking and due to the diminished capacity of intoxicated persons to respond quickly and effectively to fire (National Committee for Injury Prevention and Control, 1989). Environmental conditions also contribute to burns, with higher rates among poor people, probably as a result of less adequate housing, outdated wiring, heating systems in bad repair, greater reliance on space heaters, over-crowding, lack of fire alarms, and increased cigarette smoking (McLaughlin & McGuire, 1990).

Among adolescents 10 to 14 and 15 to 19, drowning death rates declined 27% and 38%, respectively, between 1980 and 1985 (National Safety Council, 1989). This decline parallels the sharp declines in traffic crashes at a time when many states were raising the drinking age. Whether the decline in drowning was influenced by the drinking age changes warrants scrutiny. Finally, it should be noted that exper-imental and quasi-experimental studies to test strategies to prevent drowning have infrequently been conducted compared to the wealth of studies of drunk driving countermeasures. This type of research is urgently needed to increase our under-standing of how to prevent drowning.

Recreational Injuries

Recreational injuries are by far the most common type of nonfatal injury. For every injury death there are approximately 40 hospitalizations and 1,100 cases treated in emergency rooms (Runyun & Gerken, 1989). According to the National Health interview, approximately one-third of adolescents have an injury each year that requires medical attention. Forty-six percent of adolescent injuries are attributable to recreational activity. According to studies of emergency rooms in Massachusetts, 1 out of every 14 adolescents was hospitalized annually with a sports-related injury (Galleghar, Finson, & Guyer, 1984).

Compared to traffic injuries, a smaller percentage of recreational injuries are associated with alcohol use.

Organized Sports

Most recreational injuries are sports related (Goldberg, 1989). Half of all males aged 8 to 16 and one-quarter of all females are engaged in some kind of scholastic, organized, competitive sport (McLain & Reynolds, 1989). Adolescents experience considerable pressure to participate in sports. They are offered rewards in the form of friendships, fun, healthy conditioning, prestige, and, for some, valuable eco-nomic opportunities for higher education. Boys are much more likely than girls to be injured in recreational sports, primarily because they are much more likely to play contact sports. Of the various organized sports, football is the most dangerous. The National Athletic Trainers Association (1987) found that 37% of all high school football players were injured at least once in 1987. An epidemiological study of over 40 randomly selected schools and 8,700 players in North Carolina, how-ever, found that teams with older, better-educated coaches had fewer injuries. Also, the more coaches per players, the fewer injuries occurred. Training programs that reduce player contact had fewer injuries and higher winning percentages (Blyth & Mueller, 1974).

The National Committee for Injury Prevention and Control (1989) has estab-lished 20 general recommendations for reducing sports injuries. The following are illustrative. As preventive measures, players can be provided with appropriate equipment such as helmets, protective padding, and protective eyewear. They can be instructed on ways to minimize the likelihood of injury. Playing fields should be inspected and maintained. Fixed objects should be removed or padded. Playing under supervision and adhering to the rules should be encouraged, and supervisory personnel should be specially trained in the prevention and care of injuries, including cardiopulmonary resuscitation.

Play should not occur in inclement weather, or after drinking or drug use. Care should be taken to have student athletes examined medically prior to the start of each season and before returning to play after incurring an injury. Appropriate conditioning programs should be established and pursued prior to competitive sports (Stanitski, 1989). Synthetic turf results in a higher ambient temperature, with a greater chance of causing inadequate water and salt depletion, thus making heat stress and injury more likely (Waller, 1985). Health records should be kept on all participants in organized sports, and arrangements should be made to provide for emergency medical technicians and ambulance service in case of an injury.

Organized sports provide an excellent controlled environment in which intervention strategies to reduce injury can be tested. The impact of rule modification, equipment changes, additional protective gear, and so on, should all be systematically tested.

A more fundamental question that warrants exploration is whether adolescents should be encouraged to engage in high-risk contact sports such as football, boxing, and hockey. Whether alternative, less dangerous sports can be encouraged for adolescents is worth exploring. Studies of parental attitudes and behaviors that encourage adolescents to opt for more dangerous sports also need to be explored. While some studies have explored the psychological traits associated with sports injury, there is a need to study the psychological and social factors associated with the decision to choose a specific sport to play and with the decision to engage in supervised versus unsupervised sports. Many people engage in these activities because of the inherent dangers involved. Mountain climbing, hang gliding, and sky diving are sports whose danger provides the risks that some persons with sedentary or boring jobs may crave. Fundamental changes in public attitudes are needed to dissuade some from engaging in these high-risk activities. Whether such changes are feasible or advisable is subject to debate.

Conclusions

Although several significant methodological problems need to be addressed in studying adolescent injury (Runyun & Gerken, 1989), some conclusions can be drawn from the research on adolescent injury prevention. The literature on teenage drunk driving is by far the most extensive in the area of adolescent injury, and the national experience with teenage drunk driving provides numerous insights into the process of adolescent injury prevention.

First, while adolescents began the decade more likely to engage in the high-risk behavior of drunk driving (Waganaar, 1983), declines in teenage drunk driving and alcohol-related fatal crashes exceeded drunk driving declines among other age groups (National Highway Traffic Safety Administration, 1989). By the end of the decade, adolescents were less likely to drive while drunk than older drivers in their twenties and thirties. Despite their history of risky behavior, teenagers can be influenced, and their behaviors may even be more readily changed than those of older groups.

Second, multiple interventions targeted the same behavior. Those who sought to reduce drunk driving did not rely on a single change strategy. Education in schools, driver education, laws to deter drunk driving in general, and counseling programs were implemented, as were drinking age laws to restrict alcohol purchase, increased taxes, and social host and dram shop liability laws to put pressure on servers of alcohol to be careful about who they serve (Saltz, 1989).

Third, the interventions and laws were not simply a function of government initiating regulation in response to official data and scientific research on the problem. Rather, there were strong, vociferous citizen lobby groups (e.g., MADD or RID) that demanded, with indignation, that our laws become tougher when dealing with drunk driving. From 20% to 40% of those killed in drunk driving crashes are persons other than the drunk driver. It was easier to stimulate public action to deal with this issue because those who drive while drunk endanger others. As far as possible, injury prevention efforts in other areas should highlight the behaviors that place not only the perpetrators at risk, but others as well. The dangers to others, for example, of speeding drivers, intoxicated boaters, persons who break rules in sports, and people who smoke in bed should be highlighted. Not only did new laws place pressure on people not to drive after drinking, people placed informal pressure on each other not to drive while drunk. The adage "Friends don't let friends drive drunk" in many instances turned into a reality.

Fourth, a strong body of research about the dangers of drunk driving that showed how and why alcohol impairs driving was available for proponents of the anti–drunk driving movement to call on. Unfortunately, the scientific literature is not nearly so well developed in other injury areas and should be expanded. For example, we know very little about the factors that contribute to fatal teenage burn deaths, and in many instances we have not even been able to estimate the magnitude of nonfatal teenage injuries. While limited studies have examined social and psychological theories and developmental issues in traffic crashes, almost no work of this type has examined drowning, burns, or recreational, work, or home injuries.

We need survey, observational case control, and longitudinal research to assess the causes of such injuries, and both experimental and quasi-experimental studies of interventions to prevent them. Experimental and quasi-experimental studies of injury prevention strategies are particularly lacking for nonfatal and nontraffic fatal injuries.

Fifth, those opposed to the dangers of drunk driving did not restrict their energies to adolescents, even though at the start of the decade, teenagers were the group with the greatest likelihood of driving while drunk. The spate of legislation in the 1980s targeted adult drivers as well. Consequently, drunk driving did not become associated with a rite of passage into adulthood. It was a behavior targeted for reduction in all age groups. Though adolescents are more likely to be injured, prevention efforts to reduce the types of injuries that occur to adolescents should target all age groups.

Sixth, it is not inevitable that drunk driving declines in adolescence will be sustained or never reversed. In 1986, after several years of decline, drunk driving deaths increased, particularly among adolescent drivers. Each year, a new cohort of adolescent drivers enters the driving pool. These new drivers may not have been attentive to local citizen groups, media, and legislative discussion about the dangers of drunk driving earlier in the decade. Consequently, educational and legal efforts to reduce this problem should not be relaxed, as they have in part with regard to speeding.

Seventh, many risky driving behaviors are interrelated and are disproportionately exhibited by the same drivers. People who drive while drunk are more likely to speed, run red lights, make illegal turns, and not wear safety belts. Focusing attention on only one of several interrelated behaviors contributing to a problem may not achieve optimal improvements in traffic safety. The relaxation of public concerns about teenage speeding at the same time as the public targets drunk driving reduced the overall impact of the anti–drunk driving efforts among youthful drivers. Similarly, while alcohol may play a key role in drowning and aquatic injury, other factors, such as failure to wear life preservers, boat construction, standing inappropriately, and swimming or boating alone in unsupervised areas, should all be stressed.

Eighth, much of the decline in alcohol-related traffic deaths resulted from raising the legal purchase age for alcohol. We are currently seeing declines in deaths from drowning and burns. It is extremely important to develop a series of studies that test whether changes in drinking age may also influence other types of injuries involving teenagers.

New laws also need to be explored. The lowered BAC legal limits for adolescent drivers are one example. The use of provisional licensing (Williams, 1987; Williams & Lund, 1987) for teenage drivers that would permit administrative license suspension not only for drunk driving, but also for speeding, red light running, illegal turns and other risky behaviors, also warrants study. The use of provisional licensing and administrative suspension would allow the penalties associated with driving infractions to be more closely linked in time with the infraction.

Finally, efforts to reduce drunk driving deaths have mostly focused on preventive measures focused on the driver. Much more could be done to reduce drunk driving deaths by expanding attention to the crash and the measures taken immediately following the crash and by extending efforts beyond the driver to the vehicle and the environment.

Efforts to make vehicles safer in the event of accidents and changes to make roadways easier to maneuver and safer (even for intoxicated drivers) would yield benefits for all drivers. Following an accident, improvements in emergency medical services and better communication between emergency medical technicians and hospitals, as well as integration of medical care with rehabilitation, would minimize the impact of the injuries sustained in drunk driving crashes. Careful documentation of drivers' BACs and the circumstances that originally produced the crashes could help in planning the prevention of subsequent crashes.

Adolescents are disproportionately likely to incur injuries that result in death or disability. Several factors appear to cut across injury types, suggesting some commonalities in the etiology of various injuries. Males are more likely than females to be involved in most forms of injury, and much of the difference may result from increased exposure of males to more hazardous activities. Males are also encouraged to engage in greater risk taking than females, and males drink and take drugs considerably more often than females. The inexperience of adolescents contributes to the large numbers of injuries among their population group, not only in automobile accidents but also in boating, swimming, recreational, and work activities. Teenagers underestimate the risks inherent in various driving situations and then engage in more risky driving practices.

However, other than a few studies on traffic crashes, little research has explored adolescent beliefs about the level of risk associated with common behaviors that often contribute to injury (e.g., aquatic activities such as swimming alone or in unsupervised areas, use of life preservers, aquatic activities in cold water or stormy weather). Similarly, little is known about beliefs concerning other recreational activities such as football, skateboarding, basketball, baseball, track and field, or gymnastics. Studies looking at perceptions of peers of various pressures they receive from parents, friends, and coaches to engage in high-risk sports also deserve exploration.

It is possible that some of the same psychological factors that contribute to risk taking while driving also contribute to risk taking in aquatic and other recreational and work activities (Kerr & Fowler, 1988), but this has not been tested and warrants investigation. Research is needed to test, directly and comprehensively, some of the psychosocial theories and models outlined earlier in the chapter.

However, even if there are some common social and psychological antecedents, different types of injuries appear to have distinct etiologies. For example, alcohol is much more likely to be involved in traffic injuries and drowning than other recreational injuries, particularly competitive sports. Indeed, persons who pursue athletic activities may have very different drinking habits than persons likely to drive or to go boating after drinking. While it may be useful to search for common psychological and behavioral factors across injury types, the unique features of each type of injury must be recognized if we are to develop optimally effective interventions.

Further, cohorts of adolescents should be followed over time to assess whether these beliefs change as they become older and if those changes are associated with changes in injury rates.

For example, in their mid-twenties, many drivers seem to curb their risky driving behaviors because fatal crashes decline considerably for this age group, perhaps because they marry and enter the workplace. Systematic studies are needed that follow drivers throughout adolescence and their twenties to learn more about the forces that foster and then discourage risky driving. A better understanding of these factors may help contribute to the development of educational, prevention, and treatment programs that can target the drivers at highest risk and also make better use of social pressure by peers to reduce risky behavior.

Injuries are the most important immediate threat to adolescent health. Yet injury prevention research and programs are not nearly as extensive as interventions in other areas—for example, drug abuse and smoking cessation. Considerably more attention should be focused on injury. We are learning by experience with some injury problems, such as drunk driving, that substantial progress can be made with the right combination of public and private support strategies, education, law, and treatment. An important goal will be to test whether strategies and conditions that helped produce drunk driving declines, and whether the lessons derived from those efforts can successfully be applied to other areas of adolescent injury prevention.

Toward this goal, it would be useful to consider *comprehensive, coordinated, community-based* educational and enforcement efforts that (1) target not only adolescents, but all age groups in an effort to alter social norms, and (2) target not only drunk driving but also the related risky behaviors cited earlier (e.g., speeding, running red lights, illegal turns, not yielding to pedestrians). Social pressure has been shown to mediate risky behaviors in other areas. Communitywide, multistrategy interventions for changing multiple behavioral risks related to heart disease risk factors—for example, smoking, diet, alcohol consumption, and sedentary lifestyle—have demonstrated long-term success. Large-scale controlled studies in Finland, California, and Minnesota assessed programs that target high-risk groups and the total community vis-à-vis the media, schools, workplaces, and civic organizations (Botvin & Wills, 1985; Farquhar, 1978; Farquhar & Fortman, 1990; Perry, Murray, & Klepp, 1987; Puska, Salonen, & Nissinen, 1983). Significant, positive behavioral changes were reported across socioeconomic and risk factor strata in the target communities relative to the comparison communities. These studies indicate the potential for sustaining behavioral changes by developing a community-based consensus about a problem, particularly when the problem is not defined in terms of a single risk behavior (e.g., diet or smoking). A World Health Organization Committee on Traffic Safety (1980) has advocated a centralized organization within communities to coordinate the activities of schools, police, health delivery organizations, and so on, in reducing traffic accidents. The Institute of Medicine (1989) has also called for programs like this to reduce alcohol abuse and related problems such as drunk driving.

Establishing this type of program requires a substantial commitment of time, energy, and resources, not only from federal and state governments, but also from grass-roots public and private organizations and local communities. Whether such programs can successfully achieve long-term change in social norms about drunken drivers and related risky driving behaviors warrants investigation.

References

Agran, P. (1990). Childhood motor vehicle occupants. *American Journal of Diseases in Children, 144,* 653.

Andeneas, J. (1978). The effects of Scandinavia's drinking and driving laws. *Scandinavian Statutes on Criminology, 6,* 35–53.

Atkin, C. K., & Greenberg, B. S. (1980). *A portrayal of driving on prime time commercial television 1975–1979.* Washington, DC: U.S. Department of Transportation Report.

Baker, S., Neill, B., & Karpf, S. (1984). *Injury fact book.* Lexington, MA: Lexington Press.

Bandura, A. (1969). *Principles of behavior modification.* New York: Holt, Rinehart & Winsten.

Baum, H., Wells, J., & Lund, A. (1990). Motor vehicle fatalities in the second year of the 65 mph speed limit. *Journal of Safety Research, 21,* 1–8.

Becker, M., & Janz, N. K. (1984). The health belief model: A decade later. *Health Education Quarterly, 99,* 1–47.

Bergman, A., Rivera, F., Richards, D., & Roger, L. (1990). The Seattle children's bicycle helmet campaign. *American Journal of Diseases in Children, 144,* 727–731.

Bierness, D., & Simpson, H. (1988). Life-style correlates of risky driving and accident involvement among youth. *Alcohol, Drugs and Driving, 4,* 193–204.

Blyth, C. S., & Mueller, F. D. (1974). *An epidemiologic study of school football injuries in North Carolina Chapel Hill* (CPSC, pp. 1–74). Chapel Hill, NC: University of North Carolina, Department of Education.

Borkenstein, R. F., Crowther, R. F., Shumoth, P. R., Zeil, W. B., & Zylman, R. (1964). *The role of the drinking driver in traffic accidents.* Urbana, IN: Indiana University, Department of Police Administration.

Botvin, G. J., Baker, E., Renick, N. L., Filazzola, A. D., & Botvin, E. M. (1984). A cognitive behavioral approach to substance abuse prevention. *Addiction Behavior, 9,* 137–147.

Botvin, G. J., & Wills, T. L. (1985). Personal and social skills training: Cognitive behavioral approaches to substance abuse prevention. In C. Bell & R. Battjes, (Eds.), *Prevention research: Detering drug abuse among children and adolescents* (pp. 8–49). NIDA Research Monograph No. 63. Washington, DC.

Campbell, B. J., & Campbell, F. A. (1988). Injury reduction and belt use associated with occupational restraint laws. In J. Graham (Ed.), *Preventing automobile injury* (pp. 24–48). Dover, MA: Auburn House.

Coate, D., & Grossman, M. (1986). *Effects of alcoholic beverage prices and legal drinking ages on youth alcohol use.* Working Paper 1852. Cambridge, MA: National Bureau of Economic Research.

Colton, T., & Baxbaum, R. (1968). Motor vehicle inspection and motor vehicle accident mortality. *American Journal of Public Health, 58,* 1090–1099.

Cook, P. J. (1981). The effect of liquor taxes on drinking, cirrhosis, and auto accidents. In N. Moore (Ed.), *Alcohol and public policy beyond the shadow of prohibition* (pp. 255–285). Washington, DC: National Academy Press.

Dement, W. C. (1992). Personal communication.

Division of Injury Control, Center for Environmental Health and Injury Control, and Centers for Disease Control (1990). Childhood injuries in the United States. *American Journal of Diseases in Children, 144,* 627–696.

Du Mouchel, W., Williams, A. F., & Zador, P. (1985). *Raising the alcohol purchase age: Its effects on fatal motor vehicle crashes in 26 states.* Washington, DC: Insurance Institute for Highway Safety.

Farquhar, J. W. (1978). The community based model of life-style intervention trials. *American Journal of Epidemiology, 108,* 103–111.

Farquhar, J. W., & Fortman, S. P. (1990). Effects of community wide education on cardiovascular risk factors, the Stanford Five City Project. *Journal of the American Medical Association, 264,* 359–365.

Fishbein, M., & Azjen, I. (1975). *Belief attitude intervention and behavior: An introduction to theory and research,* Reading, MA: Addison-Wesley.

Galleghar, S., Finson, K., & Guyer, B. (1984). The incidence of injuries among 87,000 Massachusetts children and adolescents. *American Journal of Public Health, 74,* 1340–1347.

Goldberg, B. (1989). Injury patterns in youth sports. *The Physician and Sports Medicine Journal, 17,* 175–186.

Graham, J., & Garber, S. (1984). Evaluating the effects of automobile safety regulation. *Journal of Policy Analysis and Management, 3,* 206–224.

Greenfield, L. A. (1988). *Drunk driving.* Statistics Special Reports NCJ 109945. Washington, DC: U.S. Department of Justice, Bureau of Justice.

Grossman, M., Coate, D., & Arluck, G. (1987). Price sensitivity of alcoholic beverages in the United States. In H. D. Holder (Ed.), *Central issues in alcohol abuse prevention: Strategies for communities* (pp. 169–198). Washington, DC: JAI Press.

Haddon, W. J., & Baker, S. P. (1981). Injury control. In D. Clark & B. MacMahon (Eds.), *Preventive medicine* (2nd ed) (pp. 109–140). Boston: Little, Brown.

Hingson, R., & Howland, J. (1990). Use of laws to deter drunk driving. *Alcohol, Health and Research World, 14,* 36–44.

Hingson, R., Howland, J., Heeren, T., & Winter, M. (1991). Effects of lowered legal BAC limits for adolescent drivers. *Alcohol, Drugs and Driving, 7,* 117–127.

Hingson, R., Howland, J., & Levenson, S. (1989). Effects of legislative reform to reduce drunken driving and other related traffic fatalities. *Public Health Reports, 103,* 659–667.

Hingson, R., Howland, J., Schiavone, T., & Damiata, M. (1991). The Massachusetts saving lives program: Six cities widening the focus from drunk driving to speeding, reckless driving and failure to wear safety belts. *Journal of Traffic Medicine, 18,* 123–132.

Hingson, R., Scotch, N., Mangione, T., Meyers, A., Glantz, L., Heeren, T., Lin, N., Mucatel, M., & Pierce, G. (1983). Impact of legislation raising the drinking age from 18 to 20 in Massachusetts. *American Journal of Public Health, 73,* 163–170.

Holt, P. L. (1981). Stressful life events preceding road traffic accidents and injury. *British Journal of Addictions, 13,* 111–115.

Howland, J., & Hingson, R. (1988). Alcohol as a risk factor for drowning: A review of the literature (1950–1985). *Accident Analysis and Prevention, 20,* 19–25.

Howland, J., Mangione, T., Hingson, R., Levenson, S., & Winter, M. (1990). Drinking and aquatic activities: Results of pilot Massachusetts survey. *Public Health Reports, 105,* 415–419.

Institute of Medicine (1989). *Prevention and treatment of alcohol problems: research opportunities.* Washington, DC: National Academy Press.

Insurance Institute for Highway Safety (1991). *Insurance Institute for Highway Safety facts.* Arlington, VA: Author.

Jessor, R. (1984). Adolescent development and behavioral health. In J. D. Matarazzo, S. M. Weiss, A. Herd, & N. E. Miller (Eds.), *Behavioral health: A handbook of health and disease prevention* (pp. 69–90). New York: Wiley.

Jessor, R. (1987). Risky driving and problem adolescent behavior: An extension of problem behavior theory. *Alcohol, Drugs and Driving, 3,* 1–11.

Job, R. (1990). The application of learning theory to driving confidence: The effect of age and the impact of random breath testing. *Accident Analysis and Prevention, 22,* 97–109.

Jonah, B., & Dawson, N. (1987). Youth and risk: Age differences in risky driving, risk perceptions and risk utility. *Alcohol, Drugs and Driving, 3,* 13–29.

Katkin, E. S., Hates, W. N., Tegor, A. I., & Pruitt, D. G. (1970). Effects of alcoholic beverages differing in congenes content on psychomotor tasks and risk taking. *Quarterly Journal of Studies on Alcohol, 31* (Suppl No 5), 105–114.

Kerr, G., & Fowler, B. (1988). The relation between psychological factors and sports injuries. *Sports Medicine, 6,* 127–134.

Kish, L. (1965). *Survey sampling.* New York: Wiley.

Klepp, K. I., Halper, A., & Perry, C. L. (1986). The efficacy of peer leaders in drug abuse prevention. *Journal of School Health, 56,* 407–411.

Klitzner, M. (1989). Youth impaired driving: Causes and countermeasures. *Surgeon General's conference on drunk driving: Background papers.* Rockville, MD: U.S. Public Health Service.

Lacey, J. H., Stewart, J. R., Marchetti, L. M., Popkin, C. L., Murphy, P. V., Luckey, R. E., & Jones, R. (1986). *Enforcement and public information strategies for general deterence: Arrest drunk driving the Clearwater and Largo Florida experience* (DOT HS 807 066). Springfield, VA: National Technical Information Service.

McCarthy, J., Wolfson, M., & Bolser, D. (1988). The founding of local citizen groups opposing drunken driving. In G. R. Caroll (Ed.), *Ecological models of organizations* (pp. 71–84). Cambridge, MA: Ballinger Press.

McCutchen, R. W., & Sherman, H. W. (1969). The influence of periodic motor vehicle inspection on mechanical conditions. *Journal of Safety Research, 1,* 184–193.

McLain, L., & Reynolds, S. (1989). Sports injury in a high school. *Pediatrics, 84,* 446–450.

McLoughlin, E., & McGuire, A. (1990). Causes, cost and prevention of childhood burn injuries. *American Journal of Diseases in Children, 144,* 677–683.

Millstein, S., & Irwin, C. (1988). Accident related behaviors in adolescents: A biopsychosocial view. *Alcohol, Drugs and Driving, 4,* 21–31.

National Athletic Trainers Association (1987). *The National Athletic Trainers Association fact sheet.* Greenville, NC: Author.

National Committee for Injury Prevention and Control (1989). Injury prevention: Meeting the challenge. Supplement to the *American Journal of Preventive Medicine, 5.* Oxford University Press: New York.

National Highway Traffic Safety Administration (1986). *Off limits: A reference guide for improving compliance with posted speed limits* (DOT HS 807 276). Washington, DC: National Highway Traffic Safety Administration.

National Highway Traffic Safety Administration (1989). *Alcohol involvement in fatal crashes* (DOT HS 807 448).

National Highway Transportation Safety Administration (1986). *National accident sampling system* (DOT HS 807 296). Washington, DC: National Highway Transportation Safety Administration.

National Safety Council. (1989). *Accident facts* (p. 83). Washington, DC: Author.

Nichols, J., & Ross, H. L. (1989). *The effectiveness of legal sanctions in dealing with drunk drivers* (pp. 93–113). Washington, DC: U.S. Public Health Service.

O'Neill, B. (1991). For under age drinkers buying beer is no problem—fatalities are. *Insurance Institute For Highway Safety Status Report, 25,* 1–2.

Pentz, M. A., Dwyer, J. H., MacKinnon, D. P., Flay, B. R., Hansen, W. B., Yu, E., Wang, M. S., & Johnson, C. A. (1989). A multi-community trial for primary prevention of adolescent drug abuse, effects on drug use prevalence. *Journal of the American Medical Association, 261,* 3259–3266.

Perry, C. L. (1980). Modifying smoking behavior of teenagers: A school based intervention. *American Journal of Public Health, 70,* 722–725.

Perry, C. L., Murray, D. M., & Klepp, K. I. (1987). Predictors of adolescent smoking and implications for prevention. *Morbidity and Mortality Weekly Reports, 36* (Suppl), 415–455.

Preusser, D., Lund, A., & Blomberg, W. (1988). Belt use by high risk drivers before and after New York's seat belt law. *Accident Analysis and Prevention, 20,* 245–250.

Preusser, D. F., Williams, A. F., Zador, P. L., & Blomberg, R. D. (1984). The effect of curfew laws on motor vehicle crashes. *Law and Policy, 6,* 115–128.

Puska, P., Salonen, J., Nissinen, J. (1983). Change in risk factors for coronary heart disease during 10 years of a community intervention program (North Karelia Project). *British Medical Journal, 287,* 1840–1844.

Quimby, P. R., & Watts, G. R. (1981). *Human factors and driving performance.* CTRRL Supplementary Report 1004. Crowthorne, England: Transport and Road Research Laboratory.

Rhodes, K., Brennan, S., & Paterson, H. (1990). Machines and microbes still serious hazards to youth on the farm. *American Journal of Diseases in Children, 144,* 707–709.

Rivera, F. (1990). Child pedestrian injuries in the United States. *American Journal of Diseases in Children, 144,* 692–696.

Robertson, L. S. (1981). Automobile safety regulations and death reductions in the United States. *American Journal of Public Health, 71,* 818–822.

Robertson, L. S., & Zador, P. L. (1978). Driver education and fatal crash involvement of teenage drivers. *American Journal of Public Health, 73,* 959–965.

Runyun, C., & Gerken, E. (1989). Epidemiology and prevention of adolescent injury. *Journal of the American Medical Association, 262,* 2273–2279.

Saffer, H., & Grossman, M. (1985). *Effects of beer prices and legal drinking age on youth in motor vehicle fatalities.* New York: National Bureau of Economic Research.

Saltz, R. (1989, December). Server intervention and responsible beverage service programs. *Surgeon General's Workshop on Drunk Driving: Background Papers* (pp. 169–179). Rockville, MD: U.S. Department of Health and Human Services, Public Health Service.

Schroer, B. J., & Peyton, W. F. (1979). The effects of automobile inspections on accident rates. *Accident Analysis and Prevention, 11,* 61–68.

Shaul, J. (1975). *The use of accidents and traffic offenses as criteria for evaluating courses in drivers education.* Salford, England: University of Salford.

Spolander, K. (1962). *Inexperienced drivers' behaviors, abilities, and attitudes.* Stockholm: Swedish National Road and Traffic Institute.

Stanitski, C. (1989). Common injuries in preadolescent and adolescent athletes. *Sports Medicine 7,* 32–41.

Swisher, T. (1988). Problem behavior theory and driving risk. *Alcohol, Drugs and Driving, 4,* 205–219.

Thompson, R. S., Rivera, F. P., & Thompson, D. C. (1989). Case control study of the effectiveness of bicycle safety helmets. *New England Journal of Medicine, 320,* 1361–1367.

Trankle, U., Gelau, C., & Metkor, T. (1990). Risk perception and age specifics of accidents of young drivers. *Accident Analysis and Prevention, 22,* 119–127.

U.S. Department of Health and Human Services (1986). Types of injuries and impairments due to injuries. DHHS Publication No. 87-1578. *National Health Survey Series, 10.* (No. 15). Washington, DC: U.S. Department of Health and Human Services.

U.S. Department of Health and Human Services, Centers for Disease Control (1989). Trends and current status in childhood mortality: United States 1980–1985. *Vital and Health Statistics Analytic and Epidemiological Studies Series, 3,* 1–40.

U.S. Department of Transportation (1990). *Fatal accident reporting system (1989)* (DOT HS 80757). Washington, DC: U.S. Department of Transportation.

U.S. Department of Transportation (1991). *Fatal accident Reporting System (1990).* Washington, DC: U.S. Department of Transportation.

U.S. General Accounting Office (1987). *Drinking age laws—An evaluation synthesis of their impact on highway safety.* Publication No. GAO PEMD 87-10. Washington, DC: Author.

Voas, R. B., & House, J. H. (1987). Deterring the drinking driver: The Stockton experience. *Accident Analysis and Prevention, 19,* 81–90.

Voas, R., & Lacey, J. (1989). Issues in the enforcement of impaired driving laws in the United States. *Surgeon General's workshop on drunk driving: Background papers* (pp. 136–156). Rockville, MD: U.S. Department of Health and Human Services.

Voas, R. B., Rhodenizer, A. E., & Lynn, L. (1985). *Evaluation of Charlottesville checkpoint operations.* Technical Report Contract No. DTNH 2283605088. Washington, DC: National Highway Traffic Safety Administration.

Waganaar, A. C. (1983). *Alcohol, young drivers, and traffic accidents.* Lexington, MA: Lexington Books.

Waksberg, J. (1978). Sampling methods for random digit dialing. *Journal of the American Statistical Association, 73,* 40–46.

Waller, J. (1985). *Injury control: A guide to the causes and prevention of trauma* (pp. 18–24). Lexington, MA: Lexington Books.

Williams, A. F. (1987). Effective and ineffective policies for reducing injuries associated with youthful drivers. *Alcohol, Drugs, and Driving, 3,* 109–118.

Williams, A. F., & Lund, A. K. (1987). Teenage driver licensing in relation to state laws. *Accident Analysis and Prevention, 17,* 135–145.

Williams, A. F., & Lund, A. K. (1988). Mandatory seat belt use laws and occupant crash protection in the United States: Present status and future prospects. In J. Graham (Ed.), *Preventing automobile injury* (pp. 51–72). Dover, MA: Auburn House.

Williams, A. F., Lund, A. K., Pruesser, D. F., & Blomberg, R. D. (1987). Results of seat belt law enforcement and publicity campaign in Elmyra, New York. *Accident Analysis and Prevention, 19,* 243–249.

Williams, A. F., Zador, P. L., Harris, S. S., & Karpf, R. S. (1983). The effect of raising the legal minimum drinking age on involvement in fatal crashes. *Journal of Legal Studies, 12,* 169–179.

Wintemute, G. (1990). Childhood drowning and near drowning in the United States. *American Journal of Diseases in Children, 144,* 663–669.

World Health Organization (1980). *Technical group psycho-social factors related to accidents in childhood and adolescence.* Copenhagen: World Health Organization Regional Office for Europe.

Zador, P., Lund, A., Fields, M., & Weinberg, K. (1989). Fatal crash involvement and laws against alcohol impaired drivers. *Journal of Public Health Policy, 10,* 467–485.

COMMENTARY ON PART II

Topical Areas of
Interest for Promoting Health:
From the Perspective
of the Physician

Charles E. Irwin

Chapters 8 to 14 of this book highlight the critical problems confronting adolescents today and raise the complex issues involved in studying or trying to understand health-related behaviors. The authors note that each system that interacts with adolescents (school, health clinics, drug stores, restaurants, churches, transit systems) needs to assume responsibility for the health of our youth. Efforts must be broad-based, with the assistance of regulating agencies and clinicians. For example, in the State of California during the 1990's, there is a major effort to change the social environment regarding tobacco use through laws that restrict access to cigarette machines and prohibit smoking in all public places.

Efforts also require the participation of individuals who come into contact with adolescents. Clinicians often feel they are impotent in dealing with health promotion and disease prevention in adolescents (Report of the U.S. Preventive Services Task Force, 1989). Clinical training in the health sciences (except for nursing) focuses on the diagnostic assessment of disease processes and the treatment of those processes. Few physicians receive training in health promotion per se. In addition, the difficulty in showing the effectiveness of preventive services in brief clinical encounters may lead physicians to feel that their efforts are futile. Yet if the physician does not ask adolescents about their health-related behaviors, does this support adolescents' assumptions that the behaviors are relatively low in risk? For example, when clinicians fail to ask about cigarette smoking, does this convey the notion that cigarette smoking does not have a negative effect on the young person's health? By asking about the young person's behaviors and intentions, the physician is behaving in a manner that is consistent with an entire health-promoting environment, which may enhance the effects of the current antismoking climate.

To help clinicians develop appropriate preventive strategies, professional organizations have issued guidelines for clinical encounters. For example, the American

Academy of Pediatrics recommends four office preventive visits in addition to sick care visits for adolescents between 13 and 20 years of age (1988). These guidelines provide the framework for what to query or screen for at specific chronological ages. The American Medical Association (AMA) is developing a specific set of guidelines for adolescent preventive services (Guidelines for Adolescent Preventive Services) with greater attention to health promotion than we have seen in previous reports (AMA, 1992).

In 1989, the National Cancer Institute developed a program for physicians to help patients stop smoking; these activities include four recommendations beginning with A's: ASK, ADVISE, ASSIST, AND ARRANGE for follow-up (Glynn & Manley, 1989). A recent article by Epps and Manely (1991) has added a fifth A: ANTICIPATORY GUIDANCE. Utilizing these five A's may also serve as an effective outline for health promotion activities during adolescence.

ANTICIPATORY GUIDANCE: To be effective with adolescents, a trusting and meaningful relationship needs to be established at entry into adolescence. This relationship is not established in one brief encounter, but rather over a series of visits. Clinicians and other adults need to be willing to listen to adolescents' concerns and issues. Clinicians need to be aware that some behaviors are more prevalent at certain times during adolescence, some of which may be gender-specific. For example, females will often initiate dieting behavior with the onset of puberty and the associated increase in the amount of adipose tissue; males may experiment with dangerous athletic activities to check out their physical prowess as rapid growth in muscle mass takes place toward the completion of puberty (Millstein et al., 1992). Adolescents with fewer economic and social resources and poor mental health may be more likely to proceed along a trajectory of increasing problems (Brindis, Irwin & Millstein, 1992). Additional supervision and support may need to be provided for these groups of adolescents.

ASK: Query adolescents about their present and future behavior. Ask adolescents about their intentions over the next several months (Irwin & Millstein, 1991). In this repertoire of questions, do not focus only on health-damaging behaviors but ask about what they are doing to stay healthy, what they are doing in their leisure time, and what they are doing to feel good about themselves.

ADVISE: Most adolescents do not ask for advice. It is developmentally inconsistent for early and middle adolescents to ask for advice from authority figures. Therefore, education programs are especially effective at this time, since the peer group generally establishes the norms during middle adolescence. Peer education programs need access to information regarding health. Clinicians may want to serve as advisers to these programs and even utilize peers in clinical settings for information gathering and giving.

ASSIST: Assist adolescents in staying healthy by encouraging their participation in programs that promote skill development in problem solving, decision making, and encouraging positive peer communication and interaction.

ARRANGE: Arrange a follow-up visit with the young person to see how things are going. Keep connected with adolescents in a society in which social connections and interactions with adults are diffuse and minimum at best. The clinical encounter may be the only time that an adolescent has a responsible adult that listens to him or her.

Health Promotion at Every Encounter

Throughout this part of the book, chapter authors have focused on a specific problem, placing it in the context of health promotion. Yet adolescents rarely present to the clinician with these defined problems. Perhaps, then, it would be useful to consider health promotion in the same way that we view the delivery of health services: primary care, secondary care, and tertiary care (Irwin & Shafer, 1992). The reason for organizing promotion in this framework is to put the construct of health promotion into every interaction with the adolescent, whether it be in the health care delivery system (emergency room, hospital inpatient care, outpatient clinic), the school, or the community center. This approach has not been evaluated and its effectiveness is still uncertain. However, it would provide an opportunity to begin to measure where and what type of health promotion given by whom is most effective.

Primary Health Promotion

Primary health promotion focuses on the entire population of children in late childhood as they enter adolescence. The major goal at this point is to encourage healthy habits by fostering positive physical, social, and cognitive development. For example, sexuality would be discussed in elementary school as a normal component of science; injury prevention and violence resolution would be discussed as normative activities for playing on the playground at recess. Other forms of safety might be discussed in social science classes that would focus on the community. Since older children and adolescents often have to use some form of transportation to get to and from school, injury behavior and violence prevention lend themselves to discussion at this developmental transition. As children enter pubescence, there would be greater emphasis on the physiological functioning of males and females and the emotional responses to physical functioning (Ryan, Millstein, & Irwin, 1988; Shore, 1984). This material could be covered in either science classes or specific family life classes.

Included in these primary promotion campaigns would be a major effort to encourage family members and responsible adults (teachers, coaches, and other community leaders) to behave in a consistently healthy manner: exercising, using seat belts, wearing helmets while riding bicycles, not drinking alcohol or using substances before swimming, quitting smoking, and responsible alcohol use.

These primary promotion campaigns would also encourage communities to develop programs to facilitate healthy development: cleaning up playgrounds, doing a safety inspection of the equipment at playgrounds for younger children and themselves, developing bicycle lanes, providing free bicycle helmets for those adolescents unable to afford the necessary safety equipment, and establishing exercise programs at community centers, religious centers, or schools.

Clinicians would incorporate into their practices primary promotion that would focus on anticipating pubertal change and its physical and psychosocial effects. Since clinical encounters are private, the clinician will be able to gear each session to the individual adolescent's maturational process.

Secondary Health Promotion

Since a significant number of adolescents will engage in health-compromising behaviors, secondary promotion is the next most critical area to address. Secondary promotion begins early in adolescence with the onset of puberty, most often during the transition to middle school or late in elementary school. The major focus of secondary health promotion is to prevent the negative outcomes of the behaviors that are initiated during adolescence (e.g., injuries from substance abuse and sexually transmitted diseases and pregnancy from sexual behaviors). Critical demographic variables (age, gender, race, ethnicity, economic status) need to be considered in the development of secondary health promotion. Secondary health promotion anticipates that many of these behaviors will be initiated during adolescence, and it is the responsibility of the community to provide information and opportunities for the adolescents to delay the onset of these behaviors and minimize the negative health outcomes once the behaviors are initiated.

Within the school setting, science classes may want to focus on the physiological effects of health-promoting and -damaging behaviors; reproductive and sexual functioning; and changes in thought processes and thinking. Physician education classes in schools, community agencies, or religious organizations may want to focus on physical functioning as well as safety.

Within the clinical setting, each clinical encounter needs to explore health-damaging and -promoting behaviors. Since males will have infrequent visits in clinical settings, one may want to focus on injuries and sexual behavior, since these are the behaviors that have the most negative health outcomes.

Tertiary Health Promotion

Tertiary health promotion involves preventing further morbidity and mortality in adolescents who have experienced negative outcomes associated with health-damaging behaviors. Most of the time, tertiary health promotion occurs within the clinical setting. However, schools and places of employment may enhance or may identify the health-damaging effects before the adolescent makes it to the clinical encounter. For example, a teacher or employer may notice that a young person smokes cigarettes, or appears to be sad or tired, and might encourage the young person to seek help. School-based clinics can provide an important avenue of access in these situations.

Within the clinical setting, the clinician will need to recognize the importance of covariation of behaviors (e.g., substance use and sexual behavior). Confining the evaluation to the most obvious behavior and ignoring the other highly related behavior may place the adolescent at risk for a more immediate negative health outcome.

The dilemma in health promotion at the tertiary level is: how much. The reality is that every clinical visit in a disease-oriented encounter should be an encounter in which the young person learns something more about the self. The clinician needs to do both: to treat the patient and then to explore how the young person may prevent the outcome from happening again.

Conclusions

Throughout this book, the authors have highlighted what we need to do to expand the science of health promotion. It is critical, however, that the limitation of our current science base not dictate whether we begin to develop and implement health promotion activities for adolescents. The future needs to be one in which we make health promotion a critical component of all clinical encounters and proceed to assess the mechanisms by which it works, under which conditions, in which settings, and for whom.

References

American Academy of Pediatrics (1988). *Committee on psychosocial aspects of child and family health. Guidelines for health Supervision II.* Elk Grove Village, IL: American Academy of Pediatrics.

American Medical Association (1992). *Guidelines for Adolescent Preventive Services.* Chicago, IL: American Medical Association.

Brindis, C., Irwin, C. E., Jr., & Millstein, S. G. (1992). United States Profile. In E. McAnarney, R. Kreipe, D. Orr, & G. Comerci (Eds.), *Textbook of adolescent medicine* (pp. 12–27). Philadelphia: W. B. Saunders.

Epps, R. P., & Manley, M. W. (1991, August). Physician's guide to preventing tobacco use. *Pediatrics, 88,* 140–144.

Glynn, T. J., & Manley, M. W. (1989). *How to help your patients stop smoking.* A National Cancer Institute manual for physicians. NIH Publication No. 89-3064. Bethesda, MD: U.S. Department of Health and Human Services, Public Health Service, National Cancer Institute.

Irwin, C. E., Jr., & Millstein, S. G. (1991). Correlates and predictors of risk taking behaviors during adolescence. In L. Lipsitt & L. Mitnick (Eds.), *Self-regulatory behavior and risk taking behavior: Causes and consequences* (pp. 3–21). Norwood, NJ: Ablex Publishing Corporation.

Irwin, C. E., Jr., & Shafer, M.A.B. (1992). Adolescent sexuality: Negative outcomes of a normative behavior. In D. E. Rogers, & E. Ginzberg (Eds.), *Adolescents at risk: Medical and social perspectives* (pp. 35–79). Boulder, CO: Westview Press.

Millstein, S. G., Irwin, C. E., Jr., Adler N. E., Kegeles, S. G., Cohn, L., & Dolcini, P. (1992). Health risk behaviors and health concerns among young adolescents. *Pediatrics, 3,* 422–428.

Report of the U.S. Preventive Services Task Force (1989). *Guide to clinical preventive services.* Baltimore: Williams and Wilkins.

Ryan, S., Millstein, S. G., & Irwin, C. E., Jr. (1988). Pubertal concerns in young adolescents. *Journal of Adolescent Health Care, 9,* 267.

Shore, L. (1984). Experience of puberty development. *Social Science and Medicine, 19,* 461–465.

Topical Areas of Interest for Promoting Health: From the Perspective of a Nurse

Jeanette M. Broering

In reading these chapters, which reflect various topical areas of interest for health promotion, I am impressed with the researchers' ability to clarify and describe comprehensive approaches within individual domains such as positive mental health, sexual well-being, or optimal oral health. Yet, across these diverse areas, integration is not complete. In addition, the various disciplines lack the necessary consensus to formulate a master strategy for optimal, comprehensive, and developmentally focused health promotion programs for youth. In particular, we see a need for programs that are practice oriented and incorporate essential life experiences.

In the varied topography of professional practice, there is a high ground overlooking a swamp. On the high ground, manageable problems lend themselves to solution through the application of research-based theory and technique. In the swampy lowland, messy, confusing problems defy technical solution. The irony of this situation is that the problems of the high ground tend to be relatively unimportant to individuals or society at large, however great their technical interest may be, while in the swamp lie the problems of greatest human concern. The practitioner must choose. Shall he remain on the high ground where he can solve relatively unimportant problems according to prevailing standards of rigor, or shall he descend to the swamp of important problems of nonrigorous inquiry? (Schon, 1990, p. 3)

This professional practice dilemma of rigor versus relevance aptly describes the daily environment in which health care practitioners live and work. Operating in the trenches of health care, decisions are made daily in the "indeterminate, swampy zones of practice" out of the necessity to formulate a plan of action, often without the benefit of the most recent research findings or strategies that might remedy a particular health care problem (Schon, 1990).

Clinicians by nature are action-oriented, savvy, reflective professionals; however, when confronted with the complexities of health-related problems and the enormous impact of the environmental context, they often feel stymied in their ability to effect positive change. For example, a 17-year-old female presents to our university-based clinic for evaluation and appropriate treatment of a urinary tract infection after being seen 24 hours prior to this visit in a local emergency room for the same complaint. "The medicine they gave me wasn't working," she told the nurse. Upon entering the exam room, I observe an old resolving bruise above her left eye. When asked "Who hit you?" she reveals that the bruise occurred as the result of having been hit in the face with a gun during a street fight 2 weeks ago by a male friend who was high on cocaine at the time. She states that the injury is "no big deal" since the bruises are almost gone. While I can correct the bladder infection, I'm not so certain about the violence. What has the greatest potential for ending her life? Certainly not the bladder infection. This scenario is all too frequent. An individual seeks out the health care system for an acute, episodic complaint while unveiling an equally compelling issue that will directly influence his or her overall health status.

Three issues illustrated in this case vignette deserve further inquiry. What internal and external conditions exist that target this adolescent as a victim of violence? How is she able to experience such violence and, at the same time, maintain a restricted perspective limited to defining its meaning in the most superficial and transient terms of the bruise? What internal and external forces exist that allow for the limitation in strategies by which to avoid a potentially negative outcome? Are these research questions areas of inquiry to be understood prior to clinical intervention or both? It is at this crossroad that the intersection of research and clinical practice occurs. What are the common areas around which researchers and clinicians can begin to coalesce as they strive to build a health agenda that incorporates constructs of wellness promotion and prevention strategies? By what process should that occur? What disciplines are essential during the development phase? The overarching contextual issues for planning should include consolidation and collaboration from all perspectives of policy development, research, clinical practice, and service delivery models.

As a nation, we have no health policy or definition of optimal health for all Americans. At best, we have a mechanism for financial reimbursement that is unequally distributed among various sectors of our population. This absence of a "philosophy of health" translates into a payment system that reimburses for illness care but often does not cover health promotion or disease prevention programs. Proximal to the adolescent and in need of more development within these topical areas is the involvement of family, parents, and peers that will define community-based health values with respect to culture, lifestyle, class, and unique geographic issues. Before we are able to move into a planning mode, it is essential that a dialogue occur that defines the value of optimal health and incorporates the entire spectrum of parties and persons relevant to determining the social and cultural values of health promotion.

Acknowledgments

During the preparation of this commentary, the author was supported in part by a grant from the Bureau of Maternal and Child Health and Resources Development (MCJ 000978A).

Reference

Schon, D. A. (1990). *Educating the reflective practitioner: Toward a new design for teaching and learning in the professions.* San Francisco: Jossey-Bass Higher Education Series.

PART III

The Future of Adolescent Health Promotion: Next Steps

15

From Causal Description to Causal Explanation: Improving Three Already Good Evaluations of Adolescent Health Programs

Thomas D. Cook, Amy R. Anson,
and Suzanne Walchli

Our Purposes and a Peek at the Conclusions

This chapter is about evaluating the quality of evaluations done in adolescent health. As such, it is an attempt at metaevaluation (Cook & Gruder, 1978). A crucial concern in all evaluative activities is to specify and justify the criteria by which judgments of quality are made. In evaluating evaluations of adolescent health programs, we distinguish three such criteria: How justified are inferences about program effectiveness, about the nature of the program activities actually implemented, and about the reasons why particular program effects do or do not come about?

Effectiveness Criteria

Klein, Kotelchuck, and DeFriese (1990) have concluded that few adolescent health programs are formally evaluated and that those that are tend to be evaluated so poorly that no clear picture of their effectiveness can be gained. Though this may be the general state of the art in adolescent health evaluation, Hamburg (1990) discovered three programs that seem to have been evaluated well in the sense that changes were observed in adolescents and from the evidence presented it seems reasonable to conclude that these changes would not have occurred without the program. These are the standards generally used to claim that a relationship is descriptively causal even in the absence of full knowledge of all the contingencies which explain why the relationship occurs (Mackie, 1974).

One purpose of this chapter is to take the three evaluations that Hamburg has described and to probe her judgment about their adequacy for drawing conclusions about program effectiveness—conclusions that require an inference about causal description. We will conclude that her judgment is in general borne out by the evidence we review, though we do discuss a few ways in which each of the studies might have been improved at the margin in order to arrive at even stronger inferences about program effectiveness.

It is important to learn about program effects because the public rationale for programs is that they change adolescents' lives in ways that our society generally considers to be beneficial. To remain ignorant about impacts is, therefore, to betray a public trust. This is particularly true when programs are mature and have overcome their initial teething problems. No social program is ever fixed; each is continuously evolving as it seeks to make accommodations to new realities. But the process of accommodation is more chaotic early in the institutional learning curve of a program, reducing the relevance of outcome assessment early in a program's history.

Assessing program effects is also important because it provides some of the knowledge required for transferring a program to new sites and new populations of persons. Each site and population is unique, and so transfer can never be taken for granted. But what is the use of transferring a program to new settings if its effectiveness is still unexplored and hence in doubt? Surely one wants to transfer only programs that have been rigorously evaluated and shown to be effective.

Unfortunately, many evaluations point to the conclusion that a program is ineffective. While studies with this result are hardly ever used to eliminate a program, they are used more often to justify marginal decreases in program budgets and shifts in a program's priorities (Weiss, 1977). It would be disastrous if such important actions were taken on the basis of evaluation results that erroneously indicated that nothing positive was happening to adolescents because of a program. We need just as convincing evidence of program ineffectiveness as effectiveness—and across as wide a wide range of relevant outcomes.

Implementation Criteria

Evaluations that only describe the causal consequences of a program run the risk of being "black box" studies. They do not inform us about how well a program has been implemented or about how different levels of implementation relate to changes in adolescent health. All conceptualizations of implementation are predicated on a description of program activities, particularly to check on whether those activities built into the original program design actually occurred at local sites. Good implementation analysis requires a clear, substantive theory of the program under evaluation, and this theory should specify the components that have to be present for effects to occur. These components then have to be measured so as to assess whether they were in place in the program in the form and quantity expected. Also required for a comprehensive implementation analysis is some description of the quality and appropriateness of program services. All services should be tailored to the demonstrated needs of specific target populations and should be potentially as good as the best services specified by the professional state of the art of the day. At a minimum, no services should be included in the program that responsible professionals know to be ineffective. No explication of implementation can be restricted to the availability and quality of planned program components. Unexpected events always happen in the life of any program and can influence the pattern of results obtained. These events also need to be documented and, where possible, related to the size of any changes observed in adolescent health outcomes.

Later in this chapter we judge Hamburg's three evaluations according to the implementation criteria above, and we conclude that the studies varied considerably in how well implementation was assessed and how well implementation data were related to outcome levels. But some limitations were common across all three evaluations. In none of them were implementation criteria assigned anywhere near the same importance as adolescent outcome criteria, and in none of them did the quality of implementation assessment in control groups match that in intervention groups.

This last criticism might seem misplaced, given that the services in intervention groups are of special policy importance, and the rationale for experimentation calls for them to be different from what is found in no-treatment control groups. Why, then, assess such controls by the same implementation criteria used in intervention groups? Control groups never involve no treatment; some things always takes place between the pretest and posttest that might affect the major outcome variables. Moreover, adolescents and their teachers and health care providers do not postpone all ameliorative activities simply because an adolescent serves in an experimental control group. Indeed, they may be stimulated to do more than they would otherwise have done *because* they know the adolescents are serving in a control group (Cook & Campbell, 1979). Also, treatment components from experimental sites are often incorporated into control sites, either through a process of deliberate imitation or because particular treatment components just happen to be fashionable in a particular profession at a particular time (Cook & Campbell, 1979). Finally—and most important of all—in experimental evaluations like those that Hamburg discussed, the causal agent under analysis is always a *contrast* between what occurs in the treatment and control groups (Cronbach, 1982). Without describing what happens in the control group, there can be no adequate description of this contrast and hence of the causal agent that is actually under evaluation.

Assessing implementation is also important for reasons of public policy. Without knowledge of implementation, it will be well-nigh impossible to determine which program components are more and less important in bringing about effects, making it all the more difficult to streamline programs so that their beneficial components are highlighted and their ineffective ones eliminated. Implementation also has implications for program transfer. Unless the effect-producing components are present in transfer attempts, effects are not likely to be re-created in new settings. Experience with program evaluation in many sectors teaches us that most effects are modest in size and much smaller than program developers claim. This should not come as a surprise. Most programs target social problems that have proven to be refractory in the immediate past, and with our current ideas and resources we simply do not know how to solve them. If we did, they would already be solved and there would be little need for our programs. If it is realistic to expect only modest effects, this underscores the need to use implementation data in subanalyses that explicitly relate variation in the size of an effect to sources of variability in implementation at the site, respondent, or treatment provider level. Effects are most to be expected in contexts where implementation quality is highest, and without tests of this hypothesis we cannot know whether any overall lack of effectiveness is due to poor program theory, to poor implementation of the program particulars, or to an evaluation design that is too insensitive to detect small effects.

Explanatory Criteria

Relating variability in implementation quality to individual-level outcomes goes some way toward explaining why effects come about. But the explanatory factors involved are related to program components and unexpected perturbations from the world outside the program. They do not include explanatory factors having to do with many other individual and social processes that occur after an intervention is in place and before the major outcomes of policy importance have changed. To provide just one example of the latter type of explanation, in a successful drug abuse prevention program it might be possible to describe the temporal process of causal influence as beginning with the implementation of some program activities that then cause changes in health professionals' beliefs about their personal efficacy to influence adolescents. These then lead to changes in adolescents' beliefs about their own efficacy to say "no" to peers who want to initiate them into drugs, and to changes in the peer groups adolescents hang around with. This last factor then leads to variation in the ultimate criterion—abstinence from using illicit substances. This particular example is of a linear causal model involving five constructs, three of which are mediational—the changes in professionals' and adolescents' self-efficacy and the change in peer group affiliation. More complex relationships can also be postulated, of course. But whatever the explanation offered, the concern is always the same: to develop and test one or more substantive theories that might plausibly explain why or how a program is effective in influencing adolescent health.

Explanation is important in program evaluation because it identifies the processes that must be stimulated for effectiveness to occur. Once these processes are known, it should then be possible to set them in motion in many ways, without being limited to the particular way the processes were set in motion in past studies (Cronbach, 1982). Indeed, local practitioners should be able to instantiate the processes in ways that are tailored to the particulars of their own work settings; they need not try to copy program particulars from elsewhere. This is a desirable state of affairs in the United States, where most local programs have considerable discretion about program design and where there is little oversight other than financial. In this view, explanatory knowledge helps local practitioners decide for themselves how they should set in motion the causal processes believed to be responsible for the beneficial treatment effects demonstrated elsewhere. Understanding how or why things happen is the goal of basic science, of course, and this goal is usually justified on the grounds that explanatory knowledge will lead to unanticipated practical uses in many contexts, some unimaginable at present. The budget of the National Aeronautics and Space Administration, for example, is routinely justified this way, reflecting the same transfer rationale offered to justify an emphasis on explanation in evaluation.

But how is explanation achieved? Some attempts at explanation in the social and health sciences seek only to identify predictors of program effectiveness. No weight is attached to conceptualizing these predictors as moderator or mediator variables or to otherwise fit them into substantive theoretical frameworks. At most there is a practical emphasis on examining predictors of treatment dosage levels, or on examining the person, setting, and time factors that condition the size of a relationship. We call this the *variance accounted-for* approach to explanation, since it seeks only to predict variability with outcomes. The origins of this approach are ultimately in positivism, with its emphasis on prediction as the ultimate criterion of knowledge growth (Bridgman, 1927).

A second approach to explanation is more theory-dependent and reductionistic. It requires explicit causal models that specify (1) those treatment components from the multidimensional interventions that influence an outcome; (2) those outcome components that vary with the treatment; and especially it requires specifying (3) those mediating processes that occur after a treatment has varied and before an effect is observed (Bhaskar, 1975). Such causal models are typically path-analytic in form, as with the earlier example of program activities that influence practitioners' self-efficacy, then adolescents' self-efficacy to resist persuasion attempts, and then the adolescents' choice of friendship groups prior to reducing drug use. Many plausible causal models can usually be invoked to explain the effects of any program (Glymour, Sprites, & Scheines, 1987), and any one model can be reformulated to reflect finer differentiations of a specific process, resulting in more boxes and arrows connecting these boxes—the typical way process models are displayed. We call this the *mediational* approach to explanation because it depends so heavily on determining which intervening factors are responsible for the demonstrated link between a global intervention and an outcome.

The third approach to explanation we call the *correspondence* approach. It does not attempt to conceptualize and measure directly the mediating causal processes. Instead, it strives to achieve manipulations of the causal agent and measures of the outcome that closely correspond with substantive theoretical constructs that have implications for explaining a wide range of phenomena. Most laboratory research subscribes to this theory of explanation, relying on manipulations and outcome measures to achieve explanatory knowledge. But as Popper (1959) makes clear, it is crucial to probe a set of theory-derived hypotheses that speak to the theory's most central and unique postulates, and not just any hypotheses. This is true whether the explanatory theory is about natural selection, gravity, DNA, adolescence, social norms, life skills, or any other causal "generative powers" (Harre & Madden, 1975). The crucial assumptions in this black box theory of explanation are not just those that Kuhn (1962) has emphasized in his critique: namely, the need for both a totally explicit, substantive theory and observations that are theory-neutral, but also (1) the treatment and the outcome measures have to correspond with the cause and effect constructs specified in the explanatory theory from which the hypotheses under test were selected, and (2) these cause–effect relationships have to assess validly what is novel and effect-generating about the substantive theory under test.

The evaluations that Hamburg judged to be exemplary by the effectiveness criteria she emphasized turn out to vary both in the emphasis given to explanation and in the approach to explanation implicitly used, though the correspondence approach is most prevalent. However, none of the evaluations we examine is good at probing explanation, whatever the approach. We suspect that the explanatory models developed in adolescent health evaluations, and the methods used to test them, are behind the state of the art in other social sciences. This may be due to several factors over and above the difficulties inherent in testing any explanatory proposition in human research: first, there is the low level of substantive theory available in the health promotion field; second, there is the primacy accorded to effectiveness over explanatory criteria in evaluative health studies, given current fashion and the logical need to determine that there is an effect before learning why it occurs; and third, there are the many practical difficulties that arise when collecting high-quality process data on a large number of potential explanatory factors at different times between when an independent variable is manipulated and outcomes are measured. Whatever the reasons, the best evaluations in adolescent health seem to do a much better job of describing program effectiveness than of explaining it, and of documenting program implementation rather than relating program quality to student outcomes.

Contextualizing Our Evaluative Criteria

We have to be mindful of certain realities when criticizing research on adolescent health programs. One is that health research in general places a very high premium on experiments, and the structure of experimentation evolved to answer questions about causal description rather than implementation or explanation (Boring, 1954). It is true that measures of explanation and implementation can—and should—be added to experimental frameworks. It is also true that some experiments without intervening measures are explanatory in the sense that the treatments and outcomes have been validly deduced from a broad, substantive theory that claims to explain particular phenomena. But such explanation is rarely convincing in program evaluation because the interventions under test are usually multidimensional and have been selected for the likelihood of creating an impact on hard-to-change health outcomes rather than for their correspondence with substantive theory. Thus, more progress is to be expected from adding implementation and explanatory measures to experiments than from the way treatments and outcomes are selected.

But to add measures of implementation and explanation incurs costs. Some costs are financial. But others occur because process measurement is likely to be obtrusive and requires a level of thought and energy that cannot therefore be devoted to answering descriptive causal questions about effects. And why should these costs be incurred? What is the purpose of using resources to explain an effect of which one is not sure, or of learning how well a program is implemented if it might be ineffectual and so not worth implementing elsewhere? Such reasonable-sounding arguments place a much higher value on describing effectiveness than on studying implementation or explanation, suggesting that the costs of such study may not be worthwhile.

Added to this is the reality that experiments are imperfect vehicles for probing issues of effectiveness, even if they are better than all the available alternatives. Because of differential attrition from treatment groups, randomization is often not maintained over time even if it is initially achieved. Sometimes, there is contamination from one treatment group to another. Also, the samples lending themselves to experimental study are sometimes composed of volunteers or are otherwise unrepresentative of meaningful populations. Experimental results can also take so long to generate that they arrive too late to be useful in the policy world. And when they enter that world, they are usually treated as controversial rather than as the nuggets of truth their advocates hoped to deliver to the debate. Finally, it should be noted that experimentation evolved to mirror an abstract theory of rational choice that is empirically not warranted in its entirety. That is, treatments are supposed to represent the options among which a policy choice is to be made; the outcome variables are supposed to represent the criteria by which the decision is to be made; and the data collection and statistical analysis procedures are supposed to represent the empirical inputs that indicate which choice is optimal and so should be made. But the policy world is rarely rational in this sense. Instead, actors in that world pursue a rationality that is designed not to make the best technical decision from an array of plausible alternatives, but to protect their jobs and agency budgets and to promote their ideologies. Political criteria seem to inform their decisions at least as much as technical criteria. One has to wonder not only whether the experiment is as effective for learning about descriptive causation as its advocates claim, but also whether it might have some negative side effects or be particularly unsuited to the more political information needs of the policy-shaping community.

Thoughts like these have led social scientists from many disciplines to abandon experimental models of evaluation and to call instead for qualitative evaluations that are designed to uncover—or answer—questions about implementation or explanation rather than questions about causal description (Atkisson, Hargreaves, Horowitz, & Sorensen, 1978; Britan, 1978; Ciarlo & Reihman, 1977; Eisner, 1985; Fetterman, 1988; Guba & Lincoln, 1981; Heckman & Hotz, 1989; House, 1980; Manski, in press; Patton, 1980, 1988; Stake, 1980; Wholey, 1979). We have some sympathy with these critics of an experimental approach to evaluation. But this chapter is nonetheless designed to explore how we can conduct experimental evaluations that provide good (but still imperfect) answers to questions about program effectiveness, as well as useful information about both implementation and explanation. It is this multiplicity of purposes (Cook, 1985) that motivates our attempt to evaluate the best adolescent health evaluations in terms of a broader range of criteria than those used either by Hamburg or by the original evaluators she cited.

It is not that implementation and explanation issues are totally absent from the three studies Hamburg identified. But they are relatively neglected, and the best study for implementation purposes turned out to be the worst for causal explanation, while the best evaluation from the standpoint of causal explanation turned out to be the worst for implementation. We want to see more adolescent health evaluations conducted that responsibly explore how well a treatment has been implemented, how effective it was, and how the size of the effects relates to the quality of implementation. We also want to see evaluations that probe which of several different causal models of process offers the best explanation of effectiveness. We realize the difficulties of trying to develop high-quality information on all three criteria and their interrelationships, but we persist in believing that more can be done on all three fronts without compromising the quality of information about program effectiveness that our very best studies in adolescent health now achieve.

In what follows, we examine the three studies Hamburg identified as exemplary by effectiveness criteria and we (1) probe how well this judgment is merited; (2) describe how implementation was studied and might have been studied better; and (3) examine how treatment effects were explained and how these explanations could have been improved. We close with some general conclusions.

The School Health Education Evaluation

The School Health Education Evaluation (SHEE) was commissioned to evaluate the School Health Curriculum Project (SHCP), a widely used health instruction program sponsored by the Centers for Disease Control. The aim was to contrast SHCP with three other promising curricula: (1) the Health Education Curriculum Guide (HECG), sponsored by the Stark County (Ohio) United Way Foundation; (2) Project Prevention, founded in the Chenowith, Oregon, School District; and (3) Reading, 'Riting, 'Rithmetic and High Blood Pressure (3Rs and HBP), sponsored by the Georgia Affiliate of the American Heart Association.

The SHEE study was conducted by Abt Associates. Data collection took place from 1982 to 1984, and the results are reported in Connell, Turner, Mason, and Olsen (1986). A total of 1,071 classrooms (grades 4–7) in 20 states participated in the evaluation, with 688 of them receiving one of the four health education programs and the other 388 serving as local controls for one of the programs. Pre- and postprogram measures were taken of students' health knowledge (both general and program-specific), and also of their attitudes and reported health practices. Though random assignment did not take place, analyses with considerable statistical power indicated that at the pretest no program reliably differed from its control in health-relevant knowledge, attitudes, or reported practices.

Among the knowledge claims made in the SHEE evaluation were that (1) participants in each school health curriculum did better than its own controls on general and program-specific knowledge, attitudes, and reported practices; (2) at 1 year, effects were stronger for knowledge than for attitudes and reported practices; (3) implementation was measured as the number of hours of instruction, the percentage of curriculum activities completed, and the adherence of instruction to the original program plan, and for each program higher-quality implementation was associated with improvements in all outcomes; (4) programs with a more comprehensive curriculum achieved larger and more generalized gains in the first year; (5) 2 years of SHCP increased the size and generalization of effects; but (6) no program was more cost-effective than any other when the size of achieved effects was related to the instructional time the program required.

How Good Are the Descriptive Causal Conclusions About Program Effectiveness?

The SHEE was exemplary in controlling the threats to validity listed by Cook and Campbell (1979). For each program a pretest/posttest design was used, and no-treatment classrooms constituted the comparison group. Though there was no formal random assignment, matching occurred on many demographic attributes and pretest analyses showed no reliable differences between treatment and control classes. This was not an artifact of low statistical power, given the large sample of classes and the enhanced reliability that results when measures are aggregated to the classroom level. Thus, the classes adopting a health education program were not systematically different from the classes not adopting it. Moreover, for no program was there differential attrition relative to its own controls, suggesting that the treatment and comparison groups remained comparable over the course of the study. For these reasons, we judge that internal validity was not a problem with SHEE.

In terms of construct validity, multiple experts were used to design the outcome measurement instrument in intensive collaboration with program developers. Continuous monitoring also took place to guard against unanticipated treatment cross-overs, and parent and teacher reports were used to cross-validate student self-reports of health-relevant behaviors. Such procedures help promote the construct validity of both the treatment and the effect. The major remaining problem, as we see it, is that student self-reports of health behaviors in the treatment groups may have been biased by social desirability. The Abt researchers correlated students' self-reports with teacher and parent reports, but the correlations were low and in the major data analyses (discussed below) only students' reports were used. Additional analyses based on the adult data or a composite of both student and adult reports would have been desirable.

As far as external validity is concerned, the SHCP program is probably the most widely available health education program in the United States today. The evaluation team first stratified school districts and then selected some at random. Classrooms were next selected within districts, also at random. This is, of course, the recommended textbook procedure. The other programs were more regional, and so the selection of schools was more purposive. Across all four programs the achieved population underrepresents large urban school districts and Latino children, but it is nonetheless more heterogeneous in student attributes than adolescent health studies usually are. Indeed, when the evaluators profiled their achieved population relative to the national population of children in the target age range, a remarkable similarity emerged between the two on a large set of attributes. The scope of the SHEE evaluation is impressive, and the analyses of representativeness are exemplary.

How Good Was the Analysis of Implementation?

The starting point for any implementation assessment is a model of the intervention components and of the processes thought to bring about outcome changes. The Abt evaluators were most comprehensive and explicit on this score. The model, reproduced from Connell, Turner, Mason, and Olsen (1986), is illustrated in Figure 15.1. The sections labeled *program inputs, process,* and *context* are relevant to implementation, and within each, some lower-order variables are detailed. Under *input* these include the quantity and cost of teacher inservice training and the instructional methods and lesson plans used. Under *process* they include the number of hours of instruction and fidelity to the theory behind the program. Under *context* they include variables that might influence the quality of implementation (e.g., district fiscal and demographic characteristics and such classroom characteristics as grade level, number of students per classroom, and prior exposure to health programs).

The evaluators systematically used this model (1) to characterize the levels of implementation achieved and (2) to relate these levels to health outcomes. Important tables in the final research report describe how the four health education programs differed in training, hours of instruction, the percentage of planned program actually taught, and the fidelity of instruction to the program's philosophy. Also available are program-specific knowledge subscores that reflect the unique content actually taught in a particular program and an index of general knowledge based on the curriculum content shared by all the programs.

However, the Abt researchers presented no information on the health instruction received in control schools. Hence, we do not know whether the treatment and control classes differed in health education, and we cannot specify where such differences did or did not occur. Yet it is important to learn this. In a comparative evaluation like SHEE, we have to be able to assume that similar levels of spontaneous implementation occurred across the different control groups used with each program. If this assumption is not viable, conclusions cannot be drawn about which program was superior to any other. Rather than reflect programs that differ in effectiveness, program differences in *gains relative to their own controls* might reflect control groups that differ in the spontaneous availability of health-relevant information.

The Abt researchers related implementation to effect sizes in two ways. One was restricted to the first-year data, since the programs differed in the hours of instruction required. The data showed that programs with more class time produced larger effects. But many other things differed between programs, and no attempt

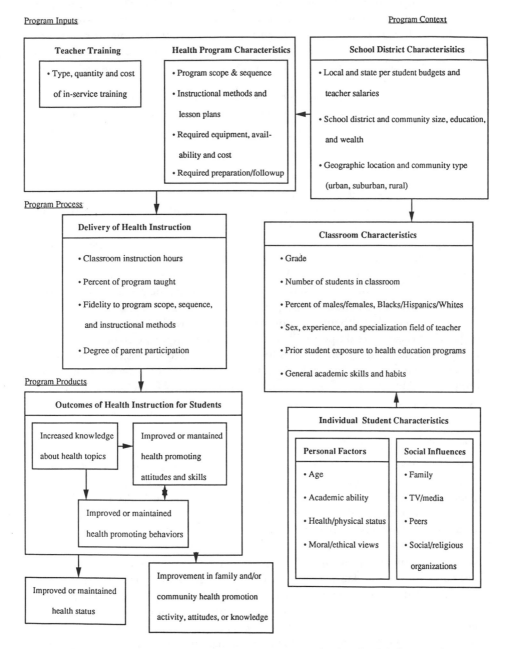

Figure 15.1. Depiction of the School Health Education Evaluation (SHEE): Intervention constructs and processes. (*Source:* Reproduced from Connell, Turner, Mason, & Olsen, 1986. School health education evaluation. *International Journal of Educational Research, 10,* p. 266.)

was made to identify them and deal with them statistically. This was probably because the major dosage analysis took another form, contrasting 1 versus 2 years of exposure to SHCP. Larger gains occurred in the 2-year classrooms for both attitude and reported behavior, implying that more instruction is needed for gains in dependent variables more removed from knowledge that is the principal component of the treatment.

The extended version of the SHEE report (Connell et al., 1986) presents correlations between implementation variables, pretest outcome variables, and residualized pretest–posttest gain scores. This was done to identify the specific implementation factors responsible for larger gains. But the analysis is not convincing. First, it is restricted to program classrooms, omitting the control classes that would have provided a greater range on the implementation predictor variables. Second, when data are combined across all four health education programs, the type of program and the level of implementation achieved are confounded, since programs differed from each other in resources, in the percentage of the total curriculum taught, and in the theoretical fidelity of what was taught. Third, simple bivariate analyses were carried out, though multivariate analyses would have been better to explore statistical interactions among the predictors and to examine process variables independently of context and input factors. Finally, the research report contains a number of puzzling and unexplained relationships—for example, previous exposure to school health information is initially negatively correlated with knowledge. The researchers' impetus to relate implementation to outcomes is praiseworthy; but the form of the analysis leaves something to be desired, as does the nonavailability of implementation data from the control groups. Otherwise, though, the Abt analyses of implementation are exemplary in technical quality and potential utility.

How Good Were the Analyses of Causal Explanation?

In terms of the correspondence approach to causal explanation, one strength of SHEE was its careful monitoring of the degree of correspondence between the planned curriculum content *as the program developers specified it* and the activities that actually took place. The high correspondence is illustrated by the fact that most of the explained variation in program effects was accounted for by the amount and fidelity of program implementation and by the unique priorities of each curriculum. Thus, Project Prevention, which emphasized decision-making and communications skills, achieved the greatest gains on items measuring just these constructs. Such correspondence suggests that it was the curriculum that caused the effects and not other components of the intervention. But since the evaluators presented no explicit substantive theory to justify any of the four interventions, there can be no question of demonstrating a high level of correspondence between a theory-based treatment and the activation of those mediational processes uniquely specified in the guiding theory.

The variance accounted-for approach to explanation seeks to increase prediction of a given health outcome. We have already seen how information about dosage levels was used to increase the prediction of outcomes, but also relevant are tests of whether a treatment effect depends on school or child-level moderator variables. Unfortunately, the Abt evaluators did not systematically examine whether the health program statistically interacts with such variables to enhance prediction. There are indeed analyses relating some of the potential moderators to residual gains. But these analyses leave out the controls, confound the program's with the moderator's variables, and combine all four programs rather than test each one singly. Thus, the SHEE evaluation does not provide us with a good example of the use of the prediction theory of explanation.

Turning to mediational approaches to explanation, Figure 15.1 represents a postulated chain of causal mediation from teacher training to changes in knowledge and attitude, and eventually to changes in physical health. But while it is a causal chain of value to practitioners, it says little about mediational processes at the individual or group level. Finally, the arrows in Figure 15.1 suggest that many contextual variables are presumed to interact with each other and with the treatment. Yet no substantive theory was advanced to explain these more complex relationships, nor were empirical analyses of them made. SHEE can be characterized as the typical practitioner's evaluation—long on measures of the fidelity of a program to its developer's plans but short on tests of the substantive theoretical links between an intervention and the outcome. SHEE was a pragmatic evaluation effort aimed more at legitimating health education and improving health education policy than at building theoretical knowledge.

Yet the SHEE evaluation is a first in evaluation. Conventional wisdom in evaluation holds that studies comparing multiple programs cannot be pulled off (Cronbach, 1982; Rivlin & Timpane, 1975). This is, first, because each program pursues unique goals and even those goals that seem to be shared turn out, on deeper analysis, to be subtly different (Cronbach et al., 1980). As a result, comparative evaluations seek to compare programs that their developers think are incommensurable, reducing whatever tenuous commitment to evaluation the developers may initially have had (Rivlin & Timpane, 1975). Second, the quality of implementation of a single program usually varies from classroom to classroom and from school to school. Indeed, in one famous comparative evaluation, the site-to-site variability for a single program was as great as the variability between different programs (Stebbins, St. Pierre, Proper, Anderson, & Cerva, 1978)! For both of these reasons, comparative studies are now downplayed in academic discussions of evaluation design. This is regrettable, since the need to choose between contending alternatives is omnipresent in social life, including public policy. According to Cook and Walberg (1985), SHEE avoided the above pitfalls (1) because of a long planning period during which each program developer's unique priorities and concerns were built into the overall study design; (2) because a common implementation metric was used to assess the implementation achieved and to relate it to the amount expected; and (3) because the written reports placed more emphasis on comparing each program with its own controls and on combining the data across all four programs than on presenting explicit contrasts between each of the four programs.

Botvin's Life Skills Training Program

The Life Skills Training program (LST) is a school-based smoking prevention program based on a theoretical analysis of the social and psychological factors believed to promote the onset of smoking among adolescents. It was primarily designed to provide young adolescents with the social and cognitive skills needed to resist peer and media influences and cope with life challenges during the preadolescent and adolescent years. The program is based on the premise that substance use is a "socially learned, and functional behavior which is . . . mediated by personal factors such as cognitions, attitudes, and beliefs" (Botvin & Tortu, 1988, p. 100).

Designed for seventh-grade students, LST was originally intended to prevent cigarette use only. But the program has sometimes been expanded to include the other "gateway" substances, alcohol and marijuana. It is taught in a specified sequence of 12 to 20 sessions covering five major components: (1) knowledge and information; (2) decision making and resistance to social influences promoting harmful substances; (3) self-directed behavior change; (4) techniques for coping with anxiety; and (5) social skills (i.e., communication skills, general interpersonal skills, and assertiveness). Botvin believes that these five components, when presented together, address the social and psychological factors that lead to smoking or other substance use.

Unlike the case with SHEE, Botvin explicitly draws upon substantive theories to explain the role that each program component plays in the overall LST strategy. He draws on Evans' (1976) social influence theory for part of the knowledge component, attributing the onset of adolescent cigarette smoking to information from peers and the media that inadvertently exaggerates the prevalence of smoking and the strength of social norms supporting it. Evans' theory also underlies the second component. Botvin assumes that students can be inoculated against social influences through awareness of peer and media pressures and by learning the social and cognitive skills necessary to resist peer pressure without becoming socially stigmatized. Communications theory (McGuire, 1964) has a role to play here by detailing both the declining acceptability of smoking and its physiological and health consequences. But Botvin creatively goes a step further, emphasizing the importance of transmitting information in ways that are appropriate to the developmental needs and capacities of adolescents. Particularly important for him in this regard is their "present-time" orientation, which weighs the perceived short-term benefits of substance use more heavily than any long-term negative consequence of such use (Botvin & Tortu, 1988).

The other three program components—self-directed behavior change, techniques for coping with anxiety, and social skills training—rely on social learning (Bandura, 1977) and problem behavior theory (Jessor & Jessor, 1977). These components distinguish LST as a skills training program designed to help students "not only resist the social influences associated with substance use, but also to teach them relatively general skills for coping with life that will have broad application rather than a situation-specific or problem-specific application" (Botvin, 1986, p. 371). To justify this last and general claim, Botvin cites findings that suggest that "differential susceptibility to social influence appears to be mediated by personality, with individuals who have low self-esteem, low self-confidence, low autonomy and an external locus of control being more likely to succumb to these influences" (Botvin, 1983, p. I-6). LST thus understands adolescents' use of tobacco or other substances as a way of coping with expected failure or social anxiety, or as a way to achieve popularity, social status or self-esteem, especially for youngsters not doing well academically. Thus, substance use becomes just an alternate route to fulfilling general adolescent needs for competence, belonging, and autonomy (Jessor, 1982).

LST is usually implemented by classroom teachers, but peer leaders have also been used. Training consists of a 1-day workshop covering the theory of the program and the skills students need to learn. Teachers or peer leaders are then provided with opportunities to practice the new teaching techniques and receive feedback and additional coaching (Tortu & Botvin, 1989). In addition to the basic seventh-grade program, Botvin and his colleagues have designed "booster" programs for eighth and ninth graders aimed at sustaining the initial program effects.

Early results from randomized experiments are impressive. Botvin, Eng, and Williams (1980) claim that there are 75% fewer new cigarette smokers among those receiving the intervention than among controls at the end of the program (and 67% fewer at 3-month follow-up (Botvin & Eng, 1982). When LST is used to prevent alcohol abuse, results at 9-month follow-up indicate that 54% fewer program students reported drinking during the past month compared to controls, that 73% fewer program students reported heavy drinking, and that 79% fewer reported getting drunk at least once a month (Botvin & Tortu, 1988). Among those in peer-led programs, 71% fewer students reported using marijuana than control groups at an immediate postprogram testing (Botvin, Baker, Renick, Filazzola, & Botvin, 1984). These findings constitute a *program* of evaluation research, and results of this magnitude have rightfully put LST in the national spotlight as an effective substance use prevention program.

How Good Are the Descriptive Causal Conclusions About Program Effectiveness?

Botvin and his colleagues are highly skilled designers of traditional experiments. The use of random assignment, control groups, pre- and posttest measurement, and statistical analyses to rule out such threats as chance or differential attrition ensure that threats to internal validity are negligible. Randomization generally occurs at the school level, so crossover effects such as compensatory equalization of treatments and compensatory rivalry are unlikely (Cook & Campbell, 1979).

Botvin himself expressed some concern about the demand characteristics in his early studies because the posttest was administered in contexts that were clearly part of the LST program. However, the later use of physiological smoking measures and "bogus pipelines" render demand characteristics less plausible as a threat to results.

LST has mostly been evaluated with homogeneous, middle-class, white populations, thus limiting its generalizability. Fortunately, more recent work has focused on urban minority populations, and we eagerly await the results from these studies. Those students who report smoking at the pretest have been excluded from presentations of results because Botvin is studying smoking onset. But this strategy prevents exploration of whether the intervention also stops smoking among those who have already begun the habit.

These minor problems aside, we believe that Botvin's summary claims about a descriptive causal connection between LST and smoking onset withstands reasonable challenge for the populations with which he has completed studies. Because of this, and because of the claim that his model is general enough to deal with all adolescent "social problems," we are inclined to accord it the same high value that Hamburg (1990) assigns it based on her criteria of policy relevance and technical quality.

How Good Were the Analyses of Implementation?

Botvin has not published a formal schema of his theory. Our best approximation, synthesized from many of his writings, is presented in Figure 15.2. The five components mentioned earlier are presented on the left. Botvin made no explicit mention of implementation in his published papers. In the best subsequent study (Botvin et al., 1989b), he had observers record on at least three occasions the number of curriculum points and objectives from the teachers' manual that were actually covered in class. The results showed that 65% of the program content was covered in the average class. These implementation data were also related to program outcomes, though on a few of the outcomes the children receiving more instruction were initially different from those receiving less.

However, implementation has not been treated as systematically in other parts of the research program. For instance, one influential paper concluded that peer-led LST reduced substance abuse more than teacher-led LST and attributed this difference to peers implementing the treatment more faithfully than teachers (Botvin, Baker, Filazzola, & Botvin, 1990). However, no implementation data were reported, so the explanation is an ex post facto conjecture based on a few unsystematic and incidental reports from members of the field staff. A more recent study by Botvin, Dusenbury, Baker, James-Ortiz, Botvin, & Kerner (in press) does the same, again "explaining" unexpected results in terms of (unmeasured) implementation factors. These interpretations would be more convincing, of course, if they were buttressed by implementation data of the kind Botvin had used just before.

It is to Botvin's credit that he has regularly examined indicators of treatment dosage, albeit through experimental design rather than measurement. For example, a once-a-week program format has been compared to an intense mini-course (Botvin, Renick, & Baker, 1983); follow-up booster sessions have been provided using both teachers and peer leaders (Botvin et al., 1983, 1990); and a 10-session booster curriculum has been used with eighth graders and a 5-session curriculum with ninth graders. By now, Botvin has the data to explore systematically the number of LST sessions or the amount of curriculum coverage that is necessary for observing effects. We eagerly await such analyses.

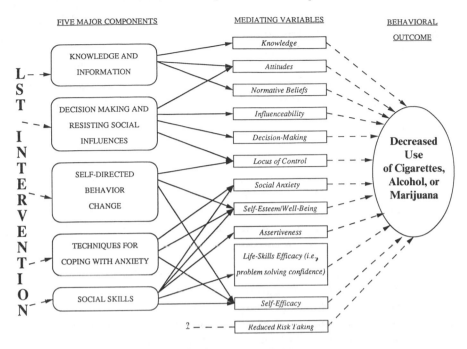

Figure 15.2. Depiction of Life Skills Training (LST): Constructs and processes.

A strength of Botvin's more recent work is his attention to ethnic and racial minority groups. He has moved beyond the primarily white, suburban, and middle-class youth of early LST research to target urban black and Hispanic populations (Botvin et al., 1989a, 1989b; Botvin et al., in press). To increase the appropriateness of program design and content for the new populations—and hence the program's implementability—the LST curriculum was extensively reviewed, and for both the Hispanic and black populations, adjustments were made to the reading level, the examples presented, and the role-play situations used. The studies with minority populations now underway are modest, but the initial results are encouraging and point to the possible involvement of some unique causal factors for each population. For Hispanics such factors include social risk variables such as the number of friends and/or family members who smoke (Botvin et al., 1989a, 1989b) and situational variables such as the level of acculturation to the United States (Botvin et al., 1989b). For blacks, the unique factors touch on some family variables (e.g., parents' education) and school performance (grades attained) (Botvin et al., 1989a).

How Good Were the Analyses of Causal Explanation?

Botvin is clearly interested in developing better substantive theory. The introduction sections of his scientific papers routinely use the language of causal mediation, and his data analyses evoke the same notion. However, unlike the Abt team, with their Figure 15.1, he has not yet created a schema for depicting the entire causal model from which he works. One is needed.

From narrative reports it is clear that the LST program is meant to be a self-contained, content-based strategy of prevention that varies only with the risk factor (alcohol, marijuana, or smoking) and population under study. Identifying effective treatment components therefore seems to be of low priority. The program is a *whole*. But there does seem to be some ambivalence on this score, since there was one early call to identify the more effective treatment components, given the obvious utility of such knowledge (Botvin et al., 1983). Temporal lags have not yet been systematically integrated into the research program to assess outcomes at different times and to probe which outcomes change before others, as the Abt researchers did. Without such knowledge it is difficult to estimate whether the outcomes Botvin typically measures are interconnected in the ways he suggests or whether some other, more complex model might fit the data better.

Botvin and his colleagues have, however, carefully measured a variety of dependent variables, mostly using self-report techniques but sometimes physiological measures. They have also assessed many of the cognitive, attitudinal, and personality variables thought to mediate drug use, and the comprehensiveness of measurement has increased over time as Botvin's theory has evolved. Even so, it is usually unclear why a particular mediator was measured (or reported on) in one study but not another. This low level of consistency in reporting from study to study precludes a cumulative analysis of the influence of particular potential mediators, undermining attempts to discover stable relationships. We believe it would be worthwhile for some scholar to collect all the (published and unpublished) data about mediators from Botvin's *program* of studies and to *review* why it is that his prevention program delays the onset of risky behaviors.

Our reading of Botvin's work suggests a conclusion about the mediation of his prevention effect that is at odds with his own claims. In his studies, statistically reliable changes are often reported for knowledge and attitude mediators but not for measures of skill-use or psychological attributes. Yet skills change and personality change are the most important and novel constructs in Botvin's theory. Is his program effective for reasons other than those that buttressed his program design? We cannot be sure about this because potential mediating constructs are measured differently from study to study and because we know nothing about the psychometric properties of any of the measures. Nonetheless, with the results available, it seems more plausible to assert that effects are due to Botvin's program causing changes in knowledge and normative expectations than to its causing changes in the social skills and personality factors that are so central to his theory (Botvin et al., in press). The need for high-quality measures and theoretical clarification is pressing.

Botvin has not attempted to construct and test formal causal models of the process whereby his program is effective. Instead, he prefers to examine in separate analyses whether a potential mediator is related first to the treatment and then to the effect. This procedure correctly supposes that a mediator must be correlated with both the cause and the effect, but it fails to take into account that the essence of mediation is influence flowing from the cause to the mediator and then from the mediator to the effect. More is involved than two correlations. Though they are not perfect for the mediational task, explicit causal models are better suited than simple correlations because they allow the exploration of direct and indirect causal paths from a set of potential and interrelated causes. Adopting an explicit causal modeling framework might have two further advantages. It might persuade Botvin and his colleagues of the crucial importance of obtaining multiple high-quality measures of each construct, and it might force him to be totally explicit about his model and perhaps see the desirability of developing several variants on it.

Though Botvin's theoretical writings reveal a preference for explanation as causal mediation, his actual research practices attest to his reliance for explanation on the correspondence theory. His argument takes the following form: The program was designed to stimulate social skills, so any experimental results not due to initial group nonequivalence or chance must be due to these skills. Logic aside, this argument overlooks the reality that (1) disappointing results were obtained when direct measures of social skills were gathered in later studies; (2) an alternative interpretation in terms of revised norms about substance use is empirically viable; and (3) the skills-training program is so multidimensional and the smoking onset effect is so multiply determined that it is difficult to infer any single mediating process from the cause–effect relationship alone. Botvin needs to move toward more high-quality, direct measurement of the life skills constructs he uses to explain his findings.

Botvin has not attempted to follow an explanatory strategy based on accounting for variance in changes in substance use. Thus, he has not systematically explored whether program effects depend on such individual demographic attributes as gender, race, income level, and so on. In some journal articles, he has reported analyses of one or two of these moderators, but rarely are the same ones analyzed in the same way from study to study. His most recent work with minority groups provides a welcome exception, for he has explored a wide range of parental attributes that might moderate effects, including education, grades, acculturation in the United States, and the smoking behavior of friends and family. Unlike the case with whites, the gains for black and Latino adolescents are only marginally reliable to date and are restricted to measures of smoking in the last month as opposed to the last week. Future research should explore more explicitly race and class differences in effect sizes, preferably within the same comparative study.

Midwestern Prevention Project

The Midwestern Prevention Project (MPP) is presented schematically in Figure 15.3. The project seeks to combine school, family, and community factors into a coordinated program aimed at bringing about sustained reductions in drug use among adolescents. It is based upon the assumption that these environmental forces must work in concert if they are to reinforce the resistance and counteraction skills emphasized in school prevention curricula and promote consistent community norms about abstinence. The rationale for MPP stems from the research team's observation that, while school-based programs in resistance skills and social competency are effective in reducing drug use, their *sustained* effectiveness has

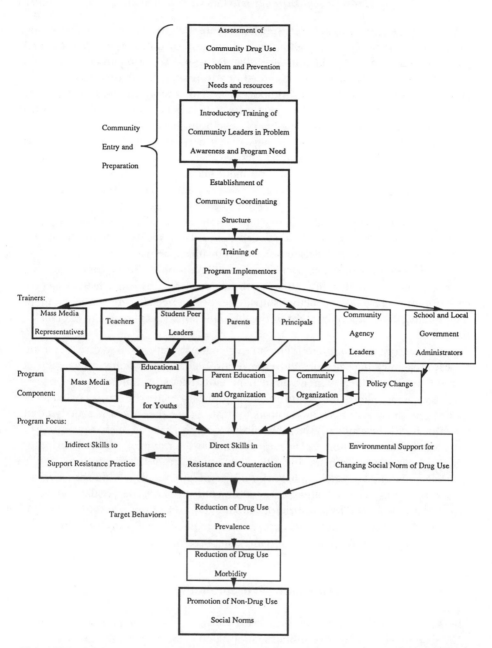

Figure 15.3. Depiction of proposed process of change resulting from Midwestern Prevention Project (MMP) intervention. (*Source:* Reproduced from Pentz, Dwyer, MacKinnon, et al., 1989. A multicommunity trial for primary prevention of adolescent drug abuse. *Journal of the American Medical Association, 261*(22), p. 3261.)

rarely been documented. Specifically, Pentz et al. (1989a) note that effects from past school-based programs have been variable with respect to the size, duration, and generalizability of effects across all the substances studied. They want to see MPP evaluated in terms of its potential to achieve effects that are comprehensive, temporally persistent, and explainable.

MPP was first implemented in the Kansas City metropolitan area in 1984. The program (known as *Project STAR,* or *Students Taught Awareness and Resistance*) is now being evaluated using a 6-year quasi-experiment. Forty-two middle and junior high schools participated—24 in the intervention condition and 18 in the delayed intervention, or control, condition. The original implementation plan called for the key components of the overall program to be introduced sequentially at approximately 1-year intervals: first, the mass media and school-based instructional components were to be introduced; then the parent education and organization components; next, the community organization element; and finally, policy interventions. Control schools were supposed to receive these same components, but with a 1-year lag after the experimental schools. Annual assessments of outcome and process variables were to be made, but with a pretest at the beginning of the first year.

A replication is underway in the Indianapolis metropolitan area that includes both public and private middle and junior high schools. Assignment to treatment is at random. The Indianapolis replication is crucial for interpreting the Kansas City results, both because of the random assignment and because the major developer and advocate of STAR lives in Kansas City. However, at present, results are available only for Kansas City, and then only for the first-year school-based intervention condition (with mass media) that was contrasted with control schools exposed only to the mass media component. Based on the 1-year follow-up results, prevalence rates were reliably lower in the intervention schools for all three "gateway" drugs: 11% versus 16% of students consuming more than two alcoholic drinks in the last month, 17% versus 24% of students using cigarettes within the last month, and 7% versus 10% using marijuana within the last month (Pentz et al., 1989a). It is not clear from these results, of course, whether the same students reduced use across one or more substances or whether the effects were independent. This is an important issue worth exploring under the assumption that the persons at greatest risk are those involved with multiple substances. It is also important to discuss how large these effects are for policing purposes, whether they are statistically significant or not. There is undoubtedly too much practical significance assigned to statistical significance in health research, given that statistical significance depends on such conceptual irrelevancies as sample size and reliability of measures, not to speak of more conceptually important matters such as the length of the delay period over which effects are measured.

How Good Are the Descriptive Causal Conclusions About Program Effectiveness?

MPP has a very strong methodological design, particularly in Indianapolis. But there is every reason to believe in the validity of the descriptive results from the first school-based year of intervention in Kansas City. Detailed analyses with reasonable levels of statistical power have revealed little evidence of pretest nonequivalence between the test and control groups in Kansas City. Additional analyses suggested little differential attrition. Moreover, the same pattern of results was obtained with and without correction for such key covariates as race, grade, father's occupation, and urbanicity. Hence, we judge the internal validity of the first-year Kansas City results to be high.

External validity is, of course, a different matter. Currently, it is limited to public schools in a single city, raising the stakes for the Indianapolis replication. Having the second city should also enhance the capacity to break the data down by more school and child attributes. Assessing the use of several different substances—and each in multiple ways—obviously improves the construct validity of the effect. Hence, in Kansas City we can confidently speak of effects on substance use in general rather than, say, on tobacco use in particular. Indeed, the questionnaire smoking items were cross-validated against an expired-air measure of carbon monoxide, producing comparable results. Thus, the smoking measures tap more than just social desirability. All in all, then, the Kansas City results provide great confidence that substance use was prevented over a 1-year period because of the school- and media-based STAR intervention.

How Good Were the Analyses of Implementation?

Two research groups took part in the evaluation. Researchers at the University of Southern California (USC) were primarily responsible for analyses of program impact on substance use. Program developers in Kansas City were primarily responsible for managing and studying program implementation. Separating implementation and outcome assessment in this way tends to have unfortunate consequences, since program developers typically study implementation to improve program operations rather than to provide data that can be used for statistically analyzing the conditions under which an intervention's effectiveness varies. Moreover, many program employees who study implementation are inclined to rely on impressions gleaned from unsystematic conversations and classroom observations rather than on systematic ethnographic data or the quantitative assessment of implementation.

Fortunately, the USC researchers did collect some implementation data directly from teachers. With these data—plus the less systematic data from program developers—it should be possible to conduct a multimethod description of implementation quality. But none is yet available. Nor has the correlation between teacher and observer reports of implementation been published, though note has been made that the correlation, while positive, was not high. This is an important issue, though, since teacher reports are potentially open to an alternative interpretation in terms of social desirability in responding, particularly among the most "invested" teachers, who may also elicit larger gains from students.

Analyses of the teacher data (Pentz et al., 1990), show that (1) all classes in the treatment group taught some of the material; (2) an average of 8.76 sessions lasting about 40 minutes was devoted to the curriculum; (3) few teachers reported deviating from the curriculum; and (4) when they did, they reported adding materials rather than substituting their own materials for program ones. To the extent that we can trust these teacher reports, they suggest high levels of implementation. The researchers related implementation levels to substance use in an analysis where schools were categorized into high or low implementers, though more levels of implementation (and more school-level covariates) would have been desirable. However, the small number of treatment schools (27) precluded such analyses.

Unfortunately, we know nothing about the level of implementation in the control schools. Since experiments are meant to assess the consequences of treatment *contrasts,* information about program-relevant activities in control groups is nearly always necessary—not just desirable. Also missing are tests of the relationship between drug use and implementation quality that use classroom observation data (rather than the more rudimentary teacher ratings) to measure implementation quality. Finally, no measures were made of individual curriculum components to see how often and how well they were taught to children. Yet the curriculum is clearly specified and is covered in teacher training sessions (Pentz, Cormack, Flay, Hansen, & Johnson, 1986). Would it not be useful to learn whether effects are larger for those curriculum components taught most often, as was the case with SHEE?

The total MPP program is more comprehensive than the school component alone. The mass media component consists of newspaper and broadcast coverage designed to create greater publicity about the project, greater public recognition for program participants and implementers, and greater awareness of drug prevalence in the community. It is therefore an integral part of the effort to create environmental forces supporting what the school program is doing. But because the mass media component is available to the entire Kansas City community, it is not—strictly speaking—part of the intervention. Rather, it is part of the context in which the intervention is embedded, making it impossible to assess either the media's unique effects or whether their citywide availability dampens the impact of other components. Furthermore, while the amount and content of media presentations are measured, no outcome variables have yet been specifically tied to media delivery. For example, no awareness or attitude surveys have been carried out to determine the salience of the media or their impact on general community knowledge or attitudes (norms) about drug use. A similar situation exists at present for the parent, community, and policy components. We do not know how the researchers propose to measure their implementation or how such measures might be conceptually linked in unique ways to particular outcomes.

How Good Were the Analyses of Causal Explanation?

In its origins, the MPP program package is more pragmatic than theoretical, using past theories and programs to borrow an array of social change techniques that seem to have worked well for their original developers. As described in Pentz et al. (1989a), the theoretical bases for MPP are eclectic, encompassing several different theories of adolescent behavior (e.g., social learning theory and problem behavior), ecological models of social influence, and theories of mass and interpersonal communication in community settings. The school-based program elements abstracted from these theories are most explicitly presented in MacKinnon, Johnson, Pentz, Dwyer, and Hansen (1991). However, no papers by the USC group make clear which theories generated which program elements, and the school intervention is not unitary in any obvious conceptual sense. Without additional analyses it would not be clear, therefore, which elements or processes explained the prevention of drug use that was found. Thus, the correspondence theory of explanation cannot help elucidate why the school-based part of the program had the effects it did.

The complete process of change for MPP is illustrated in Pentz et al. (1989a). The schools, mass media, parents, community organizations, and policy change are all expected to instill in adolescents resistance and counteraction skills and to create environmental support for changed local norms about drug use. Lower drug use and morbidity should be the result, as well as greater acceptance of antidrug norms. Testing such a model would not be easy, in part because the constructs indexing program components are so broad that few observers would agree about how they should be operationalized. Furthermore, little ingenuity is required to come up with other forces that might have mediated the Kansas City results; for example, did the intervention influence adolescents' social networks, with experimental students coming to choose different friends? Direct measures of hypothesized mediating processes—*and of alternative plausible processes*—are required for any responsible analysis of causal mediating processes. Careful intervention design is not enough. (Fortunately, the USC team did measure some potential mediators, and we discuss these later.)

Even if the researchers were to succeed in adding a fresh component each year, as planned, this would not help much in separating out the effects of individual program components for the following reasons: (1) Anticipated interactions between program elements are not specified; nor are the conditions under which they are expected to be effective. One could therefore not tell whether a later-added component was effective by itself or only in the context of the other components implemented earlier. (2) If drug use prevalence rates were to decline due to effective earlier components, the incremental program effects might well become more difficult to achieve, "penalizing" program components put in place later. (3) Finally, as secular changes occur in the national and local prevention environments over the planned 6-year research period, this could affect the relative effectiveness of various program components, confounding any attempt to interpret their sequential impact. For all these reasons, it will be very difficult to determine which set of program components is responsible for any global effects achieved.

Turning now to the theory of explanation based on accounting for variance, published reports on MPP have mostly emphasized how the intervention influenced students on the average. However, regression analyses stratified by grade level and race also showed that with both the school and the individual as the unit of analysis, statistically reliable program effects occurred in all grade and race combinations

(Pentz et al., 1989c). Also, Johnson et al. (1990) explored whether the program differentially affected students as a result of various individual risk factors (e.g., one's own history of substance use or one's friends' and parents' use). Thus, there has been some exploration of moderator variables at the *individual* level. However, few tests of *school-level* moderator variables are currently available, and it is still too early to know how well the results replicate across Kansas City and Indianapolis. Though greater geographic and cultural dispersion between these two cities might have been desirable, the total number of schools (99) and community units (26) involved is substantial. Tests can therefore be made of whether the program differs in effectiveness when it is implemented in sixth- or seventh-grade classrooms and in private versus public schools. But such analyses of program robustness are not yet available; nor are analyses exploring replication in settings where the program developers are less visible than in Kansas City or where the student population is less middle class and white (Pentz et al., 1989b).

The MPP research team has tried to move away from exclusive reliance on the black box theory of experimentation and has directly measured and analyzed some potential mediating variables. In the discussion that follows, we rely on the one published paper explicitly concerned with causal mediation (MacKinnon et al., 1991). In this paper, eight change variables are invoked as potential mediators, having been measured at two time points. They are changes in adolescents' (1) intentions to use drugs; (2) knowledge of the negative consequences of drug use; (3) belief in the positive consequences of drug use; (4) knowledge of external influences on drug use; (5) resistance skills; (6) communication skills; (7) perceived peer norms; and (8) anticipated peer reactions to drug use. While some of these variables are in the program model in Pentz et al. (1989a), it is surprising that many are not.

MacKinnon et al. first tested whether these eight change variables were related to the MPP treatment, discovering that four were. They then took these four and used a regression technique that contrasts coefficients from analyses with and without a potential mediator to probe how each of them was related to drug use. Changes in peer reactions turned out to be the only consistent predictor of changes in cigarette and alcohol use—but not marijuana. The authors then developed a covariance structure model to explore cigarette use further, and in their measurement model employed three items to assess peer reactions. They do not explain the rest of their model, but claim that when peer reactions are better measured (as in the structural equation analysis), they account for as much as 95% of the cigarette use effect. Thus, the claim is made that MPP reduced cigarette use *because* of changes in students' perceptions of how their friends would react if they smoked, implying a social norm explanation of cigarette smoking.

Commendably, MacKinnon et al. went well beyond normal practice and examined more than one mediating model. In another analysis, they reversed the causal links, postulating that drug use might have changed first and then caused a later change in students' perceptions of their friends' reactions to drugs. In yet another analysis they probed whether a change in drug use might have mediated changes in any of the seven other variables originally conceived as mediators. The authors discovered that a model with drug use mediating friends' reactions fit the data, though not as well as a model with peer reactions preceding changes in drug use.

Though the explanatory efforts of the USC authors are superior to those in the two other evaluation projects, they are not without limitations. The authors do not seem to have explored whether more reliable measurement might have enhanced the role of any of the seven original mediators. Nor did they explore other factors that might play an important mediational role, such as the program causing changes in personal self-efficacy to resist smoking. Nor did they attempt to reconcile the variables measured in MacKinnon et al. with the only partially overlapping list of mediators in Pentz' work (e.g., Pentz et al., 1989a). And finally, they did not discuss in detail the fact that some of the variables that played no causal role were the very variables that, in the original program model, Pentz had hypothesized would play a role—for example, resistance skills. Nonetheless, the preliminary process analyses now available from only one MPP site suggest the same conclusions as our reinterpretation of Botvin's data on causal mediators. Resistance skills have not yet been demonstrated to play the crucial mediating role commonly ascribed to them in theories about preventing drug use, and accurate knowledge of social norms might play a major mediational role. Sophisticated studies of these hypotheses are urgently needed.

Conclusions

Descriptive Causation and Program Effectiveness

Are the three evaluation studies examined here as good as Hamburg (1990) claims? The answer is a resounding "Yes" when judged by the criterion of providing convincing evidence of some program effectiveness—that is, information about a descriptive causal link from the program to desired adolescent health changes. It is therefore regrettable that most adolescent health programs are evaluated poorly when they are evaluated at all. The studies examined here clearly show that better evaluation practice is possible and that descriptive causal studies can be completed with the following five desirable criteria: (1) random assignment (or closely matched quasi-experiment groups), (2) valid outcome measures, (3) powerful treatments, (4) high statistical power, and (5) large samples of somewhat heterogeneous respondents.

But we have to note that the studies in question based their conclusions of effectiveness on three questionable latent assumptions. The first is that effects are important if they are statistically significant. But statistical and policy significance should never be confused, since the former depends on such policy irrelevancies as sample size and reliability of measures.

The second latent assumption is that the time periods over which prevention was demonstrated are adequate. Yet most initial effects decay with time, so that cogent justification has to be offered for the delay periods used. No such justifications are available in these studies.

And third, though many of the effects demonstrated involved preventing use of more than one substance, it was not clear whether the treatments influenced different individuals for each substance or whether the individuals who would have used multiple substances were prevented from doing so. The latter effect is of special policy importance, given the links between multiple substance use and a variety of serious negative social outcomes.

Program Implementation

How well do the three exemplary studies describe the quality of implementation, explore its determinants, and relate implementation quality to outcome changes? Connell et al. (1986) showed that the four health education programs they evaluated differed both in time spent teaching the curriculum and in the health changes obtained, but that the differences in health changes disappeared when the time spent teaching the curriculum was statistically controlled. Thus, it seems that the various curricula were equally efficient. An evaluation that provides local school districts with knowledge about multiple curricula that vary in both costs and gains—but not in their relative efficiency—has obvious policy relevance. In particular, it can help districts decide which program to acquire for themselves in light of their own (highly variable) resources and local priorities.

The USC researchers had the best theoretical analysis of implementation, stressing the importance of three attributes: theoretical integrity, local reinvention, and the amount of time spent teaching the experimental curriculum. But the quality of implementation measures did not match the quality of the theoretical analysis, since a single item was used to measure each attribute.

Botvin had the best implementation measure, using classroom observations to measure curriculum coverage and the amount teachers added to what the program developers requested of them. Unfortunately, classroom observations are more expensive than questionnaires, and this may explain why Botvin has used classroom observations only once. But it is surprising that questionnaire measures have not been used more often in his research program because implementation has twice been invoked to explain unexpected prevention outcomes. Quality measures of implementation are indispensable to support such an explanation.

Three problems beset all the analyses of implementation we have seen. The first is the absence of measures of what transpires in the no-treatment control groups. In some ways, *no-treatment* is a misnomer, for health-relevant treatments are always occurring spontaneously in schools, at home, in the media, and elsewhere. Since experiments test treatment *contrasts* rather treatments in some abstract void, it is crucial to collect implementation measures in control groups in exactly the same way as in treatment groups. A conundrum is involved here, since the wording of some implementation items may seem strange because the treatment and control groups will have undergone different experiences. The evaluator's art is to minimize any inappropriateness that might result, even if it is never completely eliminated.

The second recurrent deficiency with respect to implementation analysis in adolescent health studies is the absence of credible, comprehensive theories of implementation. There has been considerable research in evaluation designed to understand implementation in terms of many different attributes of program theory (Boruch & Gomez, 1977; Chen & Rossi, 1987; Sechrest, West, Phillips, Redner, & Yeaton, 1979). But such writings are hardly ever referenced in the adolescent health literature. There have also been considerable theoretical advances in the conceptualization of implementation in both public policy and political science. Among other things, this research stresses why difficulties occur at the local level, how local practitioners see central directives for change, and how dependent change is on many interdependent levels within an organization (Bardach, 1977; Berman & McLaughlin, 1977; Fullan, 1982; Pressman & Wildavsky, 1984; Williams, 1975). None of this literature is cited in adolescent health studies either. Such provincialism is not productive, and the designers and evaluators of health education programs would do well to enlarge their disciplinary horizons on this matter.

A third limitation of all the evaluations we considered is the absence of analyses of determinants of implementation quality. Implementation levels are described in the research, as are attempts to relate these levels to changes in outcomes. But none of the projects probes the likely determinants of implementation quality. None presents us with rich ethnographic data from school sites, and none measures the quality of even such obvious implementation determinants as the quality of teacher training, of curriculum materials, of school district commitment to health education, of principal support for a program, and so on. In adolescent health research, studying the determinants of implementation quality seems to be unimportant. This is regrettable.

Causal Explanations of Treatment Effects

The Abt evaluators did not make much effort to explain their results other than to describe the temporal sequence of change in the knowledge, attitude, and behavior domains. Their work epitomizes a pragmatic orientation to evaluation that is predicated on describing what works—especially what works better than something else—and on relating implementation quality to effectiveness. Explanation is not a priority here. Nor is it with those evaluation theorists (e.g., Campbell 1979, 1987; Scriven, 1980) who see causal explanation as intrinsically more complicated than causal description, as achieving less uncertainty reduction, and as providing little information about how to improve a program in the short term. Yet causal explanation is the Golden Fleece of conventional science, and in this one regard the theorists above are "outsiders" even among evaluation theorists. In adolescent health—unlike other topic areas—most evaluators have academic appointments. They therefore subscribe to traditional scholarly standards, and it is no surprise to note that their grant proposals and scholarly publications emphasize explanation as a research goal.

But to promote explanation, the authors we reviewed relied most heavily on what we called the correspondence approach to explanation. This is unfortunate, since this black box approach was developed for the more closed and controlled world of the laboratory sciences where explanation is achieved through the correspondence between the specifics of a substantive theory and the specifics of what was actually manipulated or measured, with many irrelevant causes kept out of the explanatory system. In adolescent health studies the most pressing current need is probably not for explanation. It is to achieve impacts in schools, homes, and communities. To improve explanation is not trivial, but it is difficult to do via the correspondence approach, given that substantive theories in adolescent health are so underspecified, that treatments have to be so multidimensional in order to achieve a practical impact, that the health outcomes of interest to policymakers are multiply determined, and that irrelevant causes of these effects cannot be controlled by means of physical isolation, as they can in the laboratory.

Botvin's basic causal relationship between life skills training and substance use has been well replicated. But the programmatic nature of the research has not been used to vary, or even measure, the components of the global intervention and has hardly been used to explore mediating processes. Instead, emphasis in the later studies in the program has been placed on demonstrating even greater robustness for the intervention, especially by showing its applicability to urban minority populations. Heterogeneity of replication takes precedence over explanation, and for explanation Botvin's team continues to rely on the correspondence approach. That is, they assert that their results are due to skills training because the treatment was designed to vary skills training.

Pentz and her associates also have a complex, multidimensional treatment that was designed to be implemented in a number of different settings—the school, the community, the mass media, and the policy world. Since obtaining effects logically precedes explaining them, and since changing the recalcitrant real world probably requires powerful rather than theoretically elegant interventions, the USC team has rightly concentrated on obtaining descriptive causal effects rather than explaining them. But this priority has probably led them to rely most heavily for explanation on the correspondence between the processes their complex treatment was designed to activate and the (unknown) processes it actually set in motion. In adolescent health research we cannot be sanguine about much explanation resulting only from knowledge of treatment particulars or from researchers' claims about the causal processes their treatments were designed to activate.

Explanation is better promoted through a prediction approach that requires direct measurement of key moderator or mediator variables—such as grade, sex, race, prior smoking history, or implementation quality—and then assessing how well these variables account for variance in the outcome either by themselves or in statistical interaction with the treatment. All the researchers discussed in this chapter used multivariate analysis for this purpose. Usually the analyses were post hoc, designed to discover patterns of relationships. But in some cases policy-relevant rationales were offered for the choice of contingency variables—especially when data were used to see how implementation quality was related to outcome changes. Even so, some failures to conduct contingency analyses were striking. For instance, Botvin's theory clearly postulates that substance use among early adolescents serves the purpose of bolstering self-esteem and other personality attributes. But measures of the relevant constructs were rarely reported on in the relevant research.

Though the variance accounted-for approach to explanation is useful, it has significant limitations. It equates explanation with prediction. In actual research practice, it tends to emphasize moderator variables more than mediators, and it usually involves simple multiple regression techniques that are problematic because of errors in variables and rigidity when it comes to probing complex models with multiple direct and indirect causal paths. For these reasons, we would prefer to see explanation in the adolescent health field depend more on our third approach to explanation, which requires tests to identify the causally efficacious components of global treatments, the causally impacted components of outcomes, and—especially—the processes set off by the treatment that are causally responsible for the effect.

This approach requires high-quality measures of treatment components. This is the major reason why studying implementation is so important for explanation. It also requires generating multiple substantive theories about the processes that might link a treatment and an outcome, as well as multiple measures of each of the constructs specified in these theories (Cook, 1985). Armed with such data, several explanatory models can then be pitted against each other, using a data-analytic program like LISREL, whose maximum likelihood factor analytic procedures reduce the risks of bias from measurement error and whose flexibility allows tests of the relative goodness of fit of several different causal models. None of the evaluations considered in this chapter were even close to the state of the art in causal modeling, though Hansen and Graham (1991) of the USC team were far superior to the others.

Future explanatory studies might do well to measure each construct in a causal model using multiple items and—where possible—several different modes of measurement. This minimizes bias from measurement error. Also needed are analyses of the psychometric properties of the measures used. Such analyses were missing from all the results reviewed in this chapter, and without them we cannot estimate what it means if a potential mediator is not related to a treatment or outcome. Is it not related in general, or has it been so poorly measured in the research under review that no reliable results could ever have been obtained? Similarly, if one mediator is related to a treatment or outcome but another is not, we would like to be able to distinguish whether this pattern reflects a genuine difference in causal mediation or the irrelevant fact that one construct was measured more validly than another.

However regrettable, the low quality of explanatory analyses in adolescent health studies is understandable. First, there is a logical primacy to knowing that a descriptive causal relationship exists before embarking on its explanation. Second, there is a strong rationale for wanting to demonstrate the robustness of an intervention along many policy-relevant dimensions before seeking to explain why it is effective. Third, trade-offs arise if researchers invest much time and effort in measuring implementation and process; for example, fewer resources are available for measuring effects. Fourth, trade-offs arise whenever process measurement is obtrusive and threatens to modify the phenomenon under study. Fifth, the exploration of mediator (and moderator) variables requires larger sample sizes for a given level of statistical power. Sixth, some evaluation theorists argue in favor of emphasizing the description of effects, leaving explanation to scientists who traditionally value it rather than to evaluators who they believe should place the highest value on describing effects relevant to pending policy issues. Seventh, the major rationale for explanation in evaluation is that it facilitates transfer to other settings, treatments, populations, and so on. Yet it is not clear how often explanation promotes such transfer, even though many basic researchers claim this in order to justify their budgets. And finally, explanation may not be the only route to knowledge about the transfer of research findings. Meta-analysis offers another such route— albeit one that is predicated on discovering descriptive causal relationships that are demonstrably robust rather than on causally explaining such relationships (Cook, 1990, 1991).

Our argument for greater emphasis on implementation in adolescent health evaluations and transfer is not the same as the argument offered by critics of the randomized clinical trial. They want to see explanation (or understanding) take precedence over causal description. But we only want to see explanation gain greater attention within a research strategy that retains the description of novel findings as its primary goal. We want to see *both* descriptive *and* explanatory causal purposes achieved *within experimental frameworks*. For this to happen, we will need substantive theories that are more explicit, better measures of implementation and process, and better statistical tests of causal models. We will also need to deemphasize theories of explanation that claim that mediating processes can be probed through treatment design alone (as in the black box, Popper-like approach we called the correspondence theory) or through the use of multivariate data analytic techniques that were developed primarily for prediction (as with the variance accounted-for approach). We suggest that causal explanation will be most advanced by the explicit modeling of plausible theories, even though the level of uncertainty reduction achieved will rarely match that achieved from descriptions of implementation or treatment effectiveness. Nonetheless, the payoffs for both theory and policy are likely to be worth the effort it will take to develop an experimental tradition in adolescent health evaluation that values, and routinely implements, process measurement and analysis based on explicit causal models.

Skills Training versus Norm Changes as Effective Causal Processes

What surprised us most in this review is how poorly the notion of social skills training fared by itself in explaining prevention results and how much better social norm concepts fared. Botvin's own work shows that, when mediating variables are measured, those that speak to skills acquisition do not predict outcomes as well as those that speak to changed perceptions of norms. The USC work also suggests the important role of the latter. We cannot be definitive on this issue, though, given the quality of the measures and data analyses available. The matter urgently needs further investigation.

One line of attack would be to take the concept of social skills and relate it more closely to current theory in social cognition. In particular, Bandura (1992) now maintains that acquiring such skills will change behavior only if knowledge of the skills is accompanied by a strong sense of motivation to perform them and by the individual's sense of self-efficacy to perform them in the situations where the behaviors are required. This reformulation suggests two things: On the one hand, we should not expect social skills to be related to behavior change in the simple way presumed in the past; and on the other hand, practical procedures need to be developed for teacher training and classroom instruction that will change students' cognitions and affect related to self-efficacy. However, while self-efficacy is important in its own right, it is only one example of a larger principle: that social skills may need to be integrated into a theory of behavior change that is more complex and contingent than Botvin's theory.

Another line of attack would be to take the concept of social norms and explicate it better. It is a notoriously slippery concept and can be used ex post facto to explain almost any social outcome. Moreover, it does not seem to have quite the same meaning in the Botvin and USC research projects whose outcomes suggested its importance for explaining adolescent health outcomes. Botvin's normative measures refer to the prevalence of substance use among students, while in the USC work the measures refer to fellow students' anticipated disapproval of substance use. (The larger USC research design—with its media, community, and policy components—is probably predicated upon a third conception of norms that emphasizes general societal disapproval.) While all the concepts above relate to norms, they are far from identical. More effort needs to be put into identifying the causally most efficacious attributes of social norms and analyzing the conditions under which various conceptions of norms are related to prevention.

Summary

In adolescent health studies today, the needs are (1) for substantive theories about mediating processes that are more specific; (2) for a larger number of such theories; (3) for better measurement of all the constructs in these theories; and (4) for improved analyses of the measures and relationships in these theories. Demonstrating descriptive causal relationships about program effectiveness is still the number one need, however, and this requires experiments. But since such experiments are likely to involve complex, multivariate treatments and to take place in open-field settings, they are not likely to advance substantive theory much or to facilitate the transfer of research findings to contexts where they have never been studied before. Hence we counsel the use of experiments to which quantitative measures of two kinds have been added—of implementation quality and of all the constructs from all the substantive theories that might plausibly explain why and how a particular program impacts on some health-relevant outcomes. This will not be an easy task and probably reflects an ultimately unattainable goal. But better approximations than we see today are possible, and they are worth pursuing if the yield from adolescent health evaluations is to be even greater tomorrow.

Acknowledgments

This work has been partly supported by the MacArthur Foundation Research Network on Successful Adolescent Development Among Youth in High-Risk Settings. Thanks are due to Brian R. Flay and Richard Jessor for a critical reading of a prior draft of this chapter.

References

Attkisson, C. C., Hargreaves, W. A., Horowitz, M. J., & Sorensen, J. E. (1978). *Evaluation of human service programs.* New York: Academic Press.

Bandura, A. (1977). *Social learning theory.* Englewood Cliffs, NJ: Prentice-Hall.

Bandura, A. (1992). Self-efficacy mechanism in psychobiological functioning. In R. Schwarzer (Ed.) *Self-efficacy: Thought control of action.* Washington, DC: Hemisphere.

Bardach, E. (1977). *The implementation game: What happens after a bill becomes a law.* Cambridge, MA: MIT Press.

Berman, P., & McLaughlin, M. W. (1977). *Federal programs supporting educational change: Volume 8: Factors affecting implementation and continuation.* Santa Monica, CA: Rand Corporation.

Bhaskar, R. (1975). *A realist theory of science.* Leeds, England: Leeds.

Boring, E. G. (1954). The nature and history of experimental control. *American Journal of Psychology, 67,* 573–589.

Boruch, R. F., & Gomez, H. (1977). Sensitivity, bias, and theory in impact evaluations. *Professional Psychology: Research and Practice, 8,* 411–434.

Botvin, G. J. (1983). *Life skills training: Teacher's manual.* New York: Smithfield Press.

Botvin, G. J. (1986). Substance abuse prevention research: Recent developments and future directions. *Journal of School Health, 56,* 369–374.

Botvin, G. J., Baker, E., Filazzola, A. D., & Botvin, E. M. (1990). A cognitive-behavioral approach to substance abuse prevention: One-year follow-up. *Addictive Behaviors, 15,* 47–63.

Botvin, G. J., Baker, E., Renick, N., Filazzola, A. D., & Botvin, E. M. (1984). A cognitive-behavioral approach to substance abuse prevention. *Addictive Behaviors, 9,* 137–147.

Botvin, G. J., Batson, H. W., Witts-Vitale, S., Bess, V., Baker, E., & Dusenbury, L. (1989a). A psychosocial approach to smoking prevention for urban Black youth. *Public Health Reports, 104,* 573–582.

Botvin, G. J., Dusenbury, L., Baker, E., James-Ortiz, S., Botvin, E. M., & Kerner, J. (in press). Smoking prevention among urban minority youth. *Health Psychology. Vol. II.*

Botvin, G. J., Dusenbury, L., Baker, E., James-Oritz, S., & Kerner, J. (1989b). A skills training approach to smoking prevention among Hispanic youth. *Journal of Behavioral Medicine, 12,* 279–296.

Botvin, G. J., & Eng, A. (1982). The efficacy of a multicomponent approach to the prevention of cigarette smoking. *Preventive Medicine, 11,* 199–211.

Botvin, G. J., Eng, A., & Williams, C. L. (1980). Preventing the onset of cigarette smoking through life skills training. *Preventive Medicine, 9,* 135–143.

Botvin, G. J., Renick, N., & Baker, E. (1983). The effects of scheduling format and booster sessions on a broad spectrum psychosocial approach to smoking prevention. *Journal of Behavioral Medicine, 6,* 359–379.

Botvin, G. J., & Tortu, S. (1988). Preventing adolescent substance abuse through life skills training. In R. H. Price, E. L. Cowen, R. P. Lorion, & J. Ramos-McKay (Eds.) *Fourteen ounces of prevention* (pp. 98–110). Washington, DC: American Psychological Association.

Bridgman, P. W., (1927). *The logic of modern physics.* New York: Macmillan.

Britan, G. M., (1978). Experimental and contextual models of program evaluation. *Evaluation and Program Planning, 1,* 229–234.

Campbell, D. T. (1979). Assessing the impact of planned social change. *Evaluation and Program Planning, 2,* 67–90.

Campbell, D. T. (1987). Guidelines for monitoring the scientific competence of preventive intervention research centers: An exercise in the sociology of scientific validity. *Knowledge: Creation, Diffusion, Utilization, 8,* 389–430.

Chen, H., & Rossi, P. H. (1987). The theory-driven approach to validity. *Evaluation and Program Planning, 10,* 95–103.

Ciarlo, J., & Reihman, J. (1977). The Denver community mental health questionnaire: Development of a multidimensional program evaluation instrument. In R. D. Coursey (Ed.) *Program evaluation for mental health: Methods, strategies, participants* (pp. 131–167). New York: Grune & Stratton.

Connell, D. B., Turner, R. R., Mason, E. F., & Olsen, L. K. (1986). School health education evaluation. *International Journal of Educational Research, 10,* 245–345.

Cook, T. D. (1985). Post-positivist critical multiplism. In R. L. Shotland & M. M. Mark (Eds.), *Social science and social policy* (pp. 21–62). Beverly Hills, CA: Sage.

Cook, T. D. (1990). The generalization of causal connections: Multiple theories in search of clear practice. In L. Sechrest, E. Perrin, & J. Bunker (Eds.), *Research methodology: Strengthening causal interpretation of non-experimental data* (pp. 9–31). Rockville, MD: Agency for Health Care Policy and Research.

Cook, T. D. (1991). Meta-analysis: Its potential for causal description and causal explanation within program evaluation. In Albrecht, G., & Otto, H. (Eds.), *Social prevention and the social sciences: Theoretical controversies, research problems, and evaluation strategies* (pp. 245–285). Berlin-New York: Walter de Gruyter.

Cook, T. D., & Campbell, D. T. (1979). *Quasi-experimentation: Design and analysis issues for social research in field settings.* Boston: Houghton Mifflin.

Cook, T. D., Cooper, H., Cordray, D., Hartmann, H., Hedges, L., Light, R., Louis, T., & Mosteller, F. (Eds.) (1992). *Meta-analysis for explanation: A casebook.* New York: Russell Sage Foundation.

Cook, T. D., & Gruder, C. L. (1978). Metaevaluation research. *Evaluation Quarterly, 2,* 5–51.

Cook, T. D., & Walberg, H. J. (1985). Methodological and substantive significance. *Journal of School Health, 55,* 340–342.

Cronbach, L. J. (1982). *Designing evaluations of educational and social programs.* San Francisco: Jossey-Bass.

Cronbach, L. J., Ambron, S. R., Dombusch, S. M., Hess, R. D., Homik, R. C., Phillips, D. C., Walker, D. F., & Weiner, S. S. (1980). *Towards reform of program evaluation: Aims, methods and institutional arrangements.* San Francisco: Jossey-Bass.

Eisner, E. (1985). *The educational imagination: On the design and evaluation of school programs.* New York: Macmillan.

Evans, R. I. (1976). Smoking in children: Developing a social psychological strategy of deterrence. *Preventive Medicine, 5,* 122–127.

Fetterman, D. F. (1988). *Qualitative approaches to evaluation in education: The silent scientific revolution.* New York: Praeger.

Fullan, M. (1982). *The meaning of educational change.* New York: Teachers College Press.

Glymour, C., Sprites, P., Scheines, R., & Kelly, K. (1987). *Discovering causal structure: Artificial intelligence, philosophy of science, and statistical modeling.* Orlando, FL: Academic Press.

Guba, E. G., & Lincoln, T. S. (1981). *Effective evaluation: Improving the usefulness of evaluation results through responsive and naturalistic approaches.* San Francisco: Jossey-Bass.

Hamburg, B. A. (1990). *Life skills training: Preventive interventions for young adolescents.* Working paper prepared for the Carnegie Council on Adolescent Development, Washington, DC.

Hansen, W. B., & Graham, J. W. (1991). Preventing alcohol, cigarette and marijuana use among adolescents: Peer pressure resistance training versus establishing conservative norms. *Preventive Medicine, 20,* 414–430.

Harre, R., & Madden, E. H. (1975). *Causal powers: A theory of natural necessity.* Oxford: Basil Blackwell.

Heckman, J. J., & Hotz, J. (1989). Choosing among alternative nonexperimental methods for estimating the impact of social programs: The case of manpower training. *Journal of the American Statistical Association, 84,* 878–880.

House, E. R. (1980). *Evaluating with validity.* Beverly Hills, CA: Sage.

Jessor, R. (1982). Critical issues in research on adolescent health promotion. In T. Coates, A. Petersen, & C. Perry (Eds.) *Promoting adolescent health: A dialog on research and practice* (pp. 447–465). New York: Academic Press.

Jessor, R., & Jessor, S. L. (1977). *Problem behavior and psychosocial development: A longitudinal study of youth.* New York: Academic Press.

Johnson, C. A., Pentz, M. A., Weber, M. D., Dwyer, J. H., Baer, N., MacKinnon, D. P., Hansen, W. B., & Flay, B. R. (1990). Relative effectiveness of comprehensive community programming for drug abuse prevention with high-risk and low-risk adolescents. *Journal of Consulting and Clinical Psychology, 58,* 447–456.

Klein, J. D., Kotelchuck, M., & DeFriese, G. H. (1990). *Critical evaluation of comprehensive multiservice delivery systems for adolescents: A framework for evaluation of effectiveness and a feasibility analysis.* Paper prepared for the Carnegie Council on Adolescent Development, Washington, DC.

Kuhn, T. S. (1962). *The structure of scientific revolutions.* Chicago: University of Chicago Press.

Mackie, J. L. (1974). *The cement of the universe.* Oxford: Oxford University Press.

MacKinnon, D. P., Johnson, C. A., Pentz, M. A., Dwyer, J. H., & Hansen, W. B. (1991). Mediating mechanisms in a school-based drug prevention program: First year effects of the midwestern prevention project. *Health Psychology, 10,* 164–172.

Manski, C. (in press). The selection problem. In C. Sims (Ed.), *Advances in Econometrics: Proceedings of the Sixth World Congress of Econometrics.* New York: Cambridge University Press.

McGuire, W. J. (1964). Inducing resistance to persuasion: Some contemporary approaches. In L. Berkowitz (Ed.), *Advances in experimental social psychology, Volume 1* (pp. 192–227). New York: Academic Press.

Patton, M. Q. (1980). *Qualitative evaluation methods.* Beverly Hills, CA: Sage.

Patton, M. Q. (1988). The evaluator's responsibility for utilization. *Evaluation Practice, 9,* 5–24.

Pentz, M. A., Cormack, C., Flay, B., Hansen, W. B., & Johnson, C. A. (1986). Balancing program and research integrity in community drug abuse prevention: Project STAR approach. *Journal of School Health, 56,* 389–393.

Pentz, M. A., Dwyer, J. H., MacKinnon, D. P., Flay, B. R., Hansen, W. B., Wang, E.Y.I., & Johnson, C. A. (1989a). A multicommunity trial for primary prevention of adolescent drug abuse. *Journal of the American Medical Association, 261,* 3259–3266.

Pentz, M. A., MacKinnon, D. P., Dwyer, J. H., Wang, E.Y.I., Hansen, W. B., Flay, B. R., & Johnson, C. A. (1989b). Longitudinal effects of the Midwestern Prevention Project on regular and experimental smoking in adolescents. *Preventive Medicine, 18,* 304–321.

Pentz, M. A., MacKinnon, D. P., Flay, B. R., Hansen, W. B., Johnson, C. A., & Dwyer, J. H. (1989c). Primary prevention of chronic disease in adolescents: Effects of the Midwestern Prevention Project on tobacco use. *American Journal of Epidemiology, 130,* 713–724.

Pentz, M. A., Treban, E. A., Hansen, W. B., MacKinnon, D. P., Dwyer, J. H., Johnson, C. A., Flay, B. R., Daniels, S., & Cormack, C. (1990). Effects of program implementation on adolescent drug use behavior: The Midwestern Prevention Project (MPP). *Evaluation Review, 14,* 264–289.

Popper, K. R. (1959). *The logic of scientific discovery.* New York: Basic Books.

Pressman, J. L., & Wildavsky, A. (1984). *Implementation* (3rd ed.). Berkeley: University of California Press.

Rivlin, M., & Timpane, P. M. (Eds.) (1975). *Planned variation in education.* Washington, DC: Brookings Institution.

Scriven, M. (1980). *The logic of evaluation*. Inverness, CA: Edgepress.

Sechrest, L., West, S. G., Phillips, M., Redner, R., & Yeaton, W. (1979). Some neglected problems in evaluation research: Strength and integrity of treatments. In L. Sechrest & Associates (Eds.), *Evaluation studies review annual, Volume 4* (pp. 15–35). Beverly Hills, CA: Sage Publications.

Shadish, W. R., Jr., Cook, T. D., & Leviton, L. C. (1991). *Foundations of program evaluation: Theories of practice*. Newbury Park, CA: Sage.

Stake, R. E. (1980). Program evaluation, particularly responsive evaluation. In W. B. Dockrell & D. Hamilton (Eds.) *Rethinking educational research* (pp. 72–87). London: Hodder & Stoughton.

Stebbins, L. B., St. Pierre, R. G., Proper, E. C., Anderson, R. B., & Cerva, T. R. (1978). An evaluation of follow-through. In T. D. Cook & Associates (Eds.), *Evaluation studies review Annual, Volume 3*. Beverly Hills, CA: Sage.

Tortu, S., & Botvin, G. J. (1989). School-based smoking prevention: The teacher training process. *Preventive Medicine, 18*, 280–289.

Weiss, C. H. (1977). Research for policy's sake: The enlightenment function of social research. *Policy Analysis, 3*, 531–545.

Wholey, J. S. (1979). *Evaluation: Promise and performance*. Washington, DC: Urban Institute.

Williams, W. (1975). Implementation analysis and assessment. *Policy Analysis, 1*, 531–566.

16

Adolescent Health Promotion in the Twenty-first Century: Current Frontiers and Future Directions

David A. Hamburg, Susan G. Millstein,
Allyn M. Mortimer, Elena O. Nightingale,
and Anne C. Petersen

The Onset of Adolescence in a Time of Dramatic Transition

Adolescence is different than it once was. Although the dramatic biological changes that usher in this great transition are essentially the same as they have been for millennia, our society provides a very different context, even if we compare it to just a generation ago, and it is still changing rapidly. These changes offer remarkable opportunities, but they also complicate the tasks of adolescent development, particularly the ways in which behavior is shaped. This is a crucial time, since it is in these years that youngsters establish healthy lifestyles that are likely to endure throughout their adult years.

Human societies evolved slowly over vast periods of time in ways that tended to foster adaptive development during childhood and adolescence—the essence of survival. This occurred mainly in the context of a cohesive family, a small community, small societies with shared values, slow technological and social changes, and great vulnerability to the vicissitudes of nature. During the past two centuries, a significant transformation in the living conditions of the human species has occurred. These changes have been especially striking in the twentieth century.

Family relationships have constituted a powerful organizing mechanism throughout human evolution. Even in the nonhuman primates, kinship is an important determinant of social interaction and mutual support. In effect, the family in one form or another has been the main locus of educational, economic, and social activity throughout human history. Indeed, the nuclear and extended family have been at the core of mutual aid and preparation for adaptive behavior for mil-

375

lennia. The Industrial Revolution brought about profound changes, and these have been accelerating in recent decades in ways that deeply influence the experience of growing up, particularly during the adolescent transition. These changes are seen in many ways, including the smaller size of nuclear families, the higher incidence of divorce, the changing roles of women, and the emergence of a youth culture.

The transition from childhood to adulthood through most of human history was steady, gradual, and cumulative. Children were given tasks from an early age that foreshadowed their responsibilities of adult life. These tasks increased in scope and complexity as the children grew older. Adaptive skills developed step by step. When children reached adolescence, they were largely familiar with what would be required of them and what their opportunities would be as adults. With some confirmation by a rite of passage, they were ready to meet the requirements of adult behavior.

Since the Industrial Revolution, children and adolescents have been given fewer opportunities to participate in the adult world. Today our youth are less certain of how to be useful and earn the respect of adults. Indeed, the time between childhood and adulthood has lengthened; and the requirements, risks, and opportunities of this period are now highly ambiguous for many adolescents.

In the modern sociotechnical context of our society, the fundamental tasks of growing up remain: to find a place in a valued group that gives a sense of belonging; to identify and master tasks that are generally recognized in the group as having value, and thereby to earn respect by acquiring skills; to acquire a sense of worth as a person; and to develop reliable relationships with other people, especially a few deep relationships—or at least one. These tasks are truly *developmental* during the adolescent years. They involve growing independence from parents, siblings, and friends—in other words, renegotiating without abandoning important prior relationships; shifting toward greater autonomy in making personal decisions, assuming responsibility for one's self, and regulating one's own behavior; establishing new friendships; moving toward greater personal intimacy and adult sexuality; dealing with more complex intellectual challenges and building new skills—cognitive, social, and technical. This interrelated set of developmental tasks is highly challenging, complex, and often difficult. The outcomes are highly variable, and many are adverse in terms of health and education.

Exploratory behavior is central to adolescence and always has been. This is a crucial feature of adolescent adaptation. Yet a large proportion of early adolescents are not well prepared to make informed decisions about the risks and opportunities they encounter. Often, they have little information or practice on which to base decisions about how to handle themselves in new situations. Further complicating adolescence today is the easy availability of activities or substances that constitute a high risk, while appearing at the same time to be recreational, tension-relieving, and gratifying. Adolescents have ready access to deadly poisons in the guise of casual experience: drugs, vehicles, weapons, and indeed the many ways in which one's body may be used dangerously. Further, sleep deprivation, common in adolescents, compounds these problems (National Commission on Sleep Disorders Research, 1993).

The vulnerability of adolescents to health and educational risks has only recently come into focus. The present casualties are excessive and will continue to produce significant cost to our society in terms of problems and their outcomes, as well as lost potential of youth. It is essential to move these problems to a higher position on the agenda of scientific researchers, public educators, and administrators who can institute innovations. Fortunately much of the damage may well prove to be preventable in light of the knowledge drawn together in these chapters and the promising lines of inquiry they describe. Especially important is the search for generic approaches that address the health, education, and social problems facing adolescents. Such interventions have the capacity to address underlying or predisposing factors that increase the likelihood that an adolescent will engage in high-risk or serious problem behaviors.

Today our children and adolescents need to find ways to develop a positive vision of the future, to formulate an image of what adulthood offers and demands, and to work out a perception of opportunity and paths toward practical implementation of such opportunity. They also need to formulate ways to earn respect and to develop self-esteem and modes of establishing a sense of belonging in at least one highly valued group.

In the profoundly transformed conditions of contemporary society, adolescents have less access to traditional social support networks than they once did. How is it possible to facilitate adolescent development by providing functions equivalent to those served in less complex societies by family, friends, and small communities? Research indicates that sustained relationships and contact with others under favorable circumstances generally promote health. Coping with stress associated with the transition of adolescence to adulthood can be greatly aided by an ethic of mutual aid among peers—aid that includes not only sufficient commonality in background to foster communication but also sufficient diversity in range of experience and coping strategies to enrich individual experience. This need is particularly acute in impoverished communities where social interactions are often limited. Such networks can be created in a wide range of existing institutions—for example, in schools and in community organizations. They can provide small-group settings that encourage a mutual aid ethic, the sharing of resources, reliable attachments, coping skills, self-esteem, and an orientation to constructive decisions about health and education. For all adolescents, in a time when they are trying out experiences with new people and situations, social support can be highly beneficial in preparing, negotiating, and making sense of these explorations. For many emerging adolescent individuals, the social support networks and life skills that might well have been taken for granted in a small, slowly changing society which characterized most human experience in past centuries are now in jeopardy. Our particular challenge is how we can find ways, especially in poor communities, to make available constructive social supports, and how to provide skills that are needed in order to take advantage of the opportunities opened up by the availability of such supports. For many young people, the changes of adolescence provide a crucial chance to acquire vital supports and to learn life skills that are essential for economic opportunity, participation in a democratic society, and the construction of healthy lifestyles.

Essential Requirements for Promoting Health of Adolescents

Over the past few decades, the medical profession has paid increasing attention to the role of lifestyle in health and illness. The Surgeon General's report on health promotion and disease prevention, *Healthy People* (1979), estimated that 50 percent of the mortality among adults is a direct result of modifiable behavioral factors, many of which have their onset during the adolescent years. Today, health-care professionals and educators, among others, have an opportunity to become catalysts for the major societal changes that will be required to promote health in the adolescent population. These changes include the following:

- Changes in social attitudes toward adolescents, with a commitment to their growth and healthy development.
- Incorporation of a life-span developmental perspective in the conception, design, and implementation of strategies employed to promote adolescent health.
- Greater consistency of messages across the different levels of the social context of adolescents' lives and the use of these multiple contexts in intervention.
- Creation of new social norms that encourage healthy development and behavior, the creation of physical environments that make it easy to be healthy, and the coordination and linkage of diverse social institutions that can interact with adolescents.
- Systematic linkage of education and health, in schools, media, and community organizations as well as health-care settings.

In responding to the challenge of promoting adolescent health, it will be necessary to utilize established knowledge bases with regard to the psychological, social, environmental, and biological world of the adolescent. Information on ways to implement and evaluate health promotion programs is also a critical part of the knowledge base needed for promoting adolescent health. Yet, there has been limited interchange among experts in the fields of behavior change, adolescent development, adolescent health care, and health promotion in various educational modalities. Furthermore, much of the relevant empirical information is not being disseminated to individuals involved in developing and implementing adolescent health promotion activities. How then is it possible during the crucially formative early adolescent years to shape behavior in healthy directions?

These concerns, along with advances in each of these fields over the past decade, stimulated the Carnegie Council on Adolescent Development to develop this volume on adolescent health promotion. The perspectives presented in the book are varied and reflect the contribution of individuals from a wide range of disciplines. Rather than taking only a problem-specific focus, this volume tackles cross-cutting themes of importance in health promotion. Themes that emerge from the chapters show much consistency across different topic areas and different disciplinary perspectives, and contribute to a major objective of this book—namely, to delineate concepts and techniques useful in constructing healthy lifestyles for adolescents.

This final chapter attempts to draw together the key ideas that have implications for the future of adolescent health vis à vis program development and implementation, research, service and training, and public policy.

Development and Implementation of Successful Programs

When we look at traditional health status measures such as morbidity and mortality, it is clear that adolescents, compared to other age groups, are relatively healthy. Their rates of mortality are low, and with the exception of a few sources of morbidity—for example, sexually transmitted diseases—their morbidity rates are also low. The focus of adolescent health, therefore, has turned to the study of behavioral risk factors, which are considered the "new morbidities" (see Chapter 1). The findings in this book clearly reveal that successful programs for adolescent health promotion are based on a number of key principles, which we detail here.

For a health promotion program to be successful, it must be acceptable to the relevant individuals, cultural groups, and communities. Programs for adolescents should reflect a theme of inclusion, not exclusion, and they need to acknowledge values of the individuals for whom they are developed. Adolescents should be a part of the process of developing and implementing adolescent health promotion programs. Because adolescents acquire increasing decision-making power during the adolescent years, it is critical to get a sense of their perceptions and beliefs. For example, by using adolescent focus groups to inform program development or by placing adolescents on advisory boards, programs may be made more acceptable. In addition, such participation by adolescents serves to develop their skills in a variety of ways.

Successful programs must also incorporate basic knowledge about adolescent development into their design, acknowledging the capabilities and needs of adolescents at different ages, capitalizing on their strengths, and recognizing their limitations. Specifically, programs must recognize and accommodate the individual needs of adolescents at different stages of development. These include needs for increased autonomy and independence, needs for peer friendship and group membership, and needs for support from interested and caring adults, especially those with whom the adolescent has extensive and ongoing contact.

Programs should be sensitive to differences in developmental issues during early and late adolescence, to individual variability within the adolescent population, and to constraints of the communities within which adolescents operate. Age-related differences in how adolescents view health and illness, for example, might suggest a two-part approach to adolescent health promotion (Chapter 6). For younger adolescents, health promotion may need to focus on physiological stimuli and visible indicators, while programs developed for older adolescents may have to stress the functional limitations and the behavioral consequences of specific actions. These two approaches are consistent with the developmental needs of early and late adolescents.

Cognitive changes during adolescence can facilitate health promotion efforts, since adolescents are better able to comprehend health risks and long-term consequences of their actions (Chapter 2). During adolescence, they become more responsive to health promotion efforts which often require a long-term perspective and attention to symbolic rewards. Although individual differences in reasoning represent a major challenge to program providers, the use of multiple approaches with varying levels of abstraction with the same adolescent population tends to improve outcomes.

The most health-enhancing environment for adolescents is one that is supportive in the long term and directs adolescents toward autonomy. The interaction of changes in family structure and employment, however, has increased the amount of time adolescents spend unsupervised by adults, alone, or with peers. These changes have also decreased the time available for communication and intimacy with parents or other supportive adults. Lack of these adult relationships may have dire consequences for the adolescent and are conducive to health-compromising behavior; these issues are discussed in Chapter 5.

Adolescents need to practice new roles and responsibilities, need a future vision worth pursuing, and need to feel competent in some area. Programs for adolescents should foster the development of skills that they will need to function effectively as adolescents and as adults. These skills include interpersonal and communication skills that allow for nonviolent conflict resolution and for support when necessary; cognitive skills that include decision-making abilities; generic employability skills that allow for entrance into the labor market; practice at functioning in productive roles; and coping skills that allow for adaptation to negative events.

Substantial progress has been made in our understanding of the nature of positive mental health during adolescence and in our ability to promote the development of adaptive functioning, including coping skills, in this developmental period (Chapter 8). Research suggests that there are multiple, different developmental paths during adolescence that can represent adaptive functioning. Health promotion efforts that foster adolescent mental health achieve change by helping adolescents develop skills for coping with stress, by involving them in personally meaningful activities, by promoting the development of healthy social environments, and by promoting positive mental health through public policy. Examples of programs that promote positive mental health are skill-building activities that teach coping and problem-solving skills, and programs that offer youth an opportunity to explore career roles, develop employment-relevant skills, make a contribution to their local communities, and experience a level of engagement and commitment that exceeds many other activities that are typically available to adolescents.

Programs will be most successful when their messages and goals are consistent with the cultural milieu of the adolescent. Promoting healthy diet and exercise habits remains one of the most challenging goals in this regard since cultural ideals for body shape are often inconsistent with healthy lifestyle (Chapter 10). As a result, adolescents are prone to develop eating disorders, to exercise excessively, or to use steroids to alter body shape. The negative influences on adolescent eating and physical activity are stronger and more numerous than the positive ones. The most potent and pervasive negative influences are from television, the food industry, peers, and family. And with the excessive use of the automobile, there is little opportunity for exercise. Effective programs that promote healthy eating and physical activity create social and physical environments that make it easy to do so; promote policies and laws consistent with healthful behaviors; ensure that adequate variety of tasteful, nutritious, low-fat, low-calorie foods are available to adolescents; encourage the media to repeat messages that are appealing and that communicate the importance of healthful diet and physical activity; and educate adolescents to analyze and resist advertisements and TV programs that try to manipulate their behavior in unhealthy ways.

Chapter 9 pointed out that interventions thus far have not focused on helping youth manage risk behavior and anticipate risky situations. Programs that promote healthy sexual development, for example, should start no later than junior high school, should be based on a combined public health and informational model, and should focus on multidimensional approaches. Interventions should pay more attention to the situations in which sex occurs; to the role of the family, peers, and schools; and to a joint community and school effort because these might work better than programs set in only the school environment. An example of a coordinated approach to reducing adolescent injuries is that of the campaign against drunk driving. Multiple interventions were used here, including joint efforts on the part of citizens' groups working with government to make changes in regulations as well as peer pressure on adolescents, their families, and society. In Chapter 14 the authors consider whether the lessons learned from the drunk driving campaign can apply to other areas of injury prevention.

Adolescent health promotion has been challenged during the past decade as the American family, the media, the economic structure, and the community have undergone tremendous changes. These changes have all affected the way adolescents live and interact with society. Programs, therefore, also need to be constituted to link adolescents to social institutions that support their healthy development. Schools are a potentially important part of an adolescent's life because they can assure access to health services and provide a health-promoting environment that includes nutritious food, regular exercise, and nonviolent methods of conflict management and resolution. Schools have also been the primary context for the delivery of formal mental health promotion programs for adolescents. On the whole, adolescents also seem to be receptive to school settings as a source of information about health. While schools should remain a primary vehicle for promotion of positive adolescent mental health, services need to be expanded to out-of-school youth and to include other settings and contexts, including the family, youth service organizations, religious institutions, and health-care settings.

Family support programs, such as those developed for parents of infants and young children, need to be instituted for parents of adolescents, especially those in disadvantaged environments. These programs should provide anticipatory guidance in addition to education about basic developmental processes. While family ties continue to be important to adolescents, peer relations take on an increasingly influential role in their lives. The potential contribution of peers to the development of health-promoting behaviors is substantial. Peers can become a positive force as peer models and tutors or as counselors on health care.

Programs must be explicit and realistic about the goals they aim to reach. Are they to delay the onset of a behavior, to maintain an existing behavior, to change an already existing behavior, or to establish lifelong patterns? Chapter 10 discusses program goals and the different strategies and intervention points that may be required to reach these goals. In considering areas for intervention, the entire array of needs and resources in the population and its subgroups should be considered so that those within the population whose needs are in the greatest jeopardy receive special attention and are targeted earlier. Care needs to be taken not to exclude youth who are poorly connected to traditional institutions—for example, out-of-school youth. Barriers to broad-based health promotion efforts are likely to be greatest where there is exceptional need, such as in disadvantaged inner-city neighborhoods, or rural communities where few resources exist and where coordination among institutions is difficult.

Poverty is frequently a barrier to health promotion, but how it influences adolescent health promotion is not entirely clear (see Chapter 3). Poor adolescents may engage in fewer health-promoting behaviors than the nonpoor, but the cumulative evidence is not very powerful. What is clear is that health promotion for poor teenagers is likely to be very difficult and is a greater challenge for the professional community than health promotion for nonpoor youth. Health promotion for poor teenagers is difficult because they often live in environments that are not conducive to health or health promotion. For example, some poor adolescents do not attend school, which is a commonly used site for health promotion efforts. Poor families may be less able to supervise the conduct of their youth, promote health behaviors, or control unhealthy behaviors. Some poor adolescents may also value membership in a peer group characterized by problem behaviors, and they may lack an orientation to the future that is sufficient to motivate positive behaviors.

Poverty also limits choices and increases stress—both factors impinge on health promotion. Oral health, for example, is an especially relevant component of adolescent health promotion. Although most prevalent oral diseases are preventable through a combination of community-based programs, accessible professional care, and a proper routine of oral self-care, the rate of untreated caries among minority and otherwise disadvantaged adolescents is almost double the national average (Chapter 11). Attempts to improve the health status of poor adolescents, therefore, will have to proceed on many levels, using both conventional and unconventional sites and methods for delivering a health promotion message.

Similarly, strategies for minority parents and teachers in guiding minority youth through the reality of reduced life opportunities and frail political power during the transition to adulthood have not been clearly defined. Minority youth must hold on to their uniqueness and at the same time develop a strategy that permits successful negotiation within the dominant group and societal institutions. The most promising health promotion programs, therefore, will try to coordinate activities for minority adolescents at four levels: public policy, community support, family functioning, and individual lifestyle. Creative solutions for minority populations may suggest alternative models for majority youth as well.

Finally, according to the authors of Chapter 15, far more attention needs to be paid to the development of theory-based programs that are well implemented, carefully evaluated, and designed to shed light on causal processes underlying at-risk behaviors. One way to enhance the development of theory-based programs is to establish mechanisms that allow for the transfer of information between researchers, program planners, and program implementors. For example, links between those implementing interventions and researchers might include a clearinghouse for information transfer, or support of research that links researchers with program staff.

Research Implications

Research on adolescent health promotion must build on what has been learned from disease prevention, emphasizing health within the context of basic adolescent development. Research on topics such as healthy lifestyle patterns, healthy sexual development, life skills, decision-making and interpersonal skills, and coping behaviors is needed. In addition, more research on contextual issues in adolescent health is needed, including research that identifies the processes by which contexts affect development and health. In this regard, the cultural context of adolescents' lives and the situational context in which health-promoting and health-damaging behaviors emerge need to be studied.

For the most part, research has been conducted on the health and development of white, middle-class adolescents. Future research should consider the health and development of nonwhite adolescents, those from poor families, and those who experience particular developmental stressors such as physical disability or variations in sexual orientation. Because minority adolescents are individuals who are not only different from the dominant group of white Americans, but also different within and among themselves, the meaning of health in their social environments may differ. Health promotion programs, therefore, should be tailored for different groups (Chapter 4).

The appropriate timing and sequence of health-promoting programs throughout the life cycle should be examined. Two important concepts are related to adolescent lifestyles: (1) how adolescents organize their lives and pattern their behavior in ways that put them at higher or lower risk for serious health problems, and (2) how these patterns develop, persist, or cease at different times during the life span. Chapter 7 summarizes research on adolescent lifestyles and the kinds of social contexts in which they emerge and are maintained. Findings indicate that most youth involved in a deviant lifestyle will terminate this behavior during late adolescence or early adulthood. In certain social environments, however, solutions that focus on the rehabilitation of individuals may be less productive than those that focus on neighborhood revitalization and reorganization. These facts should make us cautious about implementing general interventions that lack demonstrated effectiveness when we want to see an immediate or short-term impact on health.

Though costly, longitudinal research is important because it enables examination of the entire course of adolescence. In addition, community-based research must examine ways to activate communities for health promotion and how to bring state-of-the-art programs into local communities.

Research designed to identify suitable alternatives to health-damaging behaviors of adolescents should be encouraged, with a focus on identifying goals that are attractive to the adolescent. A major concern during the adolescent years is substance abuse, discussed in Chapter 12. A comprehensive, culture-wide approach will be required to promote healthy alternatives to substance abuse. Reasonable options must be made available to adolescents, such as living examples of successful nondrug lifestyles in the adolescents' local communities. Providing alternatives to substance abuse may also require cooperative action among governmental, religious, and noninstitutional organizations. Major changes in safety and housing regulations and in socioeconomic organization that separates some groups from meaningful work or learning opportunities may also be necessary.

There is a strong association between assaultive behavior and substance abuse. Chapter 13 suggested that a shift of American cultural norms toward greater restriction of firearms and less tolerance of violence may require drastic efforts, including limiting the availability of firearms, drugs, and alcohol. It may be unrealistic to expect that drug and alcohol use and abuse in adolescents or in any population can be eliminated. At best, one can hope to reduce the number of users and abusers, ideally by postponing the age of onset of use. But further research on effective preventive interventions and treatments appropriate for adolescents would be helpful.

Injuries are the most important and immediate threat to adolescent health, yet prevention research and programs in this field are less available than for drug abuse and smoking cessation (Chapter 14). Although injuries have multiple causes and different types of injuries have distinct etiologies, it might be useful to search for common psychological and behavioral factors among injuries. At the same time, the unique features of each type of injury should be identified so that optimally effective interventions can be developed.

Funding mechanisms need to be developed to support special types of research that will add important information but are currently difficult to fund. Examples include the following:

- Research using methods such as qualitative or ethnographic approaches is needed in many new or emerging areas to describe phenomena that are not currently well understood and that are therefore less amenable to more traditional quantitative approaches.
- Research using multidisciplinary teams and methods is essential because all the major problems of youth require expertise from more than one discipline.
- Research that goes beyond a single health-related behavior to examine multi-

ple cross-cutting behaviors is central since adolescents often engage in more than one unhealthy behavior, and may do so in particular combinations and sequences.
- Longitudinal research is needed to identify the shorter versus longer term significance of various risk factors and behavior patterns.

Service and Education Considerations

Professional education for all those who will interact with adolescents is extremely important and currently neglected. Such education needs to include normal development during adolescence, a multidisciplinary perspective, and professional attitudes toward adolescents.

Educating health professionals about various adolescent health issues is critical because adolescent health promotion is more effective when messages provided within schools, the community, and ambulatory health-care settings are mutually reinforcing and complementary. Currently there are only six interdisciplinary training programs in adolescent health funded by the Bureau of Maternal and Child Health (PHS). Physicians and other health-care providers have an opportunity to promote health through direct interventions with their adolescent patients as well as the manner in which they organize their office practices. The American Medical Association (AMA) is currently conducting a three-year project to develop Guidelines for Adolescent Preventive Services (GAPS; AMA, 1992). Recommendations are also being developed for health promotion and preventive interventions in an ambulatory care setting. GAPS will be comprehensive, addressing both traditional medical and psychosocial disorders as well as developmental needs.

Public Policy Considerations

Placing adolescents higher on the national agenda will require advocacy to change public perceptions of adolescents and to move appropriate legislative action forward. Initiatives on behalf of adolescents that need implementation include the following:

- The national data monitoring system needs upgrading to allow for the disaggregation of adolescent data from that of children and young adults.
- An assessment of the degree to which key institutions are functioning in ways consistent with healthy adolescent development needs to be undertaken, leading to recommendations for improved policy.
- An exploration of the mechanisms to support links between various institutions and the families of adolescents needs to be undertaken. Promising models for coordination across systems should be tested in different types of communities and using different linkage configurations.

- Funding mechanisms need to be developed for sustaining adolescent health promotion programs over lengthy periods of time so that programs can become established in communities and be part of everyday life, and subsequent cohorts of adolescents will be served.
- A social environment that limits the accessibility to substances and activities that lead to dangerous patterns of behavior and maximizes the ones that lead to healthy patterns of behavior needs to be assured in all communities. Legislation should be considered that would limit adolescents' exposure to health-damaging activities; for example, the establishment of nonsmoking policies in schools and the banning of cigarette vending machines in places where adolescents congregate.

The United States has no national body that regularly monitors and develops policy on youth issues, although the newly created office of Adolescent Health within the office of the Assistant Secretary for Health holds promise. Given the increased risks for the healthy development of youth, and the ultimate cost to the nation if their potential is unfulfilled, it seems imperative that we do more to increase the likelihood that all youth will have the opportunity to become productive citizens in our society.

Concluding Comment

Adolescence is a period of great risks and opportunities. Its onset is a crucial formative phase of development. Puberty is a profound biological upheaval, and it coincides approximately with dramatic changes in the social environment. These early adolescent years are open to the formation of behavior patterns that have lifelong significance for health. The dangerous patterns described in this volume have only recently received the research attention they deserve.

Initially, adolescents explore potentially damaging activities tentatively. They are tried on for size. Before damaging patterns are firmly established, there is a major and badly neglected opportunity for intervention to prevent casualties throughout the life span. This is best done by meeting fundamental requirements for healthy adolescent development. It is crucial to help adolescents acquire constructive knowledge and skills, inquiring habits of mind, dependable human relationships, a reliable basis for earning respect, a sense of belonging in a valued group, and a way of being useful to others.

As children experience puberty and emerge into an era in which they feel they should quickly become adults, they ask in effect, "How shall I use my body?" Any responsible education must answer that basic question with a substantial life sciences curriculum that gives adolescents accurate information about their own bodies, including the effects of various high-risk behaviors. But information is not enough.

How can adolescents make good use of accurate and personally meaningful information? Life skills training can become a vital part of education in schools and community organizations. In addition to teaching adolescents how to make informed, deliberate, and constructive decisions, such training can also enhance their people skills, their positive ways of relating to others, their learning from experience, even an unpleasant experience—for example, how to resolve a conflict without violence. Skills can be built to establish dependable friendships and participation in supportive problem-solving groups. But even this is not enough.

People also need people, especially to weather the inevitable difficulties of growing up, the stresses of education, and the turbulent search for ways to protect one's own health and the health of those one cares about. To the extent that contemporary families are unable to meet these needs, specially designed social support interventions can be exceedingly helpful.

Moreover, this conjunction of information, skills, and motivation for development, indeed for survival, can be provided through the foresight and cooperation of several pivotal institutions that powerfully shape the transition from childhood to adulthood: the family, schools, the health-care system, the media, and the community organizations that reach out to youth.

But there is still a serious unmet need for accessible health care. It may be at the school or near the school, but health care must be arranged in such a way that it is clearly recognizable to students, available and within reach, and "user friendly." Many good examples of school-linked or school-based programs exist, but their support is fragile and their emphasis on health promotion needs strengthening.

For the development of healthy lifestyles in adolescence, several factors are crucial: information, skills, motivation, and constructive human relationships. Education can contribute substantially to all of these. Through education in various settings, motivation may be strengthened and sustained, accurate information assimilated, and relevant skills developed—all in the supportive context of nurturing interpersonal relationships. Again, this must involve not only the schools, but the media, the family, churches, and community organizations. Some innovative models show that their unfulfilled potential for helping to meet the needs of healthy adolescent development are substantial.

At home and at school, indeed in a variety of settings, it is possible to build competence, to earn respect, to build a friendship group capable of fostering education and health, and to delineate a vision of an attractive future and prospects for a worthwhile life.

The research described in this volume, and the research-based interventions to promote healthy adolescent development, will in due course have a strong bearing on the health of entire populations. Although there are few complete models of successful programs that can meet the needs of adolescents, components of such programs do exist in many nations. Increasingly, these components will be put together in ways that will provide our adolescents with the full range of developmental opportunities permitted by today's knowledge and our emerging research findings. Present evidence and experience, together with highly promising research and innovative programs, suggest that sustained attention to adolescent development could greatly improve the likelihood of growing up healthy.

References

American Medical Association (1992). *Guidelines for adolescent preventive services*. Chicago: American Medical Association.

Hamburg D. A., *Today's children: Creating a future for a generation in crisis*. New York: Random House, 1992.

National Commission on Sleep Disorders Research (1993). *Wake Up America: A National Sleep Alert*, Bethesda, MD: National Institutes of Health.

U.S. Department of Health, Education, and Welfare. (1979) *Healthy People: The Surgeon General's Report on Health Promotion and Disease Prevention* DHEW (PHS) Publication No. 79-55071. Washington, D.C.: U.S. Government Printing Office.

INDEX

389